# Skills for Midwifery Practice
## Second Edition

**Ruth Johnson** (now Bowen) BA (Hons) RGN RM Supervisor of Midwives

Former Senior Lecturer, School of Nursing and Midwifery, University of Hertfordshire, Hatfield, UK

**Wendy Taylor** BSc (Hons) RN RM PGCEA PGDip

Senior Lecturer, School of Nursing and Midwifery, University of Hertfordshire, Hatfield, UK

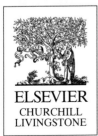

ELSEVIER
CHURCHILL
LIVINGSTONE

EDINBURGH LONDON NEW YORK OXFORD PHILADELPHIA ST LOUIS SYDNEY TORONTO 2006

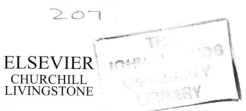

# ELSEVIER
## CHURCHILL
## LIVINGSTONE

First published 2000
Second edition 2006
  Reprinted 2006, 2007

ISBN 13: 978 0 443 10128 1
ISBN 10: 0 443 10128 0

**British Library Cataloguing in Publication Data**
A catalogue record for this book is available from the British Library
**Library of Congress Cataloguing in Publication Data**
A catalogue record for this book is available from the Library of Congress

**ELSEVIER** your source for books, journals and multimedia in the health sciences

**www.elsevierhealth.com**

Working together to grow
libraries in developing countries

www.elsevier.com | www.bookaid.org | www.sabre.org

**ELSEVIER**    **BOOK AID International**    **Sabre Foundation**

The publisher's policy is to use paper manufactured from sustainable forests

Printed in China
C/03

# Skills for Midwifery Practice

**Second Edition**

EQRE7

*For Elsevier*

*Commissioning Editor:* Mary Seager
*Development Editor:* Rebecca Nelemans
*Project Manager:* Frances Affleck
*Senior Designer:* Sarah Russell

# Contents

# Preface

We both take great delight in seeing students and midwives mature in their practice to become skilled, intuitive professionals with a complete range of skills and therefore able to offer care of the highest standards to women, families and babies in their care. We originally wrote this text with three/four year student midwives in mind, but it has become apparent that it has been useful to students of varying sorts and to midwives in various roles. This second edition has revised each chapter and added new material. We have endeavoured to search the literature thoroughly and to be as up to date as we can be.

Nevertheless, new research will come on line, debates will arise, new protocols will be developed and thinking will move on. Do be aware of the need to keep up to date and to practise accordingly. There are obviously other essential skills for midwifery practice that are not covered here (e.g. communication) that are well covered in other texts. Some subjects, such as hand hygiene, both have a dedicated chapter and are spread throughout the text, such is their importance.

The phrase 'Gain informed consent' appears in each chapter. There isn't space to discuss it in detail, but the principle is that each woman (or baby) is treated with the greatest of respect and dignity, and is supplied with (wherever possible) full, unbiased information about the procedure, before it takes place, in order that she can truly consent to it happening. As a student, assistance will be required from a midwife to achieve this. Equally, 'Document the findings and act accordingly' occurs regularly. This refers to the midwife's responsibility to maintain accurate, detailed records at the time of care and to ensure that if issues need continuing follow-up, then this occurs. Students will need to have their records countersigned by the midwife and to ensure that the midwife is fully informed of the care given and outcomes from it.

We do know that babies are both male and female, but in order to reduce confusion, babies are referred to as 'he' throughout this text, 'she' being the woman/mother.

We trust that you will enjoy learning from this text, that you will develop in your practice and that the ultimate outcome will be satisfaction for both you and those in your care.

Ruth Johnson (now Bowen) and Wendy Taylor
Hatfield, 2005

# Acknowledgements

The authors gratefully acknowledge the support of family and friends, especially Robbie, Hannah, Jean and Harold, Ian and Helen and of those who have given professional advice: Helen Buckle (Telford and Wrekin PCT), Liz Gunn (City Hospital, Birmingham), Laura Abbott, Independent Midwife (http:// www.homebirths.net), Ruth Walker and Emma Dawson-Goodey (University of Hertfordshire), Hilary Jones and colleagues (National Blood Service) and Ian Taylor.

Chapter **1**

# Principles of abdominal examination — during pregnancy

This chapter considers the skill of abdominal examination antenatally. Auscultation of the fetal heart, both intermittently and continuously, is considered, with definitions for cardiotocography (CTG monitoring) included. Please refer to the glossary for some of the terms cited.

**Learning outcomes**

Having read this chapter the reader should be able to:

- discuss when and how an abdominal examination is undertaken
- describe the stages of an abdominal examination, discussing the nature of the information sought
- discuss the role and responsibilities of the midwife when undertaking abdominal examination and when using a CTG monitor
- describe the criteria used to assess CTG tracings.

## Antenatal abdominal examination

### Rationale

Abdominal examination provides both the woman and the midwife with assurances that the pregnancy is progressing well. The woman can gain information and reassurance; she may also appreciate the benefit of therapeutic touch and the opportunity to receive holistic and individualised care. Olsen (1999) points out that a woman can believe in the ability of her own body to nurture and birth a child, as well as finding enhanced trust in the midwife. However, Olsen (1999) also discovered that many women find this an uncomfortable procedure. The NICE guideline (2003) is also clear that where the information has previously been traditionally sought, it may be of limited value at particular points during the pregnancy and that therefore there should be a good rationale for each component of the examination. It should be noted that guidelines are only for guidance, and the midwife will encounter situations in which the woman's wishes or the clinical condition requires additional or modified care – the midwife as an autonomous practitioner is fully able to make such decisions. The skill of abdominal palpation comes with practice and experience and therefore for inexperienced practitioners it remains a significant part of maternity care.

A complete antenatal examination will include abdominal examination; hence this is only one part of antenatal care. A skilled midwife will be able to detect deviations from the norm, but will also appreciate that other facilities exist to complement care (e.g. ultrasound scanning) and so will refer the woman where a deviation is found. The woman will be instrumental in knowing whether there is fetal growth, where/when the movements occur, etc. and so discussion and obtaining consent are key prior to undertaking the examination. The examination aims to:

- assess fetal growth, size, wellbeing, position and presentation
- detect deviations from the norm.

## Indications

- Each antenatal assessment, particularly after 25 weeks' gestation
- On admission to hospital (for any reason)
- Prior to auscultation of the fetal heart and use of CTG equipment.

### Contraindications

As the uterus can be stimulated when this examination is performed, it should be undertaken cautiously when there is:

- placental abruption
- preterm labour.

### Technique

Abdominal examination consists of three stages:

1. inspection
2. palpation
3. auscultation.

### Inspection

- Size: may be affected by obesity, lax abdominal muscles, multiple pregnancy, poly- and oligohydramnios, fetal size and lie, uterine fibroids and the gestation period
- Shape: may give an indication of the fetal position or presentation, e.g. a dip at the umbilicus can be indicative of an occipitoposterior position
- Skin changes may be seen, e.g. linea nigra, striae gravidarum, signs of previous abdominal surgery
- Fetal movements may be seen.

*Palpation*
This is subdivided into three aspects: fundal, lateral and pelvic palpation.

**Fundal palpation**  Fundal palpation is used to:

- assess the estimated period of gestation by assessing fundal height
- suggest an indication of the lie and presentation of the fetus, according to the presence of a fetal pole (head or buttocks).

The height of the fundus rises as the fetus grows, but maternal parity, size, a full bladder, a transverse fetal lie and the number of fetuses can influence fundal height. Fundal height can be assessed in two ways, although neither is considered to have absolute reliability:

1. Using a traditional set of indicators that consider landmarks on the abdomen (Fig. 1.1)
2. Measuring with a tape measure. A tape measure is used to measure in centimetres (cm), from the upper border of the symphysis pubis to the top of the fundus, generally along the midline of the abdomen and with the scale face down. The fundal height in centimetres generally equates with the weeks of gestation. Lindhart et al (1990) suggest this has dubious reliability, but Gardosi and Francis (1999) indicate an acceptable degree of sensitivity when the result is plotted on customised charts. NICE (2003) suggest the measuring and plotting of symphysis fundal height for each woman on each antenatal visit. Neilson (2000) recommends the practice until large scale research suggests otherwise.

**Figure 1.1**  Fundal height at different stages of pregnancy

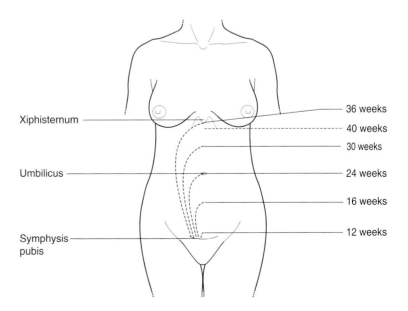

Xiphisternum

Umbilicus

Symphysis pubis

36 weeks
40 weeks
30 weeks
24 weeks
16 weeks
12 weeks

A fundal height inconsistent with gestation may indicate:

- unreliable landmarks, e.g. long abdomen
- inaccurate dates
- the fetus is larger or smaller than expected
- the amount of amniotic fluid may be greater or lesser than expected
- multiple pregnancy
- abnormal lie
- uterine mass, e.g. fibroid, cyst or tumour
- poor technique
- intrauterine death.

To find the fundus, the fingers are placed on the abdomen below the xiphisternum and moved gently downwards until the firmness of the fundus is felt. Using the palmar surfaces of both hands, palpate the fundus to identify the fetal pole (Fig. 1.2).

- Buttocks feel softer, less 'ballotable', bulkier, less clearly defined
- Head feels firmer, more rounded and 'ballotable', i.e. can be moved gently from side to side.

If a pole is not located in the fundus, the lie is not longitudinal (see Fig. 1.5). Once the fundal height is assessed and the fetal pole (if present) is identified, the palpation progresses to lateral palpation.

**Lateral palpation** Lateral palpation assesses the main body of the uterus to identify the fetal position and confirm the lie. The spine is usually firmer and smoother; the limbs on the opposing side are less

**Figure 1.2** Fundal palpation

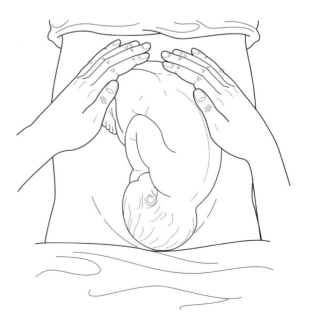

regularly defined, with that side of the uterus being softer. There are two methods of undertaking lateral palpation:

1. The hands are placed one on either side of the uterus at about umbilical level: support one side of the uterus while the other hand progresses down the length of the uterus (Fig. 1.3); palpate the other side of the uterus in the same way

Figure 1.3  (A, B) Lateral palpation. One side of the uterus is supported as the other hand progresses down the uterus. Both sides are palpated in this way

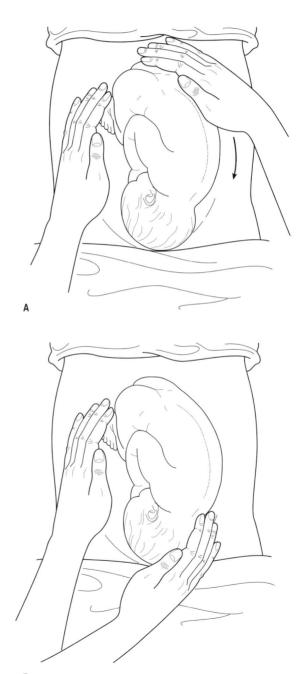

A

B

2. 'Walk' both hands across the uterus from side to side, from the fundus to the symphysis pubis (Fig. 1.4).

The lie of the fetus is determined by the relationship of the long axis of the fetal spine to the long axis of the maternal uterus. The lie is normally longitudinal, but can be oblique or transverse (Fig. 1.5).

With a longitudinal lie, the position of the fetal spine indicates the position of the fetal head. The position is defined according to the approximation of the fetal denominator (occiput for cephalic presentation) to a pelvic landmark. Figure 1.6 indicates the relevant landmarks on the pelvic brim. For example, if the occiput is in apposition with the

**Figure 1.4** (A, B) 'Walking' the fingertips across the abdomen to locate the position of the fetal back

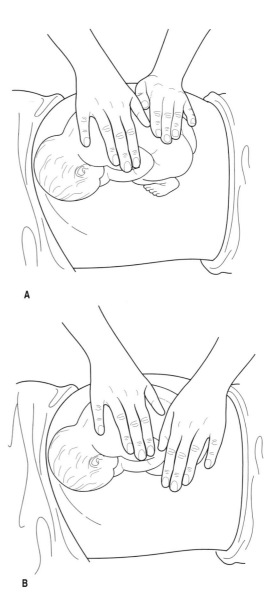

A

B

**Figure 1.5**  The lie of the fetus

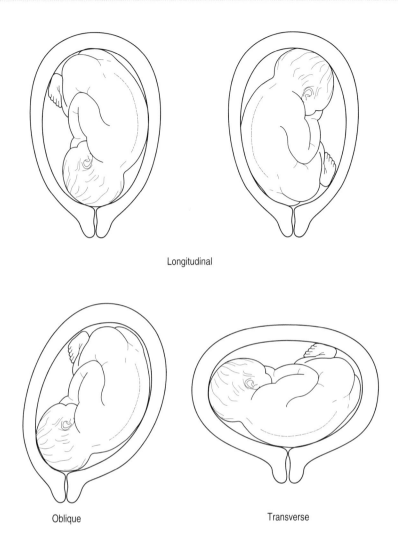

Longitudinal

Oblique

Transverse

iliopectineal eminence of the pelvis, it is described as occipitoanterior. It is further defined according to whether it is on the maternal left or right. If the occiput is in apposition with the sacroiliac joint, it is described as occipitoposterior. With occipitolateral the occiput is found midway on the iliopectineal line (Fig. 1.7). If the denominator were the sacrum (breech presentation) the same pelvic landmarks apply, and the terminology would be right or left sacroanterior, etc.

Lateral palpation also gives information about:

- fetal size
- amniotic fluid volume
- uterine tone
- fetal movements.

It should be noted, however, that NICE (2003) consider that knowledge of the fetal position is of limited relevance until after 36 weeks' gestation.

**Figure 1.6** Relevant
landmarks on the pelvic brim

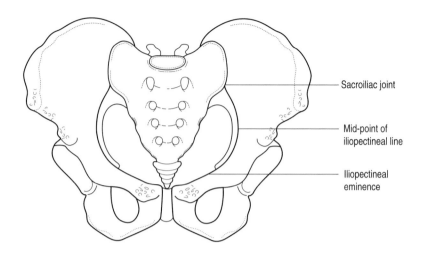

Sacroiliac joint

Mid-point of
iliopectineal line

Iliopectineal
eminence

**Figure 1.6** Relevant
landmarks on the pelvic brim

The midwife will ascertain the woman's wishes as to the need for lateral palpation prior to this gestation, along with any clinical indicators.

**Pelvic palpation** Pelvic palpation assesses the presentation, i.e. the part of the fetus lying in the lower segment of the uterus or at the pelvic brim. It can then determine:

- if the fetus is flexed
- if the presenting part has engaged in the pelvis
- how 'mobile', or moveable, the presenting part is if it has not engaged.

There are five main presentations (Fig. 1.8).

NICE (2003) rightly indicate that pelvic palpation can be uncomfortable and therefore due to its dubious value prior to 36 weeks' gestation, it should only be undertaken from 36 weeks onwards.

There are two methods of undertaking pelvic palpation:

1. Using both hands, one either side of the presentation (fingers facing towards the woman's feet), press in gently. The presentation can be felt beneath the hands, as described for fundal palpation and identified according to its features (Fig. 1.9A). It is helpful if the woman can take a deep breath and hold it for a moment while the hands are able to feel deeply around the presentation
2. Pawlik's manoeuvre can be considered. Using one hand with fingers facing the woman's head, the presenting pole is held between the fingers and thumb (Fig. 1.9B). This should be done very gently, as it is uncomfortable for the woman. Ideally it is avoided.

Engagement into the pelvis is assessed according to the passage of the widest transverse diameter through the pelvic brim. In a cephalic presentation this is the biparietal diameter (9.5 cm). Engagement is generally measured in fifths; for example, a cephalic presentation that is

**Figure 1.7** Six positions in a vertex presentation

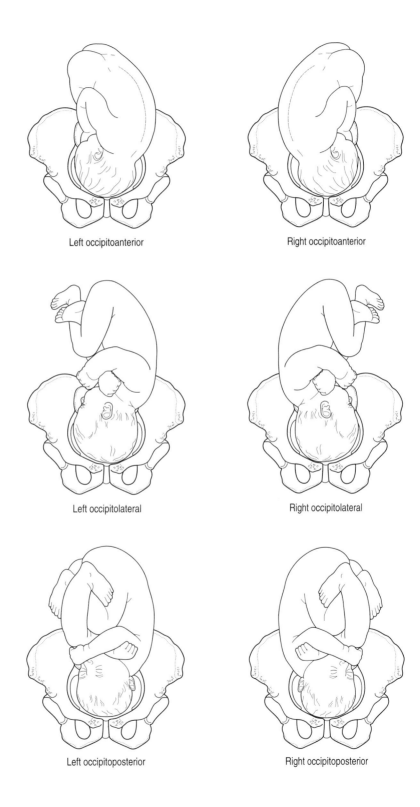

Left occipitoanterior

Right occipitoanterior

Left occipitolateral

Right occipitolateral

Left occipitoposterior

Right occipitoposterior

**Figure 1.8** Five presentations of the fetus

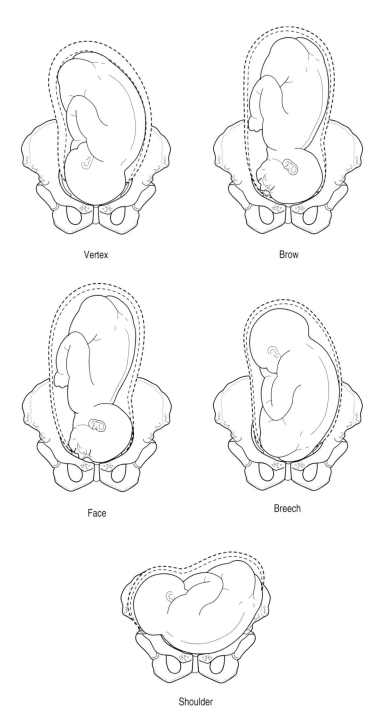

Vertex

Brow

Face

Breech

Shoulder

3/5 palpable has 3/5 of the head palpable out of the pelvis, indicating that 2/5 of the head has passed through the pelvic brim into the pelvis; 1/5 palpable would mean 4/5 have engaged, and so on. When 3/5 of the head has passed through the pelvic brim the presentation is 'engaged'. A non-engaged presentation may be referred to as 'free' or

Figure 1.9   (A) Pelvic palpation: the fingers are directed inwards and downwards; (B) Pawlik's manoeuvre

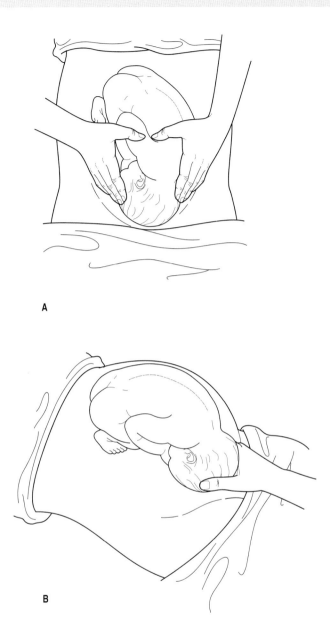

A

B

'at the brim' and may necessitate referral at term, particularly for the primigravid woman.

### Auscultation

If the fetal movements are present, then there is limited value that can be gained from auscultating the fetal heart on a routine antenatal visit. However, auscultation is often reassuring to the mother, and in other situations (e.g. labour or admission for other reasons) it is an important indicator of fetal wellbeing. The clearest fetal heart sounds are heard through the fetal shoulder (scapula). They may sometimes be heard through the chest wall, depending on the fetal position. Locating the fetal presentation and position indicates where the equipment should be placed on the woman's abdomen in order to hear the fetal heart. The sound is a rapid double beating (often rather like a tapping sound) between 110 and 160 bpm. The fetal heart is therefore assessed for:

- its presence
- rate, 110–160 beats per minute (bpm)
- regularity
- variability.

Using a Pinard stethoscope allows the midwife to confirm that it is the fetal heart that has been heard; electrical equipment can confuse the fetal and maternal heart rates. The midwife should palpate the maternal radial pulse while listening to the fetal heart to ensure confidently that the fetal heart has been heard. Using the Pinard stethoscope is a learned and practised skill; Wickham (2002a) agrees and encourages lots of practice!

Variability is assessed using a Pinard stethoscope by counting the beats over a series of 5-second intervals. A difference for each 5-second observation indicates changing variability (Wickham 2002b); no change may indicate fetal sleep and so auscultation should be repeated later.

## PROCEDURE    using a Pinard stethoscope

- Undertake abdominal examination
- Place the Pinard stethoscope over the area where heart sounds are expected (Fig. 1.10)
- Place the ear over the hole, remove the hand so that the ear, stethoscope and abdomen are in direct contact (this increases the sound variance); gentle pressure is needed
- Listen and count the fetal heart for 1 minute; simultaneously palpate the woman's radial pulse (Ch. 5)
- Discuss the results with the woman
- Document the findings and act accordingly.

# Use of the sonicaid

One advantage of using the sonicaid is that the woman can hear the fetal heartbeat and be reassured. It is useful for gestations of less than 28 weeks, when the fetal heart may not be heard clearly with a Pinard stethoscope. The sonicaid often needs to be placed directly over the fetal shoulder in order to hear the fetal heart.

**Figure 1.10**  The approximate points of the fetal heart sounds with a vertex presentation

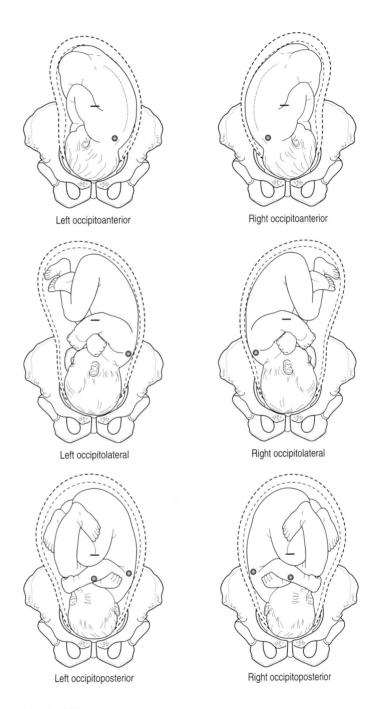

Left occipitoanterior

Right occipitoanterior

Left occipitolateral

Right occipitolateral

Left occipitoposterior

Right occipitoposterior

— Maternal umbilicus

● Positioning of sonicaid to hear fetal heart

- Undertake abdominal examination (Pinard is used if appropriate gestation)
- Lubricate the probe with a suitable conductive gel
- Place the sonicaid over the area where heart sounds are expected
- Count the heart beat for 1 minute (some sonicaids give a digital reading) while simultaneously counting the maternal pulse
- Reassure the woman about the other sounds that can be heard, such as fetal movements, uterine blood flow or cord pulsation
- Wipe off the gel with a tissue
- Discuss the results with the woman
- Document the findings and act accordingly.

### Records

An abdominal examination may be written up descriptively or recorded on an antenatal record. The NMC (2002) state that abbreviations should not be used. Observations and actions undertaken are recorded, and should include:

- the woman's thoughts and observations
- fundal height
- lie
- presentation and degree of engagement
- position
- fetal movements felt
- fetal heart rate, with equipment used
- any additional information, e.g. contractions, amniotic fluid volume, observations on inspection.

Records should be contemporaneous, legible and signed (NMC 2002).

- Gain informed consent and ensure privacy
- Gather equipment:
  — single-use tape measure
  — Pinard stethoscope, sonicaid, gel and tissues
  — watch with a second hand
  — sheet
  — antenatal record
- Encourage the woman to empty her bladder
- Ask the woman to adopt an almost recumbent position (use a wedge to avoid aortocaval occlusion if necessary), with her knees slightly bent and her arms by her side. Cover her legs with the sheet
- Wash hands

- Expose and inspect the abdomen, ensuring that her legs and upper torso remain covered
- Undertake fundal palpation and use the tape measure to assess symphysis fundal height, undertake lateral and pelvic palpations (if indicated)
- Discuss fetal movements and auscultate the fetal heart using watch and Pinard stethoscope while simultaneously palpating the maternal radial pulse; use sonicaid to allow the woman to hear also
- Replace the clothing, assist the woman into a comfortable position and discuss the findings
- Undertake other aspects of the antenatal examination, if not already completed
- Document the findings and act accordingly.

**Role and responsibilities of the midwife**

These can be summarised as:

- undertaking a competent holistic examination in which all of the information needed is gained
- recognising deviations from the norm and instigating referral
- education, explanations and support of the woman
- appropriate record keeping.

# Cardiotoco-graphy

Cardiotocography (CTG) – sometimes known as electronic fetal monitoring (EFM) – has increased the maternal intervention rates, but with no reduction in perinatal mortality or cerebral palsy (NICE 2001). NICE (2003) now recommend that for uncomplicated pregnancies routine use antenatally (including tracing on admission) is unnecessary and that for uncomplicated labours intermittent auscultation should be offered. The decision is made in conjunction with the woman. Complications antenatally or in labour and the administration of oxytocin all indicate the use of CTG.

Monitors may vary, but the principles are that the fetal heart and uterine pressure can be monitored abdominally or within the uterus (Fig. 1.11); commonly both are monitored abdominally. Electrical interference can occur, the most likely source for this being the use of a transcutaneous electrical nerve stimulation (TENS) machine. The heart rate and uterine activity are printed on graph paper, indicating the frequency, strength and length of contractions. The actual pressure changes in the uterus do not equate exactly with the printed strength of contractions, and monitoring should not replace the regular assessment

**Figure 1.11** Cardiotocography monitor

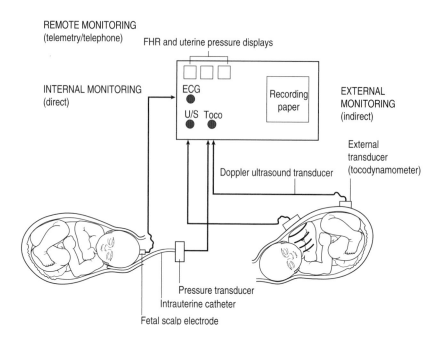

REMOTE MONITORING
(telemetry/telephone)

FHR and uterine pressure displays

INTERNAL MONITORING
(direct)

ECG

U/S  Toco

Recording
paper

EXTERNAL
MONITORING
(indirect)

External
transducer
(tocodynamometer)

Doppler ultrasound transducer

Pressure transducer
Intrauterine catheter

Fetal scalp electrode

of uterine activity by the midwife. As the fetus moves there may be loss of contact, which may be accompanied by an increase in the heart rate. The length of time that the monitor is left in situ will depend upon the condition of the woman and fetus, allowing sufficient time to make an assessment of normality.

The midwife should be trained in the correct use of the monitor, accurate interpretation of the tracing and should ensure that the machinery is serviced and maintained properly. MDA (2002) indicate that errors have occurred in which the fetus was stillborn, despite the monitor providing a tracing of wellbeing. The maternal pulse should always be assessed alongside the fetal heart rate to ensure that they are different. Further points of good practice can be found by reading the NICE guidelines (2001) and other such texts.

## Role and responsibilities of the midwife

These are summarised as:

- knowledge of current evidence-based practice
- correct application, use, supervision and servicing of the monitor
- appropriate trace interpretation and regular update of skills
- education and support of the woman
- accurate record keeping, including documentation on the printout
- referral for deviations from the norm.

PROCEDURE application of the CTG monitor

- Gain informed consent; invite the woman to empty her bladder
- Undertake an abdominal examination and auscultation of the fetal heart using a Pinard stethoscope (p. 12)
- Position the woman in a sitting or semi-recumbent position; her position may be changed once the monitor has been applied. Ensure the two belts are in position and that the woman is sufficiently covered
- Apply gel to the ultrasound transducer
- Place the transducer over the area where heart sounds are expected; the signal should indicate that the positioning is good
- Secure the transducer in position using an abdominal belt
- Place the tocodynamometer on the fundus of the uterus; secure it with an abdominal belt
- Adjust the toco setting on the machine (with the uterus relaxed) to approximately 12 mmHg, unless set automatically
- Start the paper printing (1 cm per minute); document the date, woman's name and number, time commenced and other relevant details on the trace, e.g. midwife's signature, maternal heart rate, epidural analgesia, etc.
- Check that the automatic printing of the time is correct
- Encourage the woman to record fetal movements
- Ensure that anyone else who reviews the trace should sign with the date, time and findings both on the trace and in the records
- Remove the monitor when satisfied that the tracing is within normal limits
- Wipe the gel off the abdomen
- Discuss the results with the woman
- Document the findings and act accordingly
- Clean the equipment.

## CTG interpretation

CTG interpretation begins with knowledge of the woman's history and current clinical profile and that the monitor has been correctly applied. The presence of contractions should be noted for their frequency, strength and length.

The fetal heart tracing is assessed by the:

- Baseline rate: this should be between 110 and 160 bpm and is the rate to which the fetal heart returns after accelerations or decelerations. It is determined over a period of 5–10 minutes
- Baseline variability: a variation in heart rate of between 5 and 15 bpm over a 10–20 second period of time, assessed by subtracting the lowest number of beats from the highest number

- Accelerations: a rise in the heart rate of 15 bpm from the baseline over a 15-second period at least; a reactive trace should include two or more accelerations over a 20-minute period
- Decelerations: the heart rate decelerates from the baseline, often 15 bpm and lasting for 15 seconds or more; the depth and time of recovery are observed in conjunction with the timing of the contractions.

A CTG is described as being 'reassuring' when the baseline and variability are within normal limits, there are accelerations and no decelerations (NICE 2001). Figure 1.12 shows a reassuring CTG.

In labour, decelerations are currently defined as:

- Early: decelerations occur with the contraction, often associated with head compression during the second stage of labour
- Variable: the timing and shape are variable; the fetal heart usually accelerates before and after the deceleration before returning to the baseline, referred to as 'shouldering', distinguished by a rapid fall and return to the baseline, often a result of cord compression
- Late: decelerations occur after the onset of the contraction, and recovery takes place after the end of the contraction, often a result of reduced uteroplacental blood flow
- Prolonged: occurring at any time, there is a significant decrease in heart rate for more than 2 minutes; the fetus may be compromised and delivery is generally indicated.

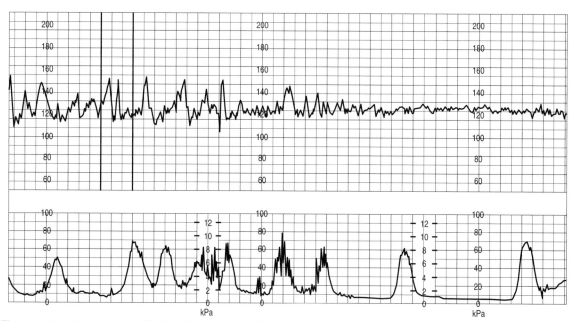

**Figure 1.12** A 'reassuring' CTG: baseline and variability are within normal limits, there are accelerations and no decelerations. This CTG shows a period of fetal activity, followed by sleep

CTG interpretation is a skill for which even experienced practitioners vary in their opinions. The principles described above confirm normality and identify deviations, instigating the need for referral if in doubt. The woman is fully informed throughout to facilitate informed choice.

## Intermittent auscultation in labour

The evidence regarding the unsuitability of continuous monitoring for uncomplicated pregnancies during labour means that midwives need the skill and confidence to use intermittent fetal heart rate assessment. This may be with a Pinard stethoscope or sonicaid. As home births, pool births and midwifery-led care increase, so does the need for intermittent auscultation (IA). The current guideline (NICE 2001) is that the fetal heart should be assessed for 60 seconds after a contraction at least every 15 minutes in the first stage, and every 5 minutes in the second stage. Beech (2001) indicates that this can be almost as invasive as continuous monitoring and that midwives should therefore exercise their autonomy and consider the wellbeing of the woman. Harrison (2004) indicates that the best protocol is actually unknown, the research being scarce and much required.

## Summary

- Abdominal examination is a skill from which significant information can be gained
- The midwife has a responsibility to undertake it competently, record the findings and make a referral if necessary
- The fetal heart is auscultated using a Pinard stethoscope, but a sonicaid or CTG monitor may be used as well where complications exist
- CTG monitors should be correctly applied and the trace interpreted accordingly
- Uncomplicated pregnancies may only require auscultation with a Pinard stethoscope throughout pregnancy and labour.

## Self-assessment exercises

The answers to the following questions may be found in the text:

1. Describe the components of an abdominal examination, discussing the rationale for each aspect.
2. Describe how the fetal heart rate is assessed.
3. Describe the procedure when applying a CTG monitor.
4. Discuss how the midwife would assess that a fetal heart tracing was within normal limits.
5. Summarise the role and responsibilities of the midwife in relation to abdominal examination and use of electronic fetal monitoring.

## REFERENCES

Beech B 2001 Electronic fetal monitoring. The Practising Midwife 4(7):31–33

Gardosi J, Francis A 1999 Controlled trial of fundal height measurement plotted on customised antenatal growth charts. British Journal of Obstetrics and Gynaecology 106(4):309–317

Harrison J 2004 Auscultation: the art of listening. Midwives 7(2):64–69

Lindhart A, Nielsen P, Mouritsen L et al 1990 The implications of introducing the symphyseal fundal height measurement: a prospective randomised controlled trial. British Journal of Obstetrics and Gynaecology 97(8):675–680

MDA (Medical Devices Agency) 2002 SN2002(23) Cardiotocograph (CTG) monitoring of fetus during labour – update. Online. Available: http://www.medical-devices.gov.uk

Neilson J P 2000 Symphysis–fundal height measurement in pregnancy. Cochrane Database Systematic Review CD000944

NICE (National Institute for Clinical Excellence) 2001 The use of electronic fetal monitoring. NICE, London

NICE (National Institute for Clinical Excellence) 2003 Antenatal care (6). NICE, London

NMC (The Nursing and Midwifery Council) 2002 Guidelines for records and record keeping. NMC, London

Olsen K 1999 'Now just pop up here, dear...'. Revisiting the art of antenatal abdominal palpation. The Practising Midwife 2(9):13–15

Wickham S 2002a Pinard wisdom tips and tricks from midwives, part 1. The Practising Midwife 5(9):21

Wickham S 2002b Pinard wisdom tips and tricks from midwives, part 2. The Practising Midwife 5(10):35

Chapter **2**

# Principles of abdominal examination — during labour

This chapter focuses on the principles of abdominal examination during labour, encompassing the abdominal examination described during pregnancy (Ch. 1) and the palpation of uterine contractions. Both of these are essential components of care during labour, and are skills in which the midwife should be competent. This chapter summarises the reasons for undertaking abdominal examination and specific issues relating to undertaking this with the labouring woman. It then considers the indications for, and the skill of, palpating contractions.

**Learning outcomes**

Having read this chapter the reader should be able to:

- discuss the indications for undertaking an abdominal examination during labour and the information that may be obtained
- discuss how uterine contractions can be palpated
- discuss the role and responsibilities of the midwife when undertaking abdominal examination and palpation of contractions.

## Abdominal examination

There are a number of reasons why the midwife may undertake an abdominal examination during labour. The information gained can help in the assessment of progress and inform care. This is therefore not undertaken in isolation, rather the information acquired should be considered with other information gained, particularly findings from the examination per vaginam and assessment of maternal and fetal wellbeing.

**Indications**

- To gain a baseline on which care is provided and subsequent progress assessed, by determining the gestation, lie, position, presentation, engagement and auscultation of the fetal heart
- To monitor progress by assessing descent and rotation of the presenting part
- Prior to auscultation of the fetal heart or commencing monitoring using cardiotocography (CTG)
- Prior to undertaking an examination per vaginam
- Multiple births, following delivery of each baby, to determine the lie, position and presentation of the remaining fetuses.

**Procedure and relevant issues**

This is the same as described earlier (Ch. 1). However, it is important to remember that women may experience heightened abdominal sensitivity during labour, resulting in the procedure being one that may cause discomfort and contraction. The midwife should ensure that the procedure is not undertaken unnecessarily and is completed promptly. The examination should be undertaken between contractions, to minimise discomfort and make it easier to palpate the fetus.

This procedure requires the woman to be in an almost recumbent position, which is not ideal for labour. Thus the midwife should ensure that the woman is encouraged to adopt a more upright position following the examination, whenever possible.

The findings from the abdominal palpation should be recorded in the relevant documentation, which should include the obstetric/midwifery notes, the partogram and CTG (NMC 2004a). Any deviations should be reported to the appropriate personnel (NMC 2004b).

**Palpation of uterine contractions**

The midwife uses the information gained from the palpation of contractions to assess progress in labour and to inform care, e.g. appropriate use of Entonox (Ch. 27). The contraction of the uterus can be felt as it hardens beneath the abdominal wall. The contraction begins in the fundus of the uterus and spreads down and across the uterus in a wave-like manner. The contraction is strongest in the fundus, becoming weaker as it spreads throughout the uterus (fundal dominance). Thus the contraction is palpated most easily by placing a hand over the area of the fundus. The midwife is able to assess the frequency of contractions by ascertaining the length of time between the onset of each contraction. Resting tone of the uterus is also observed by assessing the tone of the uterus between contractions. Noting the degree of firmness – a subjective assessment – can assess the strength of the contraction, whereas the length of the contraction is noted by timing the contraction from beginning to end. From this, the midwife can ascertain whether the contractions are increasing in length, strength and frequency, as would be expected during normal labour. As with other examinations, the findings are not taken in isolation, but form part of an overall assessment.

## Indications

- To assess progress of labour in relation to the length, strength and frequency of the uterine contractions
- Correct administration of Entonox (Ch. 27)
- During the second stage of labour – if the woman is being instructed when to push, e.g. with an epidural block
- During active management of the third stage of labour – to determine if the uterus is contracted prior to undertaking controlled cord traction to deliver the placenta and membranes (Ch. 35).

## PROCEDURE   assessing uterine contractions

- A watch/clock with a second hand is required to time the contraction
- Gain informed consent
- Wash and warm hands
- Ensure the woman is in a comfortable position, with access to the area of the abdomen beneath which the fundus is located; the abdomen can remain covered
- Place one hand on the top part of the abdomen, over the fundal region of the uterus
- Keeping the hand still, feel for the contraction along the length of the fingers (not just the fingertips)
- Note the time when the abdomen (and uterus) first contracts
- Observe the length of time the contraction lasts and the extent to which the uterus hardens
- Keeping the hand on the abdomen to await the next contraction, observe the time between contractions to assess frequency and note the relaxed, resting tone of the uterus
- If the contractions are irregular, palpate the contractions for 10 minutes to calculate the number occurring in a 10-minute period. (This is more intrusive; it may be preferable to ask the woman to note the number of contractions in a 10-minute period, provided she is aware of them)
- Discuss the findings with the woman
- Document the findings and act accordingly.

## Role and responsibilities of the midwife

These can be summarised as:

- undertaking a competent examination in which all of the information is gained
- palpating contractions sensitively and accurately
- recognising deviations from the norm and instigating referral
- education, explanations and support of the woman
- appropriate record keeping.

## Summary

- Abdominal examination during labour is an essential aspect of care, enabling the midwife to provide informed advice about care and progress
- While the procedure is the same as during pregnancy, the midwife should be aware of the heightened sensitivity of the abdomen during labour
- Palpation of uterine contractions is a simple procedure that provides information in relation to progress and informs care.

## Self-assessment exercises

The answers to the following questions may be found in the text:

1. What are the indications for performing an abdominal examination during labour?
2. How may the midwife use the information obtained during an abdominal examination?
3. Discuss how the midwife can palpate uterine contractions.
4. What are the role and responsibilities of the midwife when undertaking:
   a. an abdominal examination during labour?
   b. palpation of uterine contractions?

## REFERENCES

NMC (Nursing and Midwifery Council) 2004a
Guidelines for records and record keeping. NMC, London

NMC (Nursing and Midwifery Council) 2004b
Midwives rules and standards. NMC, London

Chapter **3**

# Principles of abdominal examination — during the postnatal period

This chapter focuses on the principles of abdominal examination during the postnatal period in relation to assessing involution of the uterus. It begins with a description of the physiology of involution, followed by a discussion of how the midwife assesses that involution is occurring normally. Palpation of the uterus forms part of the postnatal examination undertaken by the midwife.

**Learning outcomes**

Having read this chapter the reader should be able to:

- briefly outline the physiology of involution
- discuss the relevance of assessing the height, position and tone of the uterus during the postnatal period
- describe the procedure to assess involution of the uterus
- discuss the role and responsibilities of the midwife when undertaking abdominal examination during the postnatal period.

## Physiology of involution

Involution is the process by which the uterus returns to its pre-pregnant size, position and tone. This involves a reduction in weight from 1000 to 60 g and reduction in size from $15 \times 11 \times 7.5$ cm to $7.5 \times 5 \times 2.5$ cm. Autolysis refers to the digestion of excess muscle fibres by proteolytic enzymes, a process that is assisted by the continuing contraction and retraction of the uterus that began during labour. As the uterus reduces in size, the decidua is shed within the lochia (the discharges from the vagina following childbirth) and new endometrium begins to grow from the basal layer of the endometrium. New endometrial growth is evident from about the 10th day following delivery; by 6 weeks the endometrium has reformed.

Changes in the colour and amount of the lochia reflect the changes occurring within the endometrium and may vary with individual women. During the first 2–4 days following the birth of the baby, the lochia contain blood cells, necrotic deciduas, fragments of the amnion and chorion (lochia rubra), and are usually red in colour (initially bright, changing to dark red then brown as the proportion of blood cells within the lochia decreases). From around the third to fourth day, the lochia change to a pinkish-red colour (lochia serosa) and also contain leucocytes and organisms. The lochia then change to a whitish-yellow discharge, usually from the 10th to 14th postnatal day (lochia alba) (Blackburn & Loper 1992). These changes can be noted by inspecting the sanitary pad worn by the woman, and are noted in conjunction with other findings.

## Rationale for the procedure

Although involution is not complete until the end of the puerperium, much of the reduction in the size and weight of the uterus has occurred by the 10th day of the postnatal period. The rate of involution will vary from woman to woman and progress should be assessed in relation to the individual woman. This is achieved by palpating the uterus through the abdominal wall and determining whether it is decreasing in size; ideally the same midwife undertakes the palpation each time to increase reliability. The practice of measuring the height of the uterus is unreliable and has little value (Cluett et al 1997) and it is important to take into account other clinical signs.

While the effectiveness of palpating the uterus during the postnatal period in relation to preventing or predicting deviations from the norm has not been adequately researched (Montgomery & Alexander 1994), Marchant et al (2000) suggest there is benefit in undertaking assessment of postnatal uterine fundal height in relation to predicting secondary postpartum haemorrhage resulting in readmission to hospital. However, the midwife will still undertake this as part of the postnatal examination to inform the care and management until evidence suggests to the contrary.

In addition to assessing the descent of the uterus, the position and tone of the uterus are assessed. The uterus should be positioned centrally within the abdomen. A full bladder can displace the uterus, causing it to deviate to one side. This can interfere with myometrial contraction, predisposing to postpartum haemorrhage. Thus, when the uterus is deviated, the lochia should be assessed to ensure the woman is not haemorrhaging and she should be encouraged to empty her bladder. The tone of the uterus should be firm, indicating a well-contracted uterus. If the tone is poor, the uterus will feel soft, again associated with postpartum haemorrhage. A full rectum, retained products of conception or blood clots can cause the uterus to feel bulky.

Additionally, the uterus should not feel tender when palpated, and discomfort could be indicative of infection. There may be tenderness where the uterus has been incised during a caesarean section.

Palpation of the uterus during the postnatal period can assess progress. However, the findings should be considered in relation to other findings, such as the colour and amount of lochia.

### Rate of descent

Following delivery of the placenta and membranes, the uterus is found at or just below the woman's umbilicus, approximately 12 cm above the symphysis pubis; fundal height decreases approximately 1 cm each day (Blackburn & Loper 1992) (Fig. 3.1). After 6 days, the fundus is usually about halfway between the umbilicus and the symphysis pubis and should be just palpable by the end of 10 days. For many women, the fundus may not be palpable at this time, and is usually no longer palpable after the 12th postnatal day.

Involution may be slower if the uterus is unable to contract and retract effectively. This may occur following a caesarean section, uterine tear or due to the presence of retained products of conception; it could also be indicative of infection. Subinvolution of the uterus should be investigated as the woman may be predisposed to a secondary postpartum haemorrhage.

Figure 3.1    The position of the uterus during involution. (A) Following delivery; (B) 1 week following delivery – the fundal height is palpable approximately 5 cm above the symphysis pubis; (C) 2 weeks following delivery – the fundal height is usually not palpable above the symphysis pubis

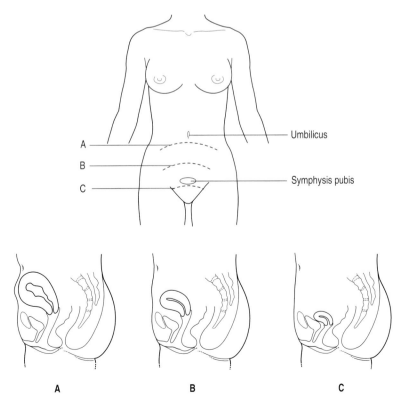

## PROCEDURE    assessing involution

- Gain informed consent
- Ask the woman to empty her bladder if she has not done so recently
- Wash and warm hands
- Ask the woman to lie down in a recumbent position with her arms by her side
- Ensure she is comfortable and privacy is maintained
- Expose the woman's abdomen
- Using the outer aspect of one hand, gently depress the abdomen to feel for the fundus. If the fundus is not found, remove the hand and reposition higher or lower and gently press down again
- When the fundus is felt, use the outer aspect of the hand to estimate the height, position and tone of the uterus
- Re-cover the abdomen, assisting the woman to a comfortable position
- Discuss the findings with the woman
- Document the findings and act accordingly.

### Role and responsibilities of the midwife

These can be summarised as:

- undertaking a competent examination in which all of the information is gained
- recognising deviations from the norm and instigating referral
- education, explanations and support of the woman
- appropriate record keeping.

## Summary

- Palpation of the uterus during the postnatal period forms part of the daily postnatal examination undertaken by the midwife
- It provides information on involution by assessing the height, position and tone of the uterus, in conjunction with other factors such as lochial loss per vaginam
- Research is required to ascertain the preventative and predictive value of undertaking this skill.

### Self-assessment exercises

The answers to the following questions may be found in the text:

1. When is involution complete?
2. What information can be gained by palpating the uterus during the postnatal period?
3. Describe the procedure for palpating the uterus during the postnatal period.
4. The lochia may be examined following abdominal palpation. What information may be gained from this in relation to involution?
5. What factors may influence the rate of involution?

## REFERENCES

Blackburn S T, Loper D 1992 Maternal, fetal and neonatal physiology: a clinical perspective. W B Saunders, Philadelphia

Cluett E R, Alexander J, Pickering R M 1997 What is the normal pattern of uterine involution? An investigation of postpartum uterine involution measured by the distance between the symphysis pubis and the uterine fundus using a paper tape measure. Midwifery 13(1):9–16

Marchant S, Alexander J, Garcia J 2000 How does it feel to you? Uterine palpation and lochial loss as guides to postnatal recovery. The Practising Midwife 3(7):31–33

Montgomery E, Alexander J 1994 Assessing postnatal uterine involution: a review and a challenge. Midwifery 10(2):73–76

Chapter **4**

# Assessment of maternal and neonatal vital signs — temperature measurement

This chapter considers the means and significance of obtaining an accurate temperature measurement. There is discussion about the different sites for temperature assessment, followed by the equipment available.

| Learning outcomes | Having read this chapter the reader should be able to: |
| --- | --- |

Having read this chapter the reader should be able to:

- discuss the midwife's role and responsibilities in relation to temperature measurement, identifying when it should be undertaken
- define normal body temperature for the childbearing woman and baby
- describe the factors that influence body temperature and the changes relating to childbearing
- discuss the suitable sites for temperature measurement, highlighting their rationale for use, normal temperature ranges and the equipment that can be used
- describe the types of thermometer and how each one is used correctly and safely
- demonstrate taking a baby's temperature.

## Definition
Body temperature is the balance between heat gain and heat loss.

## Core temperature
Humans are homoeothermic, i.e. their core temperature is maintained around 37° Celsius (C) whatever the external environmental temperature. Should the balance be altered the body may be seriously affected, as humans cannot tolerate extreme changes at either end of the temperature range. The core temperature refers to the temperature within the brain, the abdominal and the chest organs, reflecting the warmest parts of the body. Core temperatures are usually reached

about 2 cm below the body surface (Hinchliff et al 1996), with two-thirds of body mass maintained at core temperature. The most accurate measurement of the core temperature, the 'gold standard', is found in the pulmonary artery (Board 1995).

### Peripheral temperature

The peripheral temperature generated by skin and skeletal muscle is often lower than the core temperature and so helps to regulate the core temperature by assisting with heat loss and gain. Peripheral temperatures reduce proportionally as distances increase from the core.

### Effects of temperature extremes

Maintenance of the body temperature at a constant level is essential to ensure optimal functioning of the cells and their chemical reactions and consequently the body systems. Rises in body temperature increase the demands for oxygen and therefore increase the heart rate. Should the temperature rise to 40.5°C, cellular damage may begin; temperatures above 42°C may result in brain dysfunction, coma, cardiovascular collapse and death. A lowering of body temperature will result in uncoordinated muscle activity and fatigue, unconsciousness, cardiac arrhythmias and death.

### Normal values

According to Dubois (1948) the normal oral temperature is set within a range of 35.8–37.3°C; however, each person has a 'normal' temperature setting within this range. A rise in core temperature of 1°C may be difficult to detect if a person's normal temperature is 36.0°C.

## Factors influencing body temperature

Deviations may occur due to a disruption in the temperature regulating centre in the hypothalamus, resulting in a rise or decrease in the core temperature, or in response to infection or inflammation. Such factors include the following:

- Diurnal variations: circadian rhythms influence both the core and the peripheral temperature. Body temperature is lowest during the night and peaks in the evening
- Menstrual cycle: body temperature is lower during the postmenstrual period of the menstrual cycle, increasing by 0.3–0.5°C following ovulation. This rise in body temperature is maintained until

progesterone levels decrease prior to the onset of menstruation (Hinchliff et al 1996, Houdas & Ring 1982)

- Digestion: a slight increase in temperature of 0.1–0.2°C has been noted to occur with normal digestion
- Basal metabolic rate: heat is produced as a result of chemical reactions within the body. When the body is at rest, this is referred to as the basal metabolic rate (BMR). The amount of heat produced can be altered by various regulatory mechanisms to ensure the body temperature is maintained within the normal range: the higher the BMR, the more heat is produced, the higher the temperature (Houdas & Ring 1982). BMR decreases with age, with babies having a higher BMR than adults. Women also have a slightly lower BMR than men (Chinyanga 1991). Certain diseases/disorders will increase the BMR (e.g. hyperthyroidism). Exercise can also cause a rise in temperature. Closs (1987) suggests strenuous exercise may increase the core temperature to 40°C
- Hot baths: these can raise the body temperature by 0.5–1.0°C for up to 45 minutes
- Fever: leucocytes release endogenous pyrogens in response to stimulation by pyrogenic substances such as bacterial, viral and protozoal infection and necrotic tissue. This causes the thermostat within the hypothalamus to be 'reset' at a higher level. The affected person feels cold and the body attempts to raise the temperature to maintain it within its higher 'normal' range. When the level of endogenous pyrogens decreases, the thermostat returns to its original setting. The person then feels hot, with the body attempting to lower the temperature to its normal setting
- General anaesthesia: general anaesthetic drugs can interfere with the normal homeothermic mechanisms that assist with heat loss and gain, predisposing to heat loss (Schönbaum & Lomax 1991). Chinyanga (1991) proposes that the greatest decrease in body temperature will occur during the first hour of anaesthesia and that this can induce postanaesthetic shivering
- Alcohol: Kalant and Lé (1991) conclude from their review of the literature that large amounts of alcohol will lower the body temperature
- Childbearing: this is discussed in detail below.

The midwife should be aware of these factors so that inappropriate treatments are not commenced or pathologies overlooked if a false temperature reading is obtained.

# Temperature changes related to childbirth

### Pregnancy – maternal

During pregnancy, progesterone and a raised metabolic rate increase the amount of heat generated by 30–35%. Although the body attempts to compensate for this by increasing heat loss mechanisms, the maternal temperature can increase by 0.5°C (Blackburn & Loper 1992).

### Pregnancy – fetal

Intrauterine temperature is determined partly by maternal temperature and partly by the maternal–fetal gradient as the fetus is unable to regulate its own temperature. Generally, the fetal temperature is approximately 0.5°C higher than the maternal temperature. Therefore, a raised maternal body temperature will result in a higher fetal temperature and is associated with intrauterine hypoxia, fetal tachycardia, teratogenesis and preterm labour (Blackburn & Loper 1992).

### Labour

During labour, a rise in temperature can be indicative of infection, dehydration or the result of increased muscular activity from uterine contractions.

### Postnatal period – maternal

A transient rise in maternal temperature can occur within the first 24 hours following delivery. Blackburn and Loper (1992) suggest that up to 6.5% of women have a rise in temperature up to 38°C in the 24 hours following a vaginal birth. In the majority of cases, this is physiological and resolves spontaneously. However, for a small number of women, the temperature rise may be due to an infection, such as a puerperal infection, mastitis or a urinary tract infection, or may result from an inflammatory process such as the development of a deep venous thrombosis. The temperature may also rise in breastfeeding women around the second to third day as milk production occurs. This will resolve spontaneously once lactation is established although it can take several days.

### Postnatal period – baby

Babies emerge from the warmth of the uterus (37°C+) to an environment of approximately 21°C, wet and needing to establish several adaptations to extrauterine life simultaneously. Thermoregulation is difficult for the immature systems, and is further affected by:

- the large ratio of surface area to body mass with thin layers of insulating subcutaneous fat. This creates an increased opportunity to lose body heat, especially from the head
- the changeable nature of the environment, especially open doors or windows, fans, cold mattresses, etc.

Consequently, babies lose heat by evaporation, especially before thorough drying, by convection when draughts blow over them, by radiation and conduction to nearby items and surfaces. A decrease in temperature of between 1 and 2°C may occur during the first hour of birth if action is not taken to remedy this, and a normal body temperature may not be achieved for 4–8 hours (Black 1972).

Heat production comes mainly from metabolic processes, moving and shivering both being limited activities. External clothing helps, while the stores of brown fat are utilised, along with calories from milk. Metabolism requires both glucose and oxygen; a cold baby rapidly becomes hypoxic and hypoglycaemic and can have a serious metabolic acidosis. The problems are compounded significantly if the baby is preterm or small for gestational age.

Attention to careful management of the baby's temperature immediately following birth and in the first weeks of postnatal life is essential, including education of the parents. Danger exists for hyperthermia as well as hypothermia. An infected baby may display a changeable or cool temperature rather than the expected high temperature.

## Indications

Takahashi (1998) indicates that temperature measurement has been a routine part of the care given by midwives. However, although no longer a stipulated task, it is recognised to be variable in its reliability and therefore the midwife is encouraged to offer individualised care to women based on their needs. Takahashi (1998) suggests particularly that it is a limited indicator of wellbeing for postnatal women. The following list suggests the current indications:

- on admission to hospital as a baseline
- during labour, usually 4 hourly or more frequently if indicated
- after delivery initially for both the woman and baby, then as required
- as clinical condition requires for woman and baby
- preterm labour, prelabour rupture of the membranes, especially if prolonged, loin or abdominal pain (? urinary tract infection – UTI)
- blood transfusion.

Temperature assessment is rarely made in isolation, and the following factors should also be considered:

- Is it a necessary observation?
- What will the course of action be according to the findings? Has a referral been made previously?
- Are other vital signs within normal limits, e.g. pulse rate?
- Are there signs of a physiological or pathological reason for a temperature variation?

● Has it been taken in an accurate manner in an appropriate site with suitable equipment?

# Sites for temperature recording

## Choosing a site

While the presence or absence of certain equipment can automatically reduce the choice of site, the following should be considered when making a choice:

● known reliability of the site
● accessibility
● ability of the woman to comply
● safety
● local policy
● equipment available.

The reader should note that the literature is conflicting as to the accuracy and reliability of different sites, both for adults and children, and therefore regular review of the published research is necessary, along with adherence to local protocols.

## Commonly used sites

These sites are generally readily accessible and therefore are commonly used:

● oral (mouth or buccal cavity)
● tympanic (ear)
● axilla.

These three sites will be discussed in detail below. Other less common sites can also be used:

● Rectal: while some practitioners advocate its advantages (e.g. good blood supply, well insulated and good correlation with core temperature), it is now less frequently used. It is inaccessible and embarrassing for adults and vagal stimulation can be a danger in children and babies (Bailey & Rose 2000). If necessary a lubricated catheter is used to check anal patency at birth, rather than a thermometer
● Pulmonary artery: only accessible in high dependency care (e.g. intensive therapy unit), when such accuracy is essential and the readings can be safely obtained
● Oesophagus: as above
● Skin: skin probes are used in environments such as the neonatal intensive care unit.

## Oral site

**Rationale for use** Oral temperature measurement has been seen traditionally to be an accurate, almost non-invasive, technique. The
thermometer should be placed in one of the sublingual pockets, located
on either side of the tongue (Fig. 4.1). A branch of the carotid artery, the
sublingual artery, runs beneath the sublingual pocket (Closs 1987). The
blood within this vessel is travelling to the hypothalamus, therefore it
responds rapidly to changes in body temperature. It is a readily
accessible site, with little inconvenience to the woman and minimal
contact with body fluids.

**Normal values** An acceptable adult oral temperature reading is between
35.8 and 37.3°C (Dubois 1948). The temperature in other parts of the
mouth is lower than in the sublingual pocket. The temperature within
the mouth can be affected by environmental factors. Drinking hot
fluids and smoking can create an artificially high reading, while mouth
breathing, tachypnoea and drinking iced fluids can create a false low
reading.

**Safety and compliance** The woman will be required to hold the apparatus in her mouth with her mouth closed. The oral site should be
avoided due to lack of compliance and/or potential danger for:

- babies and young children
- labouring women
- anaesthetised, semi-conscious or unconscious women

**Figure 4.1** Sublingual pockets
of the mouth

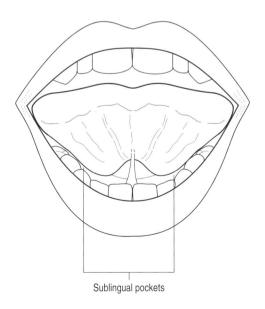

Sublingual pockets

- women likely to experience seizure, e.g. fulminating pre-eclampsia
- facial or oral impairment/injury
- known oral infection
- nausea or vomiting
- failure to gain consent.

It is therefore only a safe temperature measurement route for a coherent adult or an understanding older child.

**Suitable equipment** Electronic, mercury in glass and disposable thermometers (pp 40 and 43) are all suitable for oral use.

## Summary

- The oral site is readily accessible with a good reactive blood supply and is suitable for different thermometer types
- The woman needs to be compliant, but readings can be affected by environmental factors.

### Tympanic membrane

**Rationale for use** The tympanic membrane of the ear shares the same blood supply as the hypothalamus and is closely positioned to it. It is considered to be an accurate approximation of core temperature. The auditory canal is insulated (maintaining the temperature of the site) and easily accessible.

**Suitable equipment** Temperature recordings from the tympanic membrane can only be taken with a specific tympanic thermometer (p. 41).

**Accuracy** Accuracy is dependent upon an ambient temperature in the ear and the correct positioning of the equipment (p. 42). Any of the following factors in the ear can affect the validity of the recording:

- presence of moisture, e.g. vernix caseosa, amniotic fluid
- excessive wax
- infection
- recent surgery
- raised air temperature, e.g. an incubator.

The Medical Devices Agency (MDA 2003) has received several alerts as to the problems of incorrect use of tympanic thermometers, particularly in the home. They point out that the probe must be clean and that the ear canal must be straightened in order for the scan to be of the ear drum and not just the canal wall (see p. 42 for correct use of this thermometer).

Several studies (adult and neonatal) now suggest that tympanic thermometers (partly for their ease of use) are the most reliable (Bailey

& Rose 2001, Dowding et al 2002), but this is not by any means a consistent recommendation (Fawcett 2001, Scanga et al 2000).

**Safety** The technique uses single-use covers, eliminating the danger of cross-infection. The manufacturers suggest that it is safe for all age groups.

## Summary

- The tympanic membrane is a reactive site, minimally invasive, that uses specialised equipment with any age group. Accuracy is both advocated and questioned.

### Axilla site

**Rationale for use and normal values** Fulbrook (1993) believes that axilla temperatures are closely correlated with core temperature and therefore concludes that normal values for an adult axilla temperature equate with those of the oral route: 35.8–37.3°C. Not all authors would agree with this, but researched evidence is scarce. It is also often the site recommended for temperature measurement in babies. An inaccurate reading will be gained if the thermometer is left in situ for insufficient time or if the woman is malnourished and the skin folds of the armpit are not in good contact with the thermometer. The thermometer should be placed centrally in the axilla. The effects of sweat, deodorant and vernix on temperature measurement have not been evaluated within the literature.

**Safety and compliance** The axilla is usually accessible by moving clothes slightly and so compliance is good. The woman needs to be mindful of the fact that the thermometer is in the armpit and that mobility is restricted at that time.

**Suitable equipment** Disposable, mercury in glass and electronic thermometers are all suitable for use in the axilla.

## Summary

- Value has recently been placed on using the axilla as a reliable site in all age groups
- It is reasonably accessible and can accommodate a range of thermometers.

# Types of thermometer

Choosing the equipment for temperature measurement may depend upon the site chosen and the availability of suitable apparatus. The literature (as for site) is conflicting as to the most accurate piece of equipment to use. Training should be given and the equipment must always be used according to the manufacturer's instructions. It should also be maintained and cleaned properly. The availability of some of the equipment discussed below may depend upon finance, local policies, safety and suitability.

## Electronic thermometers

These will vary in appearance but are generally available in two designs (Fig. 4.2):

1. a digital reading at the end of the thermometer
2. a digital reading on the hand-held box attached to the temperature probe.

**Figure 4.2** (A) Electrical thermometer with digital reading (Adapted with kind permission from Jamieson et al 1997); (B) electrical thermometer with temperature probe

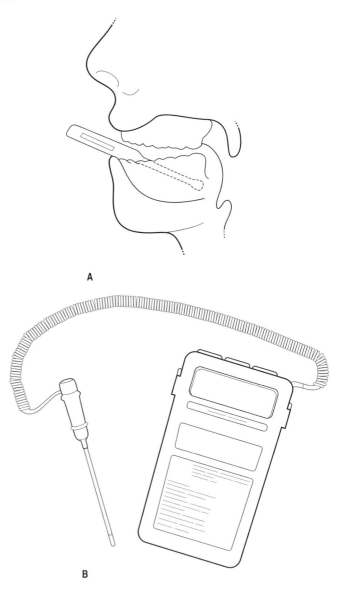

A

B

The reading usually occurs within 1 minute and an alarm sounds to indicate that this has happened. Oral, axilla or rectal sites may be used for the adult; the axilla is used for the baby. There is a danger of cross-infection, as the thermometer is often used for more than one woman. Disposable covers must be used and the thermometer must be cleaned and maintained according to the manufacturer's guidelines. Some electronic thermometers have a separate probe for rectal use.

PROCEDURE  **electronic thermometer use in oral and axilla sites**

- Gain informed consent
- Wash hands
- Take the thermometer and cover to the woman
- Clarify if any environmental factors exist that may affect the reading, e.g. a recent hot drink
- Apply a disposable cover, switch on the thermometer, allow it to self-calibrate and when ready insert correctly into the chosen site (sublingual pocket or centrally against chest wall)
- Remove and read when the alarm sounds
- Dispose of the cover correctly
- Clean the thermometer if indicated
- Discuss the findings with the woman
- Wash hands
- Document findings and act accordingly.

**Summary**

- A rapid, easy to use and read thermometer
- Attention must be paid to the prevention of cross-infection and proper maintenance.

**Tympanic thermometers**

Tympanic membrane thermometers scan the tympanic membrane using an infrared scanner to make temperature measurements. Readings are made in less than 1 minute and are displayed digitally. Clearly, the thermometer is only ever placed in the ear, but can be used with both adults and babies. As discussed earlier, some environmental conditions can affect the accuracy of the result (p. 38). It may be expensive initially and will require regular servicing and calibration. The user should be properly instructed in its use.

PROCEDURE  **tympanic thermometer use**

Due to differences in manufacturers' designs, the reader is encouraged to read the specific instructions with their thermometer. These are general guidelines:

- Gain informed consent
- Cover the thermometer tip with the supplied sheath
- Switch the thermometer on
- Aim to use the same ear for each assessment
- When it is ready to scan, insert into the ear, ensuring that the auditory canal is sealed. To do this, for adults and children over 1 year of age, the pinna is pulled gently but firmly upwards and backwards, prior to inserting the thermometer (Fig. 4.3A,B). For babies of less than 1 year of age, the pinna is pulled straight back and the tip inserted into the ear opening (Fig. 4.3C) (MDA 2003)
- Remove and read the thermometer when the alarm sounds
- Remove and dispose of the sheath
- Switch off the thermometer
- Discuss the findings with the woman
- Document the findings and act accordingly.

A baby cared for in an incubator should have the ear nearest to the sheet used (downwards ear) rather than the upper ear, which will have been exposed to the environmental heat.

**Figure 4.3** (A, B) Use of a tympanic thermometer in adults and children >1 year: the pinna is pulled up and back to straighten the auditory canal; (C) use of a tympanic thermometer in babies <1 year: the pinna is pulled straight back and the tip of the thermometer inserted into the ear opening (Adapted with kind permission from HMSO)

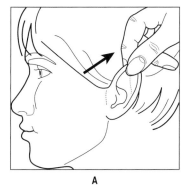
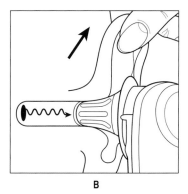

A                                    B

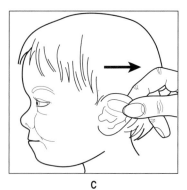

C

**Summary**

- The initial outlay may be expensive, but this is an easy, rapid technique causing minimal disruption to the woman
- Maintenance and correct positioning are necessary to ensure accuracy.

## Disposable (chemical) thermometers

Disposable thermometers are now widely available. They are considered to be accurate, cheap and comfortable to use (Board 1995). They are made of flexible plastic with a series of chemical pads at one end. As the temperature rises the pads undergo a chemical reaction and colour change. The level to which the colour change has occurred is the point at which the temperature is read (Fig. 4.4). They are suitable for oral, axilla and rectal use for the adult, axilla only for the baby. Reliability is impaired if the thermometers are stored in too hot an environment. The manufacturer's instructions should be read before the thermometer is used.

PROCEDURE    **disposable thermometer use**

The thermometer is used in the same way as an electronic thermometer (p. 41) except that:

- oral recordings can be made after 1 minute, axilla and rectal after 3 minutes (Blumenthal 1992); an accurate time source is needed
- the chemical pads should be placed against the chest wall
- the thermometer is given 10 seconds to stabilise before being read (may vary according to manufacturer)
- when reading the thermometer the first dot on the line is the same as the number next to it. The number is then counted along according to the number of dots that have changed colour (Fig. 4.4 indicates 36.8°C)
- The thermometer is disposed of correctly.

**Summary**

- Disposable thermometers are easy to use and eliminate the dangers of cross-infection
- Accuracy may be impaired under certain environmental conditions.

**Figure 4.4** Disposable thermometer indicating a reading of 36.8°C (Adapted with kind permission from Jamieson et al 2002)

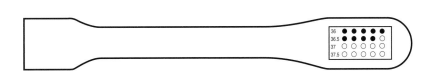

## Mercury in glass thermometers

Mercury in glass (MIG) thermometers work on the principle that the mercury enclosed in glass expands with heat. The thermometer is shaped so that the scale can be seen beneath magnified glass for ease of reading.

### Considerations for use

Mercury thermometers are now used infrequently in practice due to the hazards of mercury poisoning if breakage should occur. There are also considerable dangers of cross-infection if not cleaned or covered properly, and the time required for an accurate reading means that they are labour intensive (oral, 4 minutes; axilla, 9 minutes; Closs 1987). In the event of using a MIG thermometer, it is important that the mercury is shaken down with a firm flick of the wrist prior to inserting it. Failure to do so will create a false reading.

## Conclusion

When choosing a site for temperature recording consideration should be given to its accessibility, acceptability, known reliability and safety. The midwife needs to recognise the strengths and limitations of each site and piece of equipment available in order to make accurate recordings of a temperature. Temperature assessment can provide evidence of the clinical condition and may lead to further investigations and treatment.

## Taking a baby's temperature

Taking a baby's temperature is different from taking that of an adult. The site used is generally the axilla with a disposable or electronic thermometer. Tympanic thermometers can also be used, some of which will be a specific paediatric size and need to be inserted correctly as described on page 42. The normal values for an axilla recording are between 36.5 and 37.0°C.

## Indications

Due to immaturity and difficulties with maintaining thermoregulation, particularly in the presence of hypoglycaemia or hypoxia, babies should have their temperatures taken immediately following birth, an hour later and at any other point during the first few days of life when they appear cool or hot to the touch. The abdomen is the best guide when assessing the skin temperature. Equally, a baby that is unwell, pale, difficult to feed, preterm or needed active resuscitation will also require temperature assessment. Detailed below is the outline procedure for using the axilla site (Fig. 4.5).

**Figure 4.5** Taking a baby's temperature: axilla site using electronic thermometer

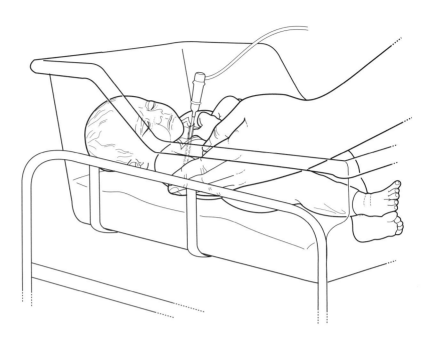

**PROCEDURE    taking a baby's temperature**

- Parents should accompany the baby, their informed consent having been gained
- The baby is placed in a safe and warm environment, e.g. in the cot
- Clothing is loosened so that the axilla is accessible; the baby is not allowed to chill, but if respiration is being counted at the same time then the chest may be exposed (Ch. 7)
- The covered or disposable thermometer is placed into the axilla and the arm held gently across the chest to keep the thermometer secure
- After the required length of time the thermometer is removed and read. The clothing is replaced and the baby returned to his parents
- Records are made and action taken according to the findings.

**Role and responsibilities of the midwife**

These can be summarised as:

- recognising the need to undertake temperature measurement
- use of appropriate equipment in the correct sites
- referral if indicated
- contemporaneous record keeping.

**Self-assessment exercises**

The answers to the following questions may be found in the text:

1. Discuss the factors that influence body temperature.
2. List the occasions when temperature assessment is undertaken for a childbearing woman and a newborn baby.
3. What is the normal temperature range for the woman and how does this alter during the ante-, intra- and postpartum periods?
4. What is an accepted normal temperature range for a newborn baby?
5. Discuss the advantages and disadvantages of each of the sites for temperature assessment.
6. Discuss how each type of thermometer currently available is used correctly.
7. Demonstrate taking a woman's temperature using a tympanic thermometer.
8. Demonstrate taking a baby's temperature using the axilla site.
9. Summarise the role and responsibilities of the midwife when undertaking temperature assessment.

## REFERENCES

Bailey J, Rose P 2000 Temperature measurement in the preterm infant: a literature review. Journal of Neonatal Nursing 6(1):28–32

Bailey J, Rose P 2001 Axillary and tympanic membrane temperature recording in the preterm neonate: a comparative study. Journal of Advanced Nursing 34(4):465–474

Black L 1972 Neonatal emergencies and other problems. Butterworth Heinemann, Oxford

Blackburn S T, Loper D 1992 Maternal, fetal and neonatal physiology: a clinical perspective. W B Saunders, Philadelphia

Blumenthal I 1992 Should we ban the mercury thermometer? Journal of the Royal Society of Medicine 85(9):533–555

Board M 1995 Comparison of disposable and mercury in glass thermometers. Nursing Times 91(33):36–37

Chinyanga H M 1991 Temperature regulation and anaesthesia. In: Schönbaum E, Lomax P (eds) Thermoregulation: pathology, pharmacology and therapy. Pergamon Press, New York, ch 9

Closs J 1987 Oral temperature measurement. Nursing Times 7:36–39

Dowding D, Freeman S, Nimmo S et al 2002 An investigation into the accuracy of different types of thermometers. Professional Nurse 18(3):166–168

Dubois E F 1948 Fever and the regulation of body temperature. C C Thomas, Springfield

Fawcett J 2001 The accuracy and reliability of the tympanic membrane thermometer: a literature review. Emergency Nurse 8(9):13–17

Fulbrook P 1993 Core temperature measurement in adults: a literature review. Journal of Advanced Nursing 18:1451–1460

Hinchliff S M, Montague S E, Watson R 1996 Physiology for nursing practice, 2nd edn. Baillière Tindall, London

Houdas Y, Ring E F J 1982 Human body temperature. Plenum Press, New York

Jamieson E M, McCall J M, Blythe R et al 1997 Clinical nursing practices, 3rd edn. Churchill Livingstone, Edinburgh

Jamieson E M, McCall J, Whyte L 2002 Clinical nursing practices, 4th edn. Churchill Livingstone, Edinburgh

Kalant H, Lé A D 1991 Effects of ethanol on thermoregulation. In: Schönbaum E, Lomax P (eds) Thermoregulation: pathology, pharmacology and therapy. Pergamon Press, New York, ch 15

Medical Devices Agency 2003 MDA/2003/010 Infra-red ear thermometer home use. Medical Devices Agency. Online. Available: http://www.medical-devices.gov.uk

Scanga A, Wallace R, Kiehl E et al 2000 A comparison of four methods of normal newborn temperature measurement. MCN 25(2):76–79

Schönbaum E, Lomax P (eds) 1991 Temperature regulation and drugs: an introduction. In: Thermoregulation: pathology, pharmacology and therapy. Pergamon Press, New York, ch 1

Takahashi H 1998 Evaluating routine postnatal maternal temperature check. British Journal of Midwifery 6(3):139–143

# Chapter 5

# Assessment of maternal and neonatal vital signs — pulse measurement

This chapter examines pulse assessment: what it is, how, when and why it is completed. Factors affecting heart rate are also discussed; other means of pulse assessment are discussed briefly. Pulse is a direct indicator of the action of the heart; the midwife should recognise the significance of it as an assessor of wellbeing. From such a straight-forward observation much information can be gained, and using the correct technique each time increases the reliability of the results. Assessment of the fetal heart is discussed in Chapter 1.

| Learning outcomes | Having read this chapter the reader should be able to: |

- discuss the midwife's role and responsibilities in relation to pulse assessment, identifying when, where and how it is undertaken
- identify the normal range for the childbearing woman and baby
- discuss factors that influence the heart rate.

## Definition

A pulse is a rhythmic expansion and recoil of the elastic arteries as the left ventricle ejects blood into the circulation (Jamieson et al 2002). The pacemaker (sinoatrial (SA) node) of the heart works to ensure that the heart meets the body's needs. The autonomic nervous system relays the cues which cause the heart to beat faster or slower to the SA node. The effects both extend to and come from the inter-relation of other body systems (e.g. the lungs). If, for example, running for a bus causes shortness of breath, one of the effects will be that the heart beats faster to supply more oxygen to the body tissues. Other factors affecting the heart rate are discussed below. These changes mean that it is necessary to assess a person's pulse for its rate, rhythm and volume. A weak or thready pulse, or a rapid or full bounding one, indicate changes in the amount of blood being pumped. An irregular pulse reflects an irregular pumping action of the heart.

## Factors influencing the heart rate

The following factors increase the rate:

- Pregnancy and labour (discussed below)
- Emotions: stress, anxiety, nervousness and excitement
- Pain
- Infection: almost any infection (with or without changes to other vital signs)
- Haemorrhage
- Shortage of red blood cells, e.g. iron deficiency anaemia
- Changes in position, e.g. from sitting to standing
- Fluid and/or electrolyte imbalances, including dehydration
- Exercise (as above)
- Allergic reactions: anaphylaxis causes the pulse to be weak, tachycardic and irregular
- Medications: drugs can cause tachycardia or bradycardia, e.g. salbutamol causes tachycardia and digoxin bradycardia
- Disease may affect heart rate, e.g. hyperthyroidism causes tachycardia.

The following factors reduce the rate:

- Rest and relaxation: calm, controlled breathing can reduce the heart rate
- Insult or injury: myocardial infarction or other injury may cause the heart to slow or stop
- Age: heart rate decreases with age.

## Normal values

A healthy non-pregnant female adult has a regular heart rate of approximately 70–80 beats per minute (bpm), with the normal range between 60 and 100 bpm.

A newborn baby has a heart rate of 110–160 bpm, with the average being approximately 130 bpm. Heart rate varies noticeably with respiration in the newborn.

## Changes related to childbirth

*Pregnancy*
During pregnancy the maternal heart rate increases from 4 weeks' gestation by approximately 15–20 bpm, peaking at 28 weeks, due to changes in cardiac output and stroke volume, corresponding with an

increase in total blood volume. The rate declines slightly during the third trimester, and positional changes are particularly obvious throughout pregnancy. The rate is higher in the sitting or supine position than the lateral recumbent position (Blackburn & Loper 1992).

Mild cardiac arrhythmias (e.g. extra beats) may occur as a result of these changes and are harmless, usually resolving without treatment. However, the presence of cardiac disease places additional stress on the cardiovascular system of a pregnant woman. Such a woman will require close observation and specialist care.

### Labour

During labour each contraction returns 300–500 mL of blood to the circulation. The heart rate rises accordingly, but this may also be due to other factors (e.g. pain, anxiety, exercise).

### Postnatal period – maternal

Blackburn and Loper (1992) suggest bradycardia occurs immediately following delivery as the circulation readjusts without the placenta. In a healthy woman without delivery complications, the heart rate then begins to stabilise, returning to its pre-pregnant level within 2–6 weeks.

# Sites for pulse measurement

A pulse can be felt anywhere in the body where an artery near to the surface can be palpated against something firm, usually bone. The heart rate can also be heard (e.g. using a stethoscope).

The most commonly used site in the adult is the radial artery, being readily accessible; other sites are indicated in Figure 5.1. The brachial artery is used in the measurement of blood pressure and the carotid or femoral arteries may be palpated in the case of collapse, where cardiac output cannot be detected in the peripheral circulation. Where there is an inconsistency between the heart beating and the pulse felt at the periphery, the two can be counted together (apical and radial) by two midwives. The midwife counting the apical assessment uses a stethoscope, placing it in the midline on the left side of the chest between the fifth and sixth ribs. Both readings are recorded using different coloured inks.

In the baby, the most usual site of pulse measurement is either apical (which can be heard or felt) or brachial (Fig. 5.2). Immediately after delivery the pulsation at the base of the umbilical cord is generally a reliable indicator of the heart rate. If this is slow the apical should be checked. The radial pulse is not a site of choice in any child under 2 years of age, the palpable area being so small and the rapidity of the pulse being hard to count (Dougherty & Lister 2004). Listening to the apical beat has greater reliability.

**Figure 5.1** Main sites for adult pulse assessment (Adapted with kind permission from Thibodeau & Patton 1999)

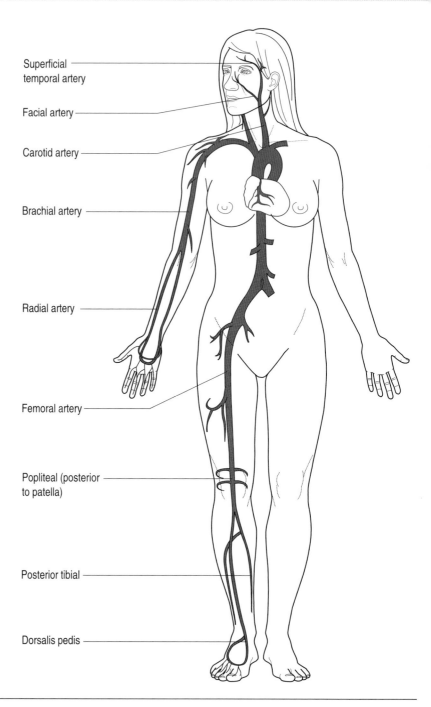

Superficial temporal artery

Facial artery

Carotid artery

Brachial artery

Radial artery

Femoral artery

Popliteal (posterior to patella)

Posterior tibial

Dorsalis pedis

## Indications

While care should be individual and according to need, indications for pulse assessment are:

### Maternal

- on admission, as a baseline recording
- any deviation from the norm or signs of illness or accident

Figure 5.2  Main sites for neonatal pulse assessment

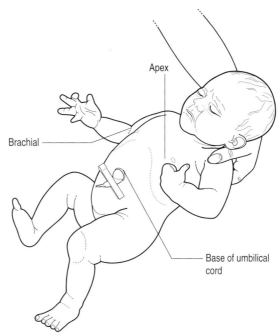

Apex

Brachial

Base of umbilical cord

- when using a Pinard stethoscope to auscultate the fetal heart
- during labour (the pulse should not be taken during a contraction) and prior to transfer of care following labour
- during and following surgery
- postnatal assessment, if indicated
- prelabour spontaneous rupture of membranes
- during blood transfusion
- treatment for preterm labour using tocolytic drugs.

### Baby

The heart rate is only generally monitored if the baby is ill or preterm, requiring intensive care. Other occasions include:

- at delivery as part of Apgar scoring and resuscitation
- any signs of cyanosis, irritability or illness.

## Documentation

Pulse assessment can be written in the woman's/baby's records as prose. However, if repeated observations are undertaken an overall picture is obtained if the findings are recorded pictorially on an observations chart or partogram. This will show at a glance if there is a pattern emerging or if the condition is changing.

PROCEDURE    **adult radial pulse**

- Obtain informed consent, ensure the woman is comfortable and if possible in the same position as the last assessment

- Locate the radial artery, placing the index and middle fingers over it, supporting the woman's wrist and arm across her chest (if the wrist is held too firmly the pulse will be occluded, if held too lightly it is difficult to count)
- Count the pulse, for either 30 seconds if it is completely regular, then double it, or 60 seconds if irregular
- Undertake respiration assessment (Ch. 7) if necessary
- Discuss the results with the woman, explaining whether it will be necessary to assess the pulse again
- Document the findings and act accordingly.

| PROCEDURE | **baby** |
|---|---|

The baby should be peaceful and not crying when undertaking pulse assessment:

- Obtain informed consent from the parents, expecting at least one parent to be present throughout
- Loosen the clothing and access the chosen site
- (a) Place the index and middle fingers over the brachial artery; or (b) place a warmed stethoscope over the apex of the heart (midline, left side of the chest); or (c) place index and middle fingers over the apex. Count the pulse for 60 seconds, noting volume and regularity
- Observe the colour, behaviour and general condition of the baby at the same time
- Replace the clothing and ensure comfort
- Discuss the results with his parents
- Document the findings and act accordingly.

# Other means of pulse measurement

ECG (electrocardiogram) monitors give a continuous or single reading, or printout of the heart rate and pattern. Pulse oximeters (Ch. 7) also give a heart rate reading, as do cardiotocograph machines for fetal heart assessment (Ch. 1).

## Role and responsibilities of the midwife

These can be summarised as:

- recognising when pulse assessment is indicated
- undertaking the assessment correctly
- referral if indicated
- contemporaneous record keeping.

## Summary

- Pulse assessment is a straightforward, non-invasive skill of considerable importance
- An accurate assessment includes the rate, volume and regularity of the pulse
- Assessment of the general condition of the woman or baby is made simultaneously.

The answers to the following questions may be found in the text:

1. Discuss the significance of pulse assessment and when it should be undertaken for the childbearing woman.
2. What changes occur to the heart rate during pregnancy and labour and why do they occur?
3. List the normal ranges for the antenatal woman, labouring woman, postnatal woman and newborn baby.
4. Discuss the factors that affect the heart rate.
5. Describe how a baby's heart rate can be measured immediately after birth.
6. Summarise the role and responsibilities of the midwife when undertaking pulse assessment.

## REFERENCES

Blackburn S T, Loper D 1992 Maternal, fetal and neonatal physiology: a clinical perspective. W B Saunders, Philadelphia

Dougherty L, Lister S 2004 The Royal Marsden Hospital manual of clinical nursing procedures, 6th edn. Blackwell Publishing, Oxford

Jamieson E, McCall J, Whyte L 2002 Clinical nursing practices, 4th edn. Churchill Livingstone, Edinburgh

Thibodeau G A, Patton K 1999 Anatomy and physiology, 4th edn. Mosby, St Louis

# Chapter 6

# Assessment of maternal and neonatal vital signs — blood pressure measurement

This chapter considers the issues surrounding the accurate measurement of arterial blood pressure, physiology, influencing factors and changes that occur during childbirth. The equipment available, technique of blood pressure measurement and factors influencing the accuracy of the recording are discussed, concluding with a discussion of venous blood pressure measurement. The midwife can confirm normality and detect deviations from the norm through the measurement of blood pressure. This is essential, as changes in blood pressure can have serious consequences for both the woman and the fetus/baby.

## Learning outcomes

Having read this chapter the reader should be able to:

- discuss the midwife's role and responsibilities in relation to the measurement of blood pressure, identifying when and how it is undertaken
- define blood pressure, identifying the difference between systolic and diastolic pressure and the normal range for the childbearing woman and baby
- discuss the factors that influence blood pressure and the changes relating to childbearing
- describe how central venous pressure is measured.

## Definition

Blood pressure is the force exerted by the blood on the vessel walls.

Blood pressure varies within the different blood vessels, being highest in the large arteries closest to the heart and decreasing gradually within the smaller arteries, arterioles and capillaries. Blood pressure continues to reduce as blood returns to the heart via the venules and veins. Blood pressure measurement (measured in millimetres of mercury – mmHg) usually reflects the arterial blood pressure although venous pressure may also be measured.

## Arterial blood pressure

This is the pressure exerted on the arterial walls. Arterial blood pressure facilitates blood flow around the body to ensure adequate oxygenation of the tissues and vital organs. It is not constant, increasing during ventricular contraction (systole) and decreasing when the ventricles relax (diastole). When recording blood pressure it is important to assess both the highest and lowest levels of pressure as these reflect differing physiological responses of the cardiac cycle.

## Mean arterial pressure

This is the average pressure needed to push the blood through the circulatory system. It can be estimated electronically or mathematically, using the formula:

Mean arterial pressure = 1/3 systolic pressure + 2/3 diastolic pressure

**Systolic pressure** This is the pressure exerted on the blood vessel walls following ventricular systole, when the arteries contain the most blood and is the time of maximal pressure. Systolic pressure is determined by the:

- amount of blood ejected into the arteries (stroke volume)
- force of the contraction
- distensibility of the arterial wall.

An increase in the first two factors, or a decrease in the third factor, raises systolic pressure and vice versa.

**Diastolic pressure** This is the pressure exerted on the blood vessel wall during ventricular diastole, when the arteries contain the least amount of blood, resulting in the least pressure being exerted on the blood vessel walls. Diastolic pressure is influenced by the:

- degree of peripheral resistance
- systolic pressure
- cardiac output.

Diastolic pressure is lower when these are reduced, particularly when the heart rate is slower as there is less blood remaining in the arteries.

**Pulse pressure** This is the difference between the systolic and diastolic pressure.

## Venous blood pressure

This is the pressure exerted on the walls of the veins, reflecting venous flow to the heart (particularly circulating blood volume) and cardiac function. Central venous pressure measures the pressure within the right atrium and is determined by:

- the volume of blood entering the right atrium (venous return)
- right ventricular function
- venous tone
- intrathoracic pressure.

### Normal maternal arterial values

The normal range for a healthy adult is 100/60–140/90 mmHg (Dougherty & Lister 2004), but varies according to age and other variables. The World Health Organization defines hypertension as a systolic blood pressure of 160 mmHg or above and a diastolic blood pressure of 95 mmHg or above. Blood pressure may vary between the right and left arm. Beevers et al (2001a) recommend that blood pressure should be measured in both arms initially to determine if significant differences are present (20 mmHg systolic pressure, 10 mmHg diastolic pressure). The same arm should be used to measure blood pressure to ensure consistency.

# Blood pressure changes related to childbirth

### Pregnancy

Haemodynamic changes occur during pregnancy primarily as a result of hormonal and anatomical changes, resulting in an increased blood volume, increased cardiac output and heart rate. While this normally causes an increase in blood pressure, these changes are counterbalanced by the effect of progesterone on the blood vessel walls, resulting in decreased peripheral resistance. Pregnancy is not normally associated with significant changes in arterial blood pressure. Blood pressure usually begins to decrease during the first trimester, as the effects of progesterone are evident before blood volume has increased to its maximum point in the third trimester. It begins to rise gradually from the middle of pregnancy, returning to pre-pregnancy levels by term. The early decrease in blood pressure is much less for systolic pressure than for diastolic pressure (Blackburn & Loper 1992).

Venous pressures do not alter significantly during pregnancy, although venous pressure below the uterus increases with gestation. This may impede venous return to the heart but does not usually create problems. However, some women may experience a transient hypotensive episode (supine hypotensive syndrome) due to the weight of the gravid uterus compressing the inferior vena cava, impeding venous return. This occurs more commonly when in a supine position and is quickly rectified by changing to a lateral or recumbent position.

### Labour

Increased anxiety and pain levels result in a rise in blood pressure. Additionally, both systolic and diastolic blood pressures increase during uterine contractions. The systolic pressure may increase by up to

35 mmHg during the first stage, rising further during the second stage. Diastolic blood pressure also increases by up to 25 mmHg in the first stage, increasing in the second stage by up to 65 mmHg (Blackburn & Loper 1992). These changes begin 5–8 seconds before the onset of the contraction and are maintained until the contraction is completed.

### Postnatal period – maternal

Increased venous return following delivery results in higher venous pressures. As the blood volume and physiological effects of pregnancy decrease, the blood pressure will return to its pre-pregnant level.

### Postnatal period – baby

Blood pressure increases with gestational age; blood pressure is lower in the preterm baby than the term baby. A rapid rise in arterial blood pressure occurs during the first week of life, with blood pressure increasing gradually with age (Walker 1993).

# Factors influencing arterial blood pressure

A variety of factors influence arterial blood pressure, including:

- Blood volume: a reduction in circulating blood volume (e.g. haemorrhage, shock), resulting in a decrease in both systolic and diastolic blood pressure
- Heart rate: blood pressure increases with an increasing heart rate providing the circulating blood volume is unaltered
- Age: blood pressure increases with age due to loss of elasticity of the arterial walls
- Diurnal variations: systolic pressure is highest in the evening, lowest in the morning and changes during rest and sleep periods
- Weight: overweight people tend to have higher blood pressure
- Alcohol: a consistently high alcohol intake is associated with higher blood pressure, although alcohol may also lower blood pressure by inhibiting the effects of antidiuretic hormone, resulting in vasodilatation
- Smoking: smoking increases blood pressure, with effects lasting up to 30–60 minutes
- Eating: blood pressure increases for 30–60 minutes following ingestion of food
- Stress, fear, anxiety: these can all raise blood pressure by stimulating the sympathetic nervous system; 'white coat' syndrome refers to anxiety-related hypertension resulting from attending a health care setting
- Exercise: exercise increases blood pressure, with effects lasting 30–60 minutes

- Distended bladder: this can increase blood pressure, with effects lasting 30–60 minutes
- Hereditary factors: some people have an inherited predisposition to raised blood pressure; Stillwell (1992) suggests this is a factor in 50% of people with raised blood pressure
- Disease: any disease process affecting stroke volume, blood vessel diameter, peripheral resistance or respiration will alter blood pressure
- Renin: high renin levels cause vasoconstriction and an increase in blood volume (due to increased salt and fluid retention within the kidneys), resulting in a rise in blood pressure.

## Indications

Blood pressure is often recorded as a matter of routine throughout pregnancy and labour, less so during the postnatal period. While the circumstances in which the estimation of blood pressure is undertaken can vary, they include:

- the initial booking history to establish a baseline
- at each antenatal visit
- during labour
- as the clinical condition dictates, e.g. shock and haemorrhage, symptoms such as headaches, visual disturbances, proteinuria
- pregnancy-induced hypertension
- preterm or sick babies
- blood transfusion
- during and following surgery.

## Equipment

*Sphygmomanometer*

The basis of measuring blood pressure is to exert a measured pressure on an artery (commonly brachial), usually with a sphygmomanometer, which comprises a manometer (pressure gauge) and an inflatable cuff. The blood flow is occluded and as the pressure is released and blood begins to flow through the artery, different sounds can be heard through a stethoscope (auscultatory). Oscillatory sphygmomanometers detect the pulsation of blood flow, avoiding the need to listen for sounds.

Different types of sphygmomanometer are available and can be divided into two categories: auscultatory (manual) and oscillatory (automated, electronic). Aneroid and mercury column manometers are the two forms of auscultatory sphygmomanometer available and are seen more commonly in the community setting. Beevers et al (2001a) consider mercury manometers to be more accurate than aneroid devices. Oscillatory systolic values tend to be higher than auscultatory values, but oscillatory diastolic values tend to be lower than auscultatory values. To ensure accurate blood pressure comparisons between different recordings, measurements should be undertaken on similar equipment. It is important to record the type of sphygmomanometer used. The use of oscillatory manometers is increasing, particularly within hospitals.

All sphygmomanometers should be maintained properly, with manometers being recalibrated every 6–12 months to maintain accuracy. The date of the last calibration should be marked on the machine. The tubing should also be checked regularly for signs of deterioration and replaced accordingly. The control valves should be able to hold a pressure of 200 mmHg for 10 seconds allowing for a rate of fall of 1 mmHg per second (Jolly 1991); it is important for the control valves to be checked regularly to ensure the free passage of air without undue force.

### Aneroid

This type of manometer has a circular gauge encased in glass, with a needle that points to numbers. Pressure variations within the inflated cuff cause metal bellows within the gauge to expand and collapse, moving the needle up and down the gauge. Prior to use, the needle should be set at zero.

These are lightweight, compact and portable but less accurate than mercury column manometers as the metal parts are liable to expand and contract with temperature changes. Aneroid manometers should undergo biomedical calibration on a regular basis to increase accuracy. Beevers et al (2001a) suggest these devices lose accuracy with time, resulting in falsely low readings.

### Mercury column manometers

This type of manometer has mercury contained within a glass column, with ascending numbers on either side of the column. The mercury should be clearly visible, have no gaps and rest at the zero level. If the mercury is below zero, the reservoir can be topped up. The column of mercury usually needs to be upright; some mercury manometers are read at an inclined angle but these are not commonly used in midwifery. The mercury should be read at eye level as looking up or down at the mercury can result in distorted readings. When examining the manometer, ensure the air vent or filter at the top of the column is clear and clean (oxidation of mercury can make it appear dirty and difficult to read, columns should be cleaned every year). If it becomes blocked, the mercury response is sluggish, leading to false results (Jolly 1991).

Mercury manometers underestimate systolic pressure by up to 10 mmHg and overestimate the diastolic (based on phase V sounds) pressure by up to 8 mmHg (Jolly 1991).

Mercury is a substance hazardous to health and should a spillage occur, appropriate steps should be taken to remove the mercury and minimise the risks of contamination. Each NHS Trust should have a policy to deal with this situation. The use of mercury-based equipment is decreasing due to the associated environmental risks. Beevers et al (2001a) refer to oscillatory devices that will measure blood pressure in both mmHg and kilopascals, suggesting these will, in time, replace mercury column manometers. The midwife will need to develop the knowledge of kilopascals as a blood pressure measurement if this becomes more commonly used in clinical practice.

### Oscillatory

These are electronic machines that measure blood pressure automatically. A cuff is placed around the arm, as with a manual manometer, and is attached to the machine. The machine can be set to record blood pressure on a regular basis, inflating and deflating the cuff at the desired time. A stethoscope is not required. The systolic and diastolic pressures are displayed visibly. The pulse is often counted and recorded at the same time.

These may reduce errors associated with auscultatory sphygmomanometers, e.g. sampling error, observer bias such as terminal digit preference, threshold avoidance (Gupta et al 1997). However, talking with the woman while blood pressure is being recorded may increase the measurement by 10–40% (Fetzer 1999).

## Summary

- There are a variety of sphygmomanometers available for use
- Aneroid manometers are lightweight and portable; however, there is a tendency to error due to expansion and contraction of the metal parts with temperature changes
- The mercury column manometer may underestimate systolic and overestimate diastolic pressure
- Automated manometers are considered more accurate and are being used increasingly in the hospital environment
- All manometers should be properly maintained and serviced.

### Cuff

The sphygmomanometer has a cuff that is placed around the upper part of the arm (Fig. 6.1), or occasionally around the forearm or lower thigh. The cuff is an inelastic cloth that encircles the arm and contains a bladder. Inside the bladder is an inflatable balloon which, when inflated to a pressure higher than the pressure within the artery, occludes the artery. At this point, blood flow ceases and the pulse is no longer palpable. The cuff is held in place either by Velcro fastenings or,

**Figure 6.1** The position of the cuff on the upper arm

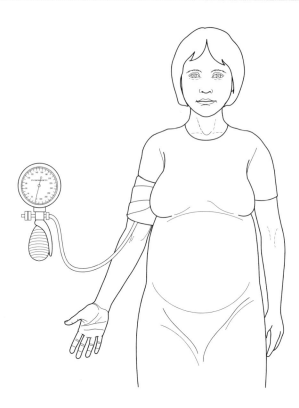

if a long tapering cuff is used, by wrapping it around the arm several times and securely tucking the end into the cuff. A loose cuff can distort the reading. The bladder is attached to tubing with a bulbous end that is squeezed to inflate the bladder. A valve on the bulb controls pressure within the bladder.

If the upper arm cannot be used, the lower arm can be used by placing the cuff centrally above the radial artery, or the lower third of the thigh with the cuff placed above the posterior popliteal artery. Systolic pressure is 20–30 mmHg higher in the leg than in the arm. The lower arm and leg are rarely used in midwifery.

It is important to use the correct cuff size; a cuff that is too small in length or depth can give falsely high readings (cuff hypertension). Conversely, a cuff that is too large can give falsely low readings (Oliveira et al 2002). The British Hypertension Society recommends the length of the inside bladder of the cuff should be at least 80% of the arm circumference and the depth should be at least 40%. The correct cuff width is 20% greater than the arm diameter (Jolly 1991, Oliveira et al 2002). Thus, standard cuff sizes (12 cm wide) are not appropriate for all adults as this is too small for large arms (use the wider 15–16 cm cuff) and too large for lean arms. Cuff lengths vary from 22 to 36 cm. Lean arms require a cuff length of 35 cm, larger arms 42 cm (Bardwell 1995).

### Stethoscope

By placing a stethoscope over the artery, the sounds of the blood flow and vibrations in the surrounding tissues can be heard. The level at which the artery is occluded and no sounds heard is equal to the systolic pressure. As the cuff is deflated, the pulse reappears and pulsating sounds are heard with each beat of the heart.

The bell-shaped part of the stethoscope head/end should be used to listen to the sounds as low pitch sounds (e.g. early and late Korotkoff sounds) can be heard more easily. When learning how to measure blood pressure, it may be easier to hear the sounds using the diaphragm (flat side) as it is often easier to hold this side of the stethoscope in place. Once the technique is mastered, the midwife should then use the bell side for greater clarity of sound.

Care should be taken not to press too hard on the stethoscope head as this compresses the brachial artery, resulting in a misleading murmur and possibly lowering the diastolic pressure reading. Bardwell (1995) suggests a pressure of 10 mmHg on the stethoscope significantly reduces the diastolic blood pressure and, of more concern, a pressure of 100 mmHg maintains the Korotkoff sounds until zero, making a recording impossible.

The stethoscope should be in good condition, particularly the earpiece, which should be clean and well fitting.

Ultrasound (Doppler) stethoscopes can be used if the arterial pulse is too weak to be heard on auscultation.

## Korotkoff sounds

The different sounds heard are named after the man who defined them in 1905. Korotkoff defined the sounds according to five phases, reflecting different stages in the measurement of blood pressure (Table 6.1).

Individual variations can occur in the sequencing of these sounds. In around 5% of hypertensive people, the phase II sounds may be absent, replaced by a short period of silence – the 'auscultatory gap'. This may last through a change of 40 mmHg. Audible Korotkoff sounds may be absent in 20–30% of obese people (Bardwell 1995).

Table 6.1  Blood pressure phases and Korotkoff sounds

| Phase | Sound |
|---|---|
| I | Faint tapping sounds that increase in intensity |
| II | Softening, swishing sounds |
| III | Crisper sounds with an intense pitch, not as intense as phase I |
| IV | Abrupt, muffled sounds, which become soft and blowing |
| V | Silence – no sounds heard |

The muffling sounds of phase IV are heard when the pressure gauge is 7–10 mmHg higher than the intra-arterial diastolic pressure. This is due to a loss of transmission of pressure from the cuff to the artery. The absence of sounds associated with phase V is considered to be more closely related to the intra-arterial diastolic pressure. However, phase V sounds may be very low or absent in some adults, particularly during pregnancy.

Whether to use phase IV or phase V sounds to record blood pressure has been the subject of debate, particularly when measuring blood pressure in pregnancy. From their analysis of the evidence, Beevers et al (2001b) recommend phase V as it is 'the most accurate measurement of diastolic pressure'. If, however, phase V continues to zero, phase IV should be used and it should be documented that this is the Korotkoff phase used.

---

PROCEDURE **blood pressure estimation using a manual manometer**

- Obtain informed consent
- Encourage the woman to empty her bladder
- Take the sphygmomanometer and stethoscope to the woman
- If the woman has been active, allow her to rest for at least 5 minutes
- Position the sphygmomanometer so that the base of the manometer is level with the woman's heart, whenever possible
- Assist the woman into a suitable position, legs uncrossed and expose her upper arm, ensuring no constriction from tight clothing
- Support her arm, and ask the woman to turn the palm of her hand upwards
- Palpate the brachial artery and position the cuff 2–3 cm above the site of brachial pulsation in the antecubital fossa, with the bladder of the cuff placed centrally above the artery to ensure even distribution of pressure during cuff inflation, and ensure the valve is closed
- Palpate the brachial or radial artery with the fingertips of one hand and, with the other hand, inflate the cuff rapidly by pumping the bulb until the pulse disappears; continue to inflate the cuff 30 mmHg above this
- Slowly deflate the cuff by opening the valve slightly, taking note of when the pulse reappears; this gives an approximate reading of the systolic pressure and prevents confusion arising from the presence of an auscultatory gap
- Quickly deflate the cuff by opening the valve fully and wait for 30 seconds then close the valve

- Place the stethoscope earpieces in your ears (allowing the angle of the earpieces to follow the angle of the external auditory canal) and the bell of the stethoscope over the brachial artery
- Inflate the cuff to a pressure 30 mmHg higher than the palpated systolic pressure
- Slowly deflate the cuff at 2–3 mmHg per second, listening for the appearance of the first clear sound
- Read the needle position or mercury level (systole) (at eye level)
- Continue to deflate the cuff slowly until the sounds become absent
- When the sounds are no longer audible, read the needle position or mercury level (diastole), deflate the cuff rapidly
- Assist the woman into a comfortable position, readjusting her clothing
- Discuss the findings with the woman
- Document the findings and act accordingly.

# Factors affecting accuracy

The whole procedure of recording blood pressure can take up to 5 minutes (Nolan & Nolan 1993). Care should be taken throughout to minimise the risk of inaccuracies occurring. Accuracy can be considered under three main headings: technique, equipment and operator bias.

# Technique

## Position

The arm should be at the level of the heart (mid-sternum). If above this level, the blood pressure may give a falsely low reading, whereas placing the arm below this level can give a falsely high reading, with differences of up to 10 mmHg (Beevers et al 2001b, Petrie et al 1986). Blood pressure is altered by 0.8 mmHg for each centimetre the arm is above or below the heart (Mallett & Bailey 1996). The arm should be horizontal and supported; if left dangling at the hip, blood pressure may increase by 11–12 mmHg (Dougherty & Lister 2004). An unsupported, extended arm may result in the diastolic pressure rising by up to 10% (Beevers et al 2001b).

The woman may adopt any position that is comfortable, although her legs should not be crossed as this can result in a falsely high recording (Nolan & Nolan 1993). If the woman changes her position immediately prior to this procedure, it is better to wait for a few minutes before recording the blood pressure to avoid erroneous results. Beevers et al (2001b) suggest waiting 3 minutes if a supine or sitting position is used, and 1 minute for a standing position.

## Cuff position

The bladder needs to be over the brachial artery and fitted properly as discussed earlier.

### Deflation of the cuff

Rapid deflation can result in the systolic pressure being underestimated and the diastolic being overestimated. The measurement should be recorded to the nearest 2 mmHg.

Never stop deflating the cuff between systolic and diastolic readings or reinflate the cuff to recheck the systolic reading. Blood will begin to flow into the lower arm, increasing the blood volume below the cuff, reducing the intensity and loudness of sounds (Hill 1980).

### Rechecking the measurement

If the reading is abnormal, it should be repeated twice more and the mean value calculated (Cook 1996). However, if multiple recordings are taken, at least 2 minutes should elapse between recordings (Hill 1980). Cook (1996) further recommends that if an abnormal blood pressure is found on the initial assessment, it should be estimated in both arms.

## Equipment

- Auscultatory and oscillatory manometers can yield different results
- Inappropriate cuff size
- Equipment not properly maintained.

## Operator bias

Operators may have an unconscious bias about what they expect to hear, influenced by knowledge of earlier recordings. If checking a woman's blood pressure that has already been recorded, accuracy is increased if previous findings are not known.

## Monitoring blood pressure in the baby

Blood pressure estimation in the baby is of particular significance as babies, especially preterm babies, are unable to tolerate fluctuations in blood pressure, predisposing them to intracranial haemorrhage.

Blood pressure can be read intermittently with a manometer system, using either auscultatory or oscillatory manometers, or continuously, using a transducer attached to an arterial line, connected to an oscilloscope. If the manometer system is used, minimal handling is required; oscillatory manometers are preferred. If the cuff is left on between measurements, it should be repositioned every 4–6 hours to reduce the risk of skin damage, nerve palsy or limb ischaemia. Blood pressure is recorded as for the adult; however, it may be difficult to auscultate the brachial artery with a stethoscope, and thus Doppler stethoscopes are often used. It is important to use the correct cuff size to obtain an accurate measurement, and neonatal cuff sizes are available. The cuff can be placed around either the arm or the leg.

*Normal range*

Blood pressure in the baby varies according to postnatal age, birthweight and state of arousal. It is lowest in babies who are sleeping, increasing during periods of wakefulness, agitation, crying and suckling. While systolic and diastolic pressures can be recorded, it is more usual to record the mean arterial pressure. The normal blood pressure for a term baby is 76/46 mmHg (mean 58 mmHg), rising to 76/48 mmHg (mean 64 mmHg) at 7 days. Roberton (1993) recommends the mean blood pressure for a baby weighing less than 1.5 kg is 30 mmHg, preferably 35 mmHg, and for larger term babies, 40 mmHg.

# Central venous pressure

Central venous pressure (CVP) is the pressure within the superior vena cava or right atrium, measured in centimetres (cm) of water ($H_2O$). The catheter is inserted via the femoral, brachial, subclavian or internal jugular vein. It is a direct measurement of blood pressure and is considered an important determinant of venous return measuring the pressure of blood filling the right atrium and cardiac output. It provides a more accurate reading of blood pressure and informs fluid management in the critically ill woman (Holloway 1993).

CVP measurement is usually read from one of two sites, both in line with the right atrium: the sternal angle, used with the supine position, and the mid-axilla site, used for a variety of positions (Fig. 6.2). There is a difference in pressure of up to 5 cm $H_2O$ between these two sites. The same site should be used for each measurement, ideally supine to reflect the pressure within the right atrium. Often an ink mark is used to mark the place used to obtain the reading. If the woman is breathless she will need to be semi-recumbent or upright. The position used should always be recorded.

Normal CVP measurements are 0–7 cm $H_2O$ at the sternal angle and 7–14 cm $H_2O$ at the mid-axilla site (Woodrow 2002). To convert from cm $H_2O$ to mmHg, multiply by 0.74 (1 cm $H_2O$ = 0.74 mmHg).

CVP readings are affected by the amount of blood in the right ventricle prior to systole, the contractility of the right ventricle and the amount of resistance to blood being ejected from the right ventricle. A low CVP reading is associated with haemorrhage, dehydration, hypovolaemia, drug-induced vasodilatation and vigorous diuresis. A high CVP reading is associated with ventricular failure, fluid overload, fluid retention in cardiac and renal disease, pulmonary obstruction, congestion and/or embolism.

# Equipment

CVP readings can be obtained via a water manometer, suitable for low pressures (less than 40 cm $H_2O$) or a pressure transducer and

**Figure 6.2**  CVP sites.
(A) Mid-axilla; (B) sternal
(The lower part of A and part B
have been adapted with kind
permission from Mallett &
Bailey 1996)

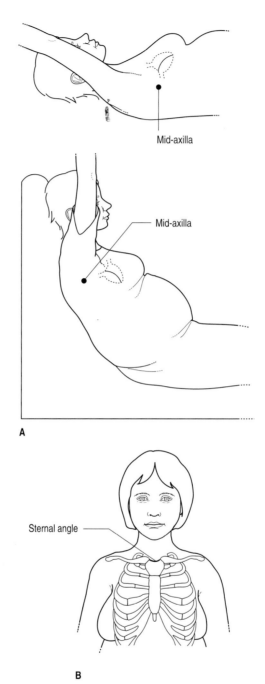

oscilloscope. The transducer converts the pressure waves to electrical
energy, displayed on the oscilloscope. It is useful when pressures are
high or where waveform depiction is required. Water manometers
provide intermittent readings, whereas pressure transducers provide
continuous readings of a CVP trace with a clear waveform that moves
up and down in line with the respiratory pattern.

**Figure 6.3** Three-way tap on the CVP line. (A) The position prior to reading or between readings, with fluid running from the fluid solution to the woman; (B) the position at the beginning of the procedure, as the manometer fills with fluid; (C) the position during the recording (Adapted with kind permission from Jamieson et al 1997)

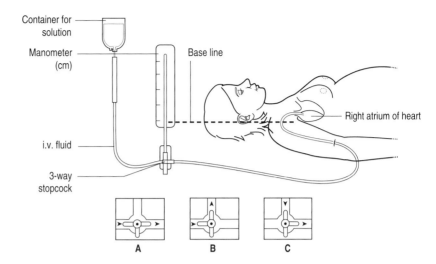

The CVP line is attached to a three-way tap, allowing for movement of fluid between the central venous line, intravenous infusion (saline, dextrose or dextrose saline) and manometer (Fig. 6.3). This allows for fluid infusion directly into the larger veins, and the tap is usually open to facilitate this. By moving the tap, the fluid can be redirected to an alternative site (e.g. the manometer) or prevented from flowing altogether. It is important to note the position of the tap prior to, during and following CVP measurement.

PROCEDURE    **measuring central venous pressure**

- Gain informed consent, gather equipment and ascertain site to be used
- Assist the woman in a supine or semi-recumbent position to allow the baseline of the manometer to be level with the woman's right atrium; with a critically ill woman, the position is usually supine with the bed flat
- Place the manometer so that the baseline is level with the woman's right atrium
- Slide the scale up or down by loosening the securing screw until the baseline figure is next to the arm of the spirit level – this should correspond to zero
- Extend the arm of the spirit level to the sternal angle or mid-axilla position to ensure the baseline and right atrium are level
- Move the manometer to position the bubble between the parallel lines of the spirit level
- Turn off all intravenous infusions running through the same site as the CVP line
- Turn the three-way tap to open the access from the intravenous infusion to the manometer, allowing the fluid to run slowly into the manometer

- Allow the manometer to fill several centimetres above the expected reading, without the upper end of the manometer becoming contaminated with fluid, then switch off the infusion line
- Remove any bubbles in the manometer as this can distort the reading
- Turn the three-way tap to direct the fluid from the manometer to the central venous line, allowing the fluid from the manometer to enter the woman's right atrium
- The column of fluid will fall rapidly and begin to oscillate with respiration between two numbers (usually 1 cm $H_2O$). The pressure in the column of fluid in the manometer is now equal to the pressure in the right atrium
- Note where the fluid is and read off the higher number
- Turn off the three-way tap to the manometer, and recommence the intravenous infusion, adjusting the infusion rate accordingly
- Assist the woman into a comfortable position, readjusting her clothing
- Document the findings and act accordingly.

## Summary

- Central venous pressure measurement provides an accurate reading of blood pressure in the critically ill woman
- Two sites may be used – the sternal angle and the mid-axilla site – with a difference in pressure of up to 5 cm of water between these two sites; consistency of site used is important.

## Role and responsibilities of the midwife

These can be summarised as:

- recognising the need to undertake blood pressure measurement
- completing the procedure correctly
- documenting the findings and acting on them accordingly
- ensuring that any equipment used is properly serviced and maintained.

## Self-assessment exercises

The answers to the following questions may be found in the text:

1. What is the difference between systolic and diastolic blood pressure?
2. What is the normal blood pressure and how is this altered during childbirth?
3. Discuss the factors that may influence blood pressure.
4. Discuss the factors that influence the accuracy of the measurement and how the midwife can minimise this.
5. What is the central venous pressure and how can it be measured?

## REFERENCES

Bardwell J 1995 For good measure...blood pressure measurement. Nursing Times 91(27):40–41

Beevers G, Lip G Y H, O'Brien E 2001a ABC of hypertension. Blood pressure measurement Part 2 – conventional sphygmomanometry: technique of auscultatory blood pressure measurement. British Medical Journal 322:1043–1047

Beevers G, Lip G Y H, O'Brien E 2001b ABC of hypertension. Blood pressure measurement Part 1 – sphygmomanometry: factors common to all techniques. British Medical Journal 322:981–985

Blackburn S T, Loper D 1992 Maternal, fetal and neonatal physiology: a clinical perspective. W B Saunders, Philadelphia

Cook R 1996 Measuring and recording blood pressure (continuing education credit). Nursing Standard 11(7):51–53

Dougherty L, Lister S 2004 The Royal Marsden Hospital manual of clinical nursing procedures, 6th edn. Blackwell Science, Oxford, p 448–455

Fetzer S J 1999 Vital signs. In: Potter P A, Perry A G (eds) Basic nursing: a critical thinking approach, 4th edn. Mosby, St Louis, p 434–477

Gupta M, Shennan A H, Halligan A et al 1997 Accuracy of oscillometric blood pressure monitoring in pregnancy and pre-eclampsia. British Journal of Obstetrics and Gynaecology 104:350–355

Hill M N 1980 What can go wrong when you measure blood pressure? American Journal of Nursing 80(5):942–946

Holloway N M 1993 Nursing the critically ill adult, 4th edn. Addison Wesley, California

Jamieson E M, McCall J M, Blythe R et al 1997 Clinical nursing practices, 3rd edn. Churchill Livingstone, Edinburgh

Jolly A 1991 Taking blood pressure. Nursing Times 87(15):40–43

Mallett J, Bailey C 1996 The Royal Marsden NHS Trust manual of clinical nursing procedures, 4th edn. Blackwell Science, Oxford

Nolan J, Nolan M 1993 Can nurses take an accurate blood pressure? British Journal of Nursing 2(14):724–729

Oliveira S M J V, Arcuri E A M, Santos J L F 2002 Cuff width influence on blood pressure measurement during the pregnant–puerperal cycle. Journal of Advanced Nursing 38(2):180–189

Petrie J C, O'Brien E T, Littler W A et al 1986 Recommendations on blood pressure measurement: British Hypertension Society. British Medical Journal 293:611–615

Roberton N R C 1993 A manual of neonatal intensive care, 3rd edn. Edward Arnold, London

Stillwell B 1992 Skills update. Macmillan, London

Walker A M 1993 Circulatory transitions at birth and the control of the neonatal circulation. In: Hanson M A, Spencer J A D, Rodeck C H (eds) Fetus and neonate physiology and clinical application, Vol 1. The circulation. Cambridge University Press, Cambridge, ch 7

Woodrow P 2002 Central venous catheters and central venous pressure. Nursing Standard 16(26):45–51

Chapter **7**

# Assessment of maternal and neonatal vital signs — respiration assessment

Respiration assessment is rarely undertaken for the healthy woman and baby, but is of significance in the event of ill health. This chapter considers the effects of pregnancy upon the respiratory system, other factors affecting respiration and the midwife's role and responsibilities in completing the observation correctly. Pulse oximetry is also discussed.

| Learning outcomes | Having read this chapter the reader should be able to: |

Having read this chapter the reader should be able to:

- define external respiration, identifying the normal ranges, factors that influence it and the principles for correct assessment
- discuss the safe and accurate use of pulse oximetry.

### Definition
External respiration is the means by which the body gains oxygen (inspiration) and excretes carbon dioxide (expiration). Assessment of respiration includes observation of the rate (number per minute), depth and regularity of breaths and any associated signs (e.g. skin colour). Breath sounds may also be heard, or the chest felt to rise and fall, as well as being visually observed.

### Normal values
A healthy adult at rest breathes regularly approximately 12–20 times per minute (Kozier et al 1998). Respiration can be consciously controlled (e.g. for swimming, singing, etc.) but is unconsciously determined by definite and precise mechanisms.

The newborn baby may breathe irregularly with a respiration rate of 40–60 breaths per minute (Michaelides 2004). Due to the weakness of the intercostal muscles, the baby may appear to be breathing abdominally, as the diaphragm is extensively used (Blackburn & Loper 1992).

## Changes related to childbirth

### Pregnancy

In supporting the fetus and the woman, the body's oxygen demands are high. The function and anatomy of the respiratory tract changes. Breathing is largely diaphragmatic, with the diaphragm being displaced upwards as the lower ribs flare. Progesterone relaxes the smooth muscle of the alveoli and despite the gravid uterus splinting the diaphragm from below, each breath is deeper. The rate of respiration is unchanged.

### Labour

The number and strength of contractions affect the pattern and depth of respiration during labour. Breath holding should be discouraged and deep breathing between contractions should be encouraged to maintain oxygenation amidst considerable muscular activity. Breathing exercises can assist the woman both physically and psychologically. The fetus is more likely to experience distress if there is maternal distress (Blackburn & Loper 1992). In the event of caesarean section, smaller ventilatory pressures may be required for the latter part of the surgery, when the diaphragm is no longer compressed (Blackburn & Loper 1992).

### Postnatal period – maternal

Respiration returns swiftly to its pre-pregnant pattern once labour is completed.

### Postnatal period – baby

Respiration is initiated as the baby is born and the fetal circulation adapts to the extrauterine circulation. A mature, patent respiratory tract is needed for oxygenation of the lungs. The first breath requires high negative intrathoracic pressure (30–40 cm $H_2O$) but thereafter, due to the action of surfactant, a pressure of only 5 cm $H_2O$ is required. Respiration is established by a number of factors:

- stimulation (light, tactile and temperature)
- compression and decompression of the chest as it passes through the vagina
- reflex stimulus of the respiratory centre from the chemoreceptors
- changes within the cardiovascular system to perfuse the lungs.

## Factors influencing normal respiration

- Exercise: an increase in oxygen demand causes an increase in respiration
- Emotions: the respiration rate and depth can be consciously controlled, which can be useful, e.g. breathing patterns in labour. Anxiety, nervousness, stress, excitement, fear and other emotions may also affect respiration

- Pain: hyperventilation is a physiological response to pain
- Insult or injury: complications such as pulmonary embolism or amniotic fluid embolism may cause infarction of the lung tissue and respiration may cease. The preterm infant may lack maturity of the respiration centre in the brain or have structural/physiological deficiencies, e.g. lack of surfactant
- Infection: infections that impair lung function cause the lungs to work harder to oxygenate the body. Fever (wherever the infection is) also increases the body's oxygen demands
- Reduced number of red blood cells: anaemia or haemorrhage reduces the oxygen-carrying capacity of the blood. In order to overcome this hypoxia the respiration rate increases to supply the body with extra oxygen
- Acidosis/alkalosis: respiration adjusts automatically to maintain acid–base balance in conjunction with other body systems. Changes in respiration can shift the balance, e.g. hyperventilation creates alkalosis
- Medications: opiate analgesics depress respiration; they are unlikely to have this effect in a healthy woman experiencing small doses, e.g. pethidine, but transplacental passage and therefore respiratory depression for the fetus/baby at birth is well documented (Siney 2004). The woman undergoing a general anaesthetic will require mechanical ventilation as paralysis of her respiratory function is induced. Mechanical ventilation controls the rate, depth and regularity according to need.

## Indications

*Maternal*

Although a recognised part of the vital signs assessment, the respiration rate is usually only counted if observed to be abnormal in rate, depth or regularity upon initial observation. The woman's colour and behaviour should also be noted – cyanosis may be seen in the mucous membranes (e.g. lips or nail beds), and shortage of oxygen can result in confused behaviour and speech. Respirations should be assessed in the following circumstances:

- admission to hospital with any respiratory complaint, e.g. asthma, chest infection, tuberculosis, etc., chest pain, breathlessness, cyanosis, after a road traffic accident or with any serious disorder, e.g. major haemorrhage, pre-eclampsia
- during active resuscitation
- before, during and following surgery (pre-surgery assessment provides a baseline against which later observations are compared)
- any signs of altered breathing pattern associated with psychological upset.

*Baby*
- at birth, as part of the Apgar score
- any signs of cyanosis, sternal recession, nasal flaring, noisy breathing, e.g. grunting, or laboured breathing, where the baby is using obvious energy to breathe
- after meconium-stained amniotic fluid or administration of naloxone at delivery
- during active resuscitation (see Ch. 60).

PROCEDURE    maternal

This is probably the only procedure when the consent of the woman is not sought. Making her aware of the action of counting her respirations will undoubtedly cause her to think about them and thus give a false reading. A respiration assessment is made at the same time as counting the pulse. If the wrist is supported across the woman's chest, it is possible to count the pulse and then to either feel the rise and fall of the chest, or observe it, counting respiration. The other factors (e.g. sound, depth, regularity, symmetry of both sides of the chest) are observed at the same time along with the woman's colour and condition. If the respiration rate is regular, it is counted for 30 seconds and doubled. If any abnormalities are detected, respiration is counted for a whole minute. Records are completed and the result is acted upon accordingly. As for pulse assessment (Ch. 5), the findings may be recorded pictorially on an observations chart or written in prose. The findings are discussed with the woman.

PROCEDURE    baby

A crying or excited baby should be calmed before respiration can be counted accurately. When assessing the respiration rate of a baby, it is better to expose the chest and abdomen, and observe/feel, listen and count for 1 minute, due to the irregularity of respiration. Informed consent is gained from the parents and the findings are recorded and discussed with them.

# Pulse oximetry

Pulse oximetry is used in conjunction with respiration assessment, particularly when a woman is seriously ill or after surgery. While technologically complicated, pulse oximetry is straightforward to use and has good reliability (Moyle 1999). Approximately 98–99% of the oxygen breathed is carried by the haemoglobin in the blood to the body tissues and organs (arterial haemoglobin saturation – $SaO_2$). The other 1–2% is dissolved in the plasma and is known as the partial pressure of oxygen ($PaO_2$). Sufficient amounts of oxygen in the plasma result in more being carried by the haemoglobin and vice versa: less in plasma = less in haemoglobin. Pulse oximetry measures the arterial saturation and is known this time as $SpO_2$. Red and infrared wavelengths of light are passed through peripheral tissue; the 'redness' of the saturated haemoglobin absorbs the light and is converted into a percentage (Chandler 2000). Normal oxygen saturation in women and babies would be in the range of 92–98% (Coull 1992), ideally over 97%, but unlikely to be 100%. It is clear, however, that $O_2$ saturation assessments do not take the place of arterial blood gas assessments (Moyle 1999). The DoH (1996) suggests that failure to use pulse oximetry postoperatively constitutes substandard care.

Informed consent is gained. In adults the monitor (Fig. 7.1A) is placed over a finger, toe or earlobe; in babies a hand, toe or foot is the most likely site for the probe (Fig. 7.1B). The light should pass from the top to the bottom of the limb (switch on and check direction before applying the monitor).

## Accuracy and safety

- Accuracy and safety are only maintained if the correct type of probe is applied correctly, hence the need to understand the different manufacturers' instructions
- Accuracy also depends on the flow of blood through the light being adequate. Poor circulation in a limb, or too much extraneous light (poorly fitted probe), can affect the reliability of the results

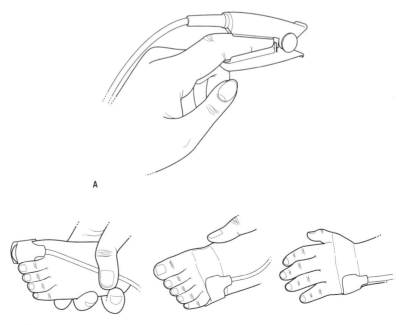

**Figure 7.1** (A) Adult pulse oximetry probe (Adapted with kind permission from Jamieson et al 2002); (B) neonatal pulse oximetry probe

A

B

- Thermal damage, possibly leading to necrosis, can occur to the skin of neonates if a probe is left in position for too long without a change of site. Anecdotally, this is believed to be 2 hourly (MDA 1988). This is particularly relevant in a preterm infant
- Accuracy is also affected by movement, dirt, dark nail polish and an inaccurately sized probe, e.g. never use an adult probe on a baby
- Neonatal probes are supplied with their fixative (tape or Velcro); applying additional tape can also affect the results
- Pulse oximetry is unaffected by skin colour or by jaundice (Moyle 1999).

The midwife must be familiar with the equipment, noting correct storage, use and maintenance, and knowing too, when to refer. Pulse oximetry use and findings must be documented.

## Role and responsibilities of the midwife

These can be summarised as:

- recognising when respiration assessment is indicated and when other interventions such as pulse oximetry are required
- undertaking the techniques correctly
- referral if indicated
- contemporaneous record keeping.

## Summary

- Assessing respiration is completed unobtrusively and includes the rate, depth, regularity and sound
- The general condition of the woman or baby is assessed simultaneously
- Pulse oximetry is an accurate, non-invasive technique that measures oxygen saturation via a correctly fitted peripheral probe.

## Self-assessment exercises

The answers to the following questions may be found in the text:

1. Discuss how pregnancy, labour and the puerperium affect respiration. What would be the accepted normal values during these times?
2. Define external respiration.
3. Describe when the midwife is likely to complete a respiration assessment:
   a. for a woman
   b. for a baby.
4. Which factors affect the accuracy of pulse oximetry?
5. Summarise the role and responsibilities of the midwife when undertaking respiration assessment.

## REFERENCES

Blackburn S T, Loper D 1992 Maternal, fetal and neonatal physiology: a clinical perspective. W B Saunders, Philadelphia

Chandler T 2000 Oxygen saturation monitoring. Paediatric Nursing 12(8):37–42

Coull A 1992 Making sense of pulse oximetry. Nursing Times 88(32):42–43

DoH (Department of Health) 1996 Report on Confidential Enquiries into Maternal Deaths in the United Kingdom 1991–1993. The Stationery Office, London

Jamieson E M, McCall J, Whyte L 2002 Clinical nursing practices, 4th edn. Churchill Livingstone, Edinburgh

Kozier B, Erb G, Blais K et al 1998 Fundamentals of nursing, 5th edn. Addison Wesley, California

Medical Devices Agency (MDA) 1988 Pulse oximeters: potential dangers during use, SIB 88 No. 46. Online. Available http://www.medical-devices.gov.uk

Michaelides S 2004 Physiology, assessment and care. In: Henderson C, Macdonald S (eds) Mayes' midwifery: a textbook for midwives, 13th edn. Baillière Tindall, Edinburgh, ch 31

Moyle J 1999 Pulse oximetry. Journal of Neonatal Nursing 5(2):24–26

Siney C 2004 Drugs and the midwife. In: Henderson C, Macdonald S (eds) Mayes' midwifery: a textbook for midwives, 13th edn. Baillière Tindall, Edinburgh, ch 71

# Chapter **8**

# Assessment of maternal and neonatal vital signs — neurological assessment

This chapter focuses on the principles of neurological assessment and the midwife's role in relation to undertaking this assessment. Neurological assessment is undertaken on any woman where there are concerns about actual or possible alterations in her levels of consciousness (e.g. post-seizure, magnesium toxicity, meningitis, head injury). A complete neurological assessment encompasses the level of consciousness, pupillary reaction, motor (including reflexes), sensory and cerebellar function and vital signs. This is the remit of the doctor with neurological experience and is completed initially and then as needed to determine the woman's condition. The midwife's involvement is to undertake a reduced assessment of level of consciousness, motor signs (limb movement), pupillary assessment and vital signs.

---

**Learning outcomes**

Having read this chapter the reader should be able to:

- describe the different components of the Glasgow Coma Scale (GCS)
- discuss how the midwife can complete the GCS
- identify the other observations that should be undertaken in conjunction with the GCS to gain a thorough neurological assessment.

---

### Frequency of observations

The midwife must be able to complete the neurological assessment competently as it provides invaluable information regarding the condition of the woman. While the observations should be completed according to the condition of the woman, Cree (2003) recommends this should be carried out every 30 minutes until her condition has stabilised or the GCS score is 15 to enable any changes in condition to be identified early. On the other hand, NICE (2003) recommends that the observations should be completed every 30 minutes for 2 hours, hourly for 4 hours, then every 2 hours, reverting to 30-minute assessments if the condition deteriorates.

## Glasgow Coma Scale

This was developed in 1974 to provide a quick and objective assessment of eye opening, verbal response and motor ability. Each of these three categories has four to six different responses and each response is scored. The three scores are totalled to score between 15 (fully conscious) and 3 (no response) to provide a rapid assessment of the woman's condition and response to treatment.

### Eye opening

The midwife should look at the woman to see if her eyes are opening spontaneously (score 4). If not, she should speak to the woman, which should provoke the eyes to open (score 3). If the eyes continue to remain closed, the midwife can apply central stimulation by applying gentle pressure on the orbital bone just underneath the inner aspect of the eyebrows (suborbital pressure) or at the angle of the jaw below the ear, where the mandible joins with the maxillary bones (jaw-margin pressure) to elicit a response (score 2). This should not be used if a traumatic head injury is present. In this instance a trapezium squeeze can be used – the trapezium muscle (at the junction of the head and neck) is squeezed between the thumb and two fingers and twisted. If the eyes remain closed a score of 1 is given.

If damage has been sustained to the eyes resulting in swelling, it is unlikely the eyes will open easily, rendering this unreliable until the swelling subsides.

### Verbal response

The midwife should ascertain the level of verbal response by asking questions that require answers to show clarity and understanding – What is your name? Where are you? What day is it? – for which an accurate answer scores 5. However, if the woman is able to speak using full sentences but the answers are incorrect a score of 4 is given. If only words and incomplete sentences are given, the score is 3 regardless of whether or not the words are appropriate. A score of 2 is given if incomprehensible sounds (e.g. grunts, groans) are made. If no sound is made in response to verbal or painful central stimuli, 1 is scored.

It is important to take into account the language spoken by the woman and if she does not speak English, an interpreter should be used.

### Motor ability

The response of the upper limbs is tested to determine brain function as the lower limbs can also be affected by spinal function. The midwife should ask the woman to bend then hold out her arms and squeeze the midwife's hands with both of her hands. The midwife can then determine that both arms can be moved, and the elbows flexed, and the power and release of grip from each hand can be noted.

A score of 6 is given if the woman is able to complete these movements and 1 if there is no response despite painful central stimuli. Scores of 2–5 are given according to the degree of movement and flexion occurring as a result of painful stimulus – the arm moving towards the stimuli to try to remove it (5), arm bends at the elbow without rotation of the wrist (4) or with wrist rotation and forearm rotation (3), the arm extends at the elbow while the wrist flexes (2).

# Pupillary assessment

The size and shape of each pupil and reaction to light are assessed by the midwife. The midwife should look at the pupils to determine if they are the same shape and whether the eyes are working together. The diameter of each pupil is then measured – the normal range being 2–6 mm (Dawson 2000) – and they are usually equal in size (unequal pupils are a late sign associated with raised intracranial pressure, but may be of little significance if the woman is alert and orientated). Pupil reaction is assessed by shining a bright light from a pen torch into one eye, then the other. The pupils should decrease in size and the speed at which this is achieved is recorded. If there is no response, the pupil is fixed. The level of sedation administered to the woman will affect pupil reaction.

The findings of the neurological assessment should be recorded on a neurological observation chart (Fig. 8.1) in conjunction with vital signs including temperature (Ch. 4), pulse (Ch. 5), blood pressure (Ch. 6) and respiratory rate (Ch. 7). Blood oxygen saturation should also be monitored (NICE 2003) (Ch. 7). While the total GCS score is recorded it is also important to record separately the scores of the three different categories, as each one is assessing different areas of the brain. A woman with a decreasing score or one of 8 or less should always be referred to the neurologist.

PROCEDURE     **neurological assessment**

- Gather equipment and take to the bedside:
  — pencil torch
  — observation chart
  — thermometer
  — sphygmomanometer
  — pulse oximeter
- Wash and dry hands

**Figure 8.1** Neurological observation chart (Adapted with kind permission from Jamieson et al 2002)

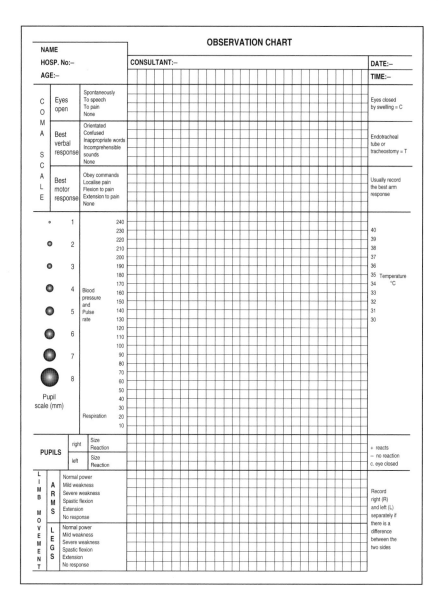

- Inform the woman of the procedure and gain consent if conscious and responsive
- Complete vital signs – temperature, blood pressure, pulse, respiration and blood oxygen saturation estimation
- Assess level of consciousness by talking with the woman and asking her who she is, what day it is and where she is; use central stimuli if no response
- Assess motor function by asking the woman to bend and lift her arms and to squeeze both your hands; use central stimuli if no response

- Assess the size and shape of the pupils and movement of the eyes
- Assess pupillary reaction by:
  - — darkening the room if necessary
  - — holding one eyelid open, move the pen torchlight towards and across the eye, moving the light from side to side
  - — assess the degree and speed at which the pupil constricts
  - — repeat with the other eye
  - — then with both eyelids held open, shine the light into one eye – the pupil in the other eye should also be observed to constrict
  - — repeat with the other eye
- Ensure the woman is covered and comfortable
- Document all findings on the observation chart
- Act on findings accordingly.

## Role and responsibilities of the midwife

These can be summarised as:

- undertaking a competent examination in which all of the information is gained
- recognising deviations from the norm and instigating referral
- appropriate record keeping.

## Summary

- Neurological assessment is undertaken where there are actual or potential altering levels of consciousness
- The Glasgow Coma Scale determines the level of consciousness by assessing the woman's response to the three categories of eye opening, verbal response and motor ability
- The midwife can undertake the Glasgow Coma Scale and estimation of vital signs as part of the woman's neurological assessment to determine any changes to her condition
- Additionally the doctor will evaluate motor and sensory function as required.

## Self-assessment exercises

The answers to the following questions may be found in the text:

1. What are the three categories of the Glasgow Coma Scale?
2. What observations should you undertake in conjunction with the Glasgow Coma Scale?
3. How does the midwife assess eye opening?
4. If there is no response, how are central stimuli applied?
5. How can the midwife determine the verbal response?
6. How does the midwife assess motor response?

## REFERENCES

Cree C 2003 Acquired brain injury: acute management. Nursing Standard 18(11):45–53

Dawson D 2000 Neurological care. In: Sheppard M, Wright M (eds) Principles and practices of high dependence nursing. Baillière Tindall, Edinburgh, p 145–182

Jamieson E M, McCall J, Whyte L 2002 Clinical nursing practices, 4th edn. Churchill Livingstone, Edinburgh

NICE (National Institute for Clinical Excellence) 2003 Clinical guideline 4: head injury. NICE, London

# Chapter 9

# Principles of infection control — standard precautions

Health care professionals are widely exposed to large numbers and varieties of microorganisms. Human immunodeficiency virus (HIV) and other blood-borne contagious infections have increased the need to protect both women and midwives from infection. The term 'standard precautions' (previously known as universal precautions) refers to the measures taken universally, i.e. by all health professionals for all women and babies, all the time, to achieve this level of protection. As an important area of care, the reader is required to keep up to date with developing protocols, both for self-protection and to provide the best possible care. The cost to the NHS of infection is also considerable (May 2000). This chapter will review the use of standard precautions and isolation nursing.

## Learning outcomes

Having read this chapter the reader should be able to:

- discuss the nature and significance of standard precautions, indicating the midwife's role and responsibilities
- describe source and protective isolation nursing
- briefly discuss the principles of protective isolation.

## Standard infection control precautions

Childbearing women are considered to be in a high risk category for standard precaution use because:

- unprotected sexual intercourse is likely to have taken place
- there is exposure to large amounts of blood and body fluid during care.

It is almost impossible to appreciate who may be infected and who is not. Applying precautions to everyone maintains safety and prevents any individual feeling isolated or 'singled out'. Confidentiality may be compromised if some procedures are perceived to be used for some women and not for others. While there may be times when wearing protective clothing is potentially disruptive to the relationship that a midwife has built up with a woman, the midwife must consider the significance of self-protection and that of other women.

Standard precautions should be used when there is contact with any of the following:

- blood
- vaginal and seminal secretions
- urine
- cerebrospinal fluid
- amniotic fluid
- saliva
- any body fluid
- breast milk
- situations in which it is difficult to differentiate between body fluids.

## Principles of standard precautions

The following principles are adapted from RCN (2004):

- Hand hygiene should be practised routinely and thoroughly, even when gloves are to be worn, and after their removal, using the recommended antibacterial soap, paper tissues and foot-operated bin (see Ch. 10 for greater detail)
- Cuts or abrasions on the skin should be covered with a waterproof dressing that is an effective barrier to viruses and bacteria
- Latex or properly fitting vinyl gloves should be worn in any situation where the hands may be contaminated with body fluids. Sterile gloves are worn for sterile procedures. Gauntlet gloves may be worn for particular procedures, e.g. manual removal of placenta. Double gloving has been shown to reduce needlestick injury by six times, but it does not prevent it (Bott 1999)
- Plastic aprons should be worn when any body fluids can be splashed; waterproof gowns may be worn in some circumstances
- Eye protection is necessary when body fluids can be splashed
- Sharps must be disposed of in a recognised sharps disposal unit, carefully and at the point of use. The sharps box should only be filled to three-quarters full and should be immediately sealed and sent for incineration; used needles must never be resheathed
- The use of newer products is encouraged, e.g. blunt-ended needles for suturing, disposable drapes, self-capping needles, etc. (May & Brewer 2001)

- Local protocols exist for issues such as sterilisation and decontamination of equipment, cleanliness of the environment, disposal of clinical waste, managing accidents and spillages and post-exposure prophylaxis, all of which the reader needs to be familiar with.

The principles can be adapted and used in every situation, in whichever venue care is being carried out. The midwife should be particularly aware of the following situations:

- examination per vaginam, use of amnihook, fetal scalp electrodes, etc.
- childbirth, of whichever type
- theatre work, including suction/aspiration of body fluids
- disposal of administration sets, blood transfusion sets, etc.
- specimens, including neonatal capillary sampling
- injections
- newborn babies prior to bathing
- postnatal observations of lochia and perineum
- perineal repair
- cannulation and venepuncture.

## Management of spills or accidents

- Skin that is accidentally exposed should be washed immediately with soap and water
- If the conjunctiva or any mucous membrane is splashed the areas should be irrigated with copious amounts of water. Avoid swallowing if the splash is into the mouth, then rinse several times with cold water
- All waste should be disposed of correctly. Clinical waste is incinerated after being placed in yellow refuse sacks; this includes placentae
- Contaminated linen is also handled separately, usually by placing it in red alginate bags specifically designed to melt in hot water, so that the linen does not have to be handled again
- In the event of a needlestick injury (or other percutaneous injury, e.g. a bite), the area should be encouraged to bleed (but do not suck the wound) under running water for at least 5 minutes (Boyle 2000). It should then be washed thoroughly (but not scrubbed) with soap and water and covered with a waterproof dressing. The agreed local protocol should be followed; this is likely to include reporting the incident to a manager and to occupational health, completing an accident form and being involved in a risk assessment
- Spillages of body fluids should be cleared up using gloves, an apron and disposable wipes as soon after the event as possible. The local protocol will suggest which detergents are to be used.

These can be summarised as:

- recognising the significance of standard precautions and the need to utilise them in every clinical situation with every woman and baby
- the ability to adapt them to each area of work, maintaining safety for all
- the need to be familiar with up-to-date reports and protocols
- universal use to protect dignity and confidentiality
- the need to report and act on spillages or accidents.

# Isolation nursing

## Source isolation

For an individual with a known infection there is a specific need to contain the transmission. In the maternity setting infections such as hepatitis B, tuberculosis, salmonella or MRSA (methicillin resistant *Staphylococcus aureus*) come into this category. Source isolation is the term used for care that aims to contain or isolate the infection – from other women, health professionals and visitors – and therefore means that the infected woman is cared for separately. The psychological stress is well recognised and therefore a multidisciplinary risk assessment should be thorough to ensure that the isolation is necessary.

## General principles

- In a hospital environment the use of an en suite sideroom is the most likely means of isolation; it is helpful if it has an anteroom where necessary items can be kept. The room should ideally have negative pressure ventilation, i.e. air is drawn in from the ward but leaves the room externally, away from the ward (Cutter & Dempster 1999)
- The room should be equipped with all the materials required, e.g. sphygmomanometer, washing equipment, water jug and glass, sharps box, antibacterial soap and disposable towels, linen skip, yellow refuse sack, Pinard stethoscope, etc. The refuse sack is sealed in the room and then removed, but otherwise none of the equipment is removed from the room until cleaned or disposed of appropriately after the woman's departure. Unnecessary furniture is removed and a visible indication is placed on the door – often a colour-coded sign – to remind all staff. Instructions should be given to friends and relatives as to how to maintain the isolation principles
- A trolley outside the room contains items that are needed when entering the room, e.g. gloves, disposable gowns, masks, goggles, overshoes, plastic aprons and antibacterial hand rub
- The midwife should recognise the value of the multidisciplinary team: the infection control nurse, microbiologist, obstetrician and

midwife will all need to work in close communication and partnership to provide appropriate care for the woman. The woman may also remain in her sideroom for delivery and additional precautions should be instigated accordingly

- The woman needs to understand the reason for isolation nursing and how she can be instrumental in upholding the philosophy of care. The midwife should ensure that the woman's psychological health is maintained as well as her physical health. Occasionally, specific members of staff may be assigned to care for infected women; they should then have restricted access to other women, especially any that may be considered vulnerable to infection.

| PROCEDURE | entering, attending the woman and leaving the room |
| --- | --- |

- Gather any necessary additional equipment
- Wash hands, apply gloves, apron and any other necessary protective clothing for the procedure
- Knock, enter the room and close the door
- Complete the necessary care, containing all of the tasks within the room:
  — crockery may be brought out of the room, providing that it will be decontaminated in a dishwasher
  — domestic services are required to clean the room and bathroom daily; other spillages should be cleaned according to standard precaution guidelines
- On preparing to leave the room, remove all protective clothing, dispose of it in the room and wash hands
- Close the door on leaving; use antibacterial hand rub once outside the room
- On discharge the room is thoroughly cleaned using approved solutions; steam cleaning may be required. All furniture and equipment is washed and dried, curtains are sent to the laundry; carpeted floor may be steam cleaned.

## Protective isolation

The midwife is unlikely to be involved in this type of care. It is usually applicable to severely immunosuppressed patients, where it is vital that they are protected from infection. All unnecessary visitors are prohibited and extreme care is taken to ensure that no infection is taken into the room. A positive pressure environment is needed where clean air is drawn into the room from outside and forced out into the general ward area. Clearly, the ventilation systems need to be properly understood so that the opposite does not happen! (Cutter & Dempster

1999). Hands are washed and protective clothing is applied before entering and removed after leaving the room.

## Summary

- Standard precautions aim to protect all staff, women, babies and visitors from potentially serious infections, by recommending hand hygiene, protective clothing, correct management of spills, accidents, waste and sharps, and protocols that cover other issues such as environmental hygiene. It is an important aspect of the midwife's role
- The midwife works with a high risk client group and should adopt standard precautions use as a matter of routine in *every* situation
- Source isolation aims to contain infection by carrying out all procedures within the woman's single room, keeping all equipment and materials within that room
- Protective isolation prevents infection from entering the room by use of protective measures before entering and after leaving; visitors are restricted.

## Self-assessment exercises

The answers to the following questions may be found in the text:

1. Describe standard precautions.
2. Discuss the significance of them and the role and responsibilities of the midwife when using them.
3. Discuss the principles of source and protective isolation nursing.

## REFERENCES

Bott J 1999 HIV health and safety practice: considerations for midwives. British Journal of Midwifery 7(10):609–612

Boyle M 2000 Blood borne infections. The Practising Midwife 3(7):48–50

Cutter M, Dempster L 1999 Cover notes. Nursing Times 95(31):25–27

May D 2000 Infection control. Nursing Standard 14(28):51–57

May D, Brewer S 2001 Sharps injury: prevention and management. Nursing Standard 15(32):45–52

RCN (Royal College of Nursing) 2004 Good practice in infection control. RCN, London

Chapter **10**

# Principles of infection control — hand hygiene

This chapter focuses on the principles of hand hygiene, an important means of infection control. Hand hygiene encompasses both hand care and hand decontamination. 'Hand decontamination is the most effective and certainly the most cost effective method of preventing health-related infection' (Gould 2002).

| Learning outcomes | Having read this chapter the reader should be able to: |

Having read this chapter the reader should be able to:

- discuss the principles of general hand care
- identify the occasions when the midwife should undertake hand decontamination
- describe the main differences between 'medical' and 'surgical' scrub
- discuss the role and responsibilities of the midwife in relation to hand hygiene.

## General hand care

- Examine the hands for cuts, grazes, torn cuticles; these increase the risk of infection to the midwife and should be covered with a plaster
- Keep nails short and filed; long or ragged nails can scratch women and babies and introduce infection; dirt and secretions may be found under the nails, which can harbour microorganisms
- Avoid using false nails as bacteria can flourish in the ridge that appears as the nail grows
- Apply moisturiser to the hands on a regular basis to prevent them from drying out and cracking.

## Hand decontamination

Handwashing refers to both social and clinical situations where hands are washed. Social handwashing is generally ineffective in destroying bacteria due to incorrect washing technique or inappropriate cleansing agents used. Hand decontamination is a more accurate term that refers to the removal of microorganisms and their debris by mechanical means or their destruction (Gould 2002).

### Cleansing agents

The use of soap and water removes almost all transient bacteria but does not reduce the number of resident bacteria (e.g. *Staphylococcus aureus*) by any significant amount (Mallett & Dougherty 2000). While this is acceptable in non-invasive situations with a low-risk population, there are many situations where the resident bacteria also need to be reduced (e.g. aseptic procedures). Antiseptics (e.g. chlorhexidine) reduce the transient and resident bacteria at the time of application, with some residual activity keeping bacterial counts low over several days (Gould 2002). Both soap and antiseptics usually involve the use of running water following one of two procedures: the 'medical/social' or the 'surgical' scrub. The former is used for normal handwashing and prior to aseptic techniques, while the latter is used when scrubbing for an operative procedure; this is a lengthier procedure involving the hands and arms. Alcohol-based hand rubs can be used without water and are applied to the hands and wrists. This is much quicker as the hand rub often dries within 15 seconds and is recommended for use when the hands are visibly clean (RCN 2000).

| | |
|---|---|
| **Indications for hand decontamination** | • Prior to and after contact with the skin of the woman or baby or body fluids<br>• Prior to undertaking an aseptic technique<br>• Prior to handling food<br>• When visibly soiled<br>• After going to the toilet<br>• After contact with soiled or potentially contaminated equipment<br>• After removing gloves. |
| **Principles of hand decontamination** | • Consider all equipment as being contaminated: minimal handling of taps, soap dispenser, sinks, drying equipment, especially after washing; the use of foot-operated pedal bins and elbow taps is advised<br>• Avoid wearing jewellery: rings increase the number of microorganisms found on the hand; jewellery also makes it difficult to clean the hands thoroughly<br>• Use warm running water, with the flow regulated for comfort: hot water opens the pores, predisposing to skin irritation; avoid splashing water, especially over clothes, as microorganisms may be transferred and multiply in moisture |

- Use appropriate soap and work up a lather: soap will emulsify fat and oil and lower the surface tension, making cleaning easier
- Use a circular motion, encouraging rubbing and friction: this loosens and removes dirt and transient microorganisms
- Use disposable paper towels to dry hands as microorganisms are removed by friction and the spread of microorganisms is minimised compared with hot air driers and towels (Blackmore 1987).

## PROCEDURE    medical/social scrub

The hands should be rubbed vigorously together under tepid running water for a minimum of 15 seconds (NICE 2003). If an alcohol hand rub is used, $2 \times 5$ mL applications should be rubbed in following the steps in Figure 10.1B–G until the hands and wrists are dry.

- Remove all jewellery (except for plain gold band), including wrist watch
- Turn the taps on and adjust the water temperature and flow, taking care not to splash the water, and wet the hands (Fig. 10.1A)
- Using an appropriate cleansing agent, rub the palms together vigorously (Fig. 10.1B), then rub the palm of one hand along the top of the other hand and along the fingers, using the fingers on the top hand to rub along the edge of the lower hand; repeat for the other hand (Fig. 10.1C)
- Wash the fingers by interlacing together, rubbing them back and forth, ensuring the inner aspects of both sides of all the fingers are rubbed together (Fig. 10.1D)
- Wash the fingertips of one hand by rubbing them against the palm of the other hand; repeat for other hand (Fig. 10.1E)
- Wash the thumb of one hand by using the fingers of other hand wrapped around it, washing in a circular motion; repeat for the other thumb (Fig. 10.1F)
- Grasp the left wrist with the right hand, rubbing around the wrist; repeat for the right wrist (Fig. 10.1G)
- Rinse all the surfaces of the hand and wrist
- Repeat handwashing if hands are heavily contaminated
- Dry each hand and wrist separately
- Turn off the taps using the elbows or the paper towel
- Dispose of the towel using a foot-operated pedal bin.

## PROCEDURE    surgical scrub

This involves washing the hands and forearms with a sterile scrubbing brush; washing should take at least 2 minutes.

- Remove all jewellery, including wrist watch

**Figure 10.1** Medical scrub.
(A) Rinsing with water;
(B) washing the palms;
(C) washing the top surfaces
of the fingers; (D) interlacing
the fingers; (E) washing the
fingertips; (F) washing the
thumbs; (G) washing the wrists

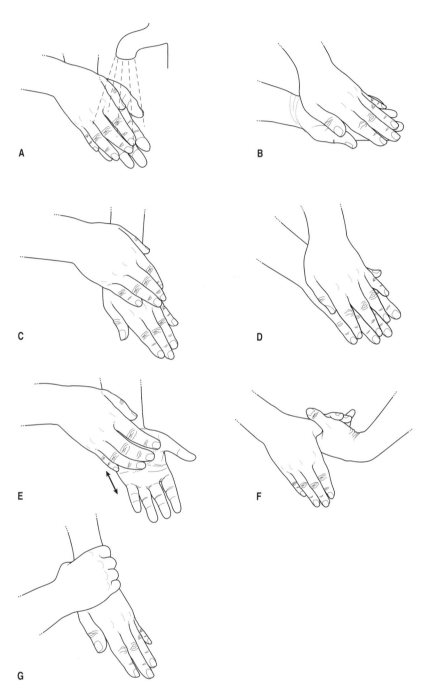

- Open the sterile scrubbing brush packet (but retain the brush in the packet) placing close to the sink, e.g. on the drainer, ensuring the brush does not come into contact with an unsterile surface
- Turn the taps on and adjust the water temperature and flow, taking care not to splash the water

- Keeping the hands above the level of the elbows, wet the hands and forearms to the elbows
- Using an antiseptic soap, e.g. 4% chlorhexidine solution, povidone–iodine, wash fingers and hands as for medical scrub
- With the brush, scrub all the skin surfaces of the fingers, thumbs, hands and forearms for 2 minutes, then discard the brush
- Rinse the soap from hands and elbows, keeping the hands above the level of the elbows, allowing the water to run from the fingertips down to the elbows
- Turn off the taps using elbows
- Dry each hand and arm separately with a disposable towel, drying from the fingertips towards the elbows, keeping the hands above waist level
- Dispose of the towel using a foot-operated pedal bin.

## Role and responsibilities of the midwife

These can be summarised as:

- recognising when hand decontamination should be undertaken
- being able to undertake a medical or surgical scrub correctly.

## Summary

- Hand decontamination is an important means of infection control
- The use of soap and water will remove almost all transient bacteria but does not reduce the number of resident bacteria
- A 'medical scrub' involves washing for a minimum of 15 seconds
- A 'surgical scrub' involves washing with a brush for at least 2 minutes, with the hands above the elbows.

## Self-assessment exercises

The answers to the following questions may be found in the text:

1. What are the general principles of hand care?
2. When should the midwife undertake decontamination?
3. Describe how the hands are washed for a 'medical' scrub.
4. What are the main differences between a 'medical' and a 'surgical scrub'?

## REFERENCES

Blackmore M 1987 Hand drying methods. Nursing Times 83(37):71–74

Gould D 2002 Hand decontamination. Nursing Times 98(46):48–49

Mallett J, Dougherty C 2000 The Royal Marsden NHS Trust manual of clinical nursing procedures, 5th edn. Blackwell Science, Oxford

NICE (National Institute for Clinical Excellence) 2003 Clinical guideline 2: infection control. Prevention of healthcare-associated infection in primary and community care. NICE, London

RCN (Royal College of Nursing) 2000 Good practice in infection control. RCN, London

Chapter **11**

# Principles of infection control – principles of asepsis

Asepsis – the absence of sepsis or infection – is a critical component of care. Infection can mean mortality, morbidity and expense, amongst other factors. In the maternity setting any invasive procedure that touches the mucous membranes or breaks the skin (examples below) requires an aseptic technique:

- venepuncture and intravenous cannulation
- urinary catheterisation
- examination per vaginam
- childbirth, of whichever mode
- perineal suturing
- siting of epidural analgesia
- any surgical procedure in theatre or on the ward.

They are, however, very different procedures and therefore it is the *principles* of asepsis that should be employed. Briggs et al (1996) indicate that the evidence for much of accepted aseptic practice is limited, but is becoming more evidence based. This chapter reviews aseptic principles and summarises the role of the midwife. Elements of aseptic principles are included in almost every chapter of this text, such is its importance.

---

**Learning outcomes**

Having read this chapter the reader should be able to:

- discuss the principles of asepsis, including equipment used, no-touch technique and establishing a sterile field
- summarise the role of the midwife.

---

# Medical and surgical asepsis

There are two suggested levels of asepsis: medical (clean) and surgical (sterile). Surgical asepsis refers to the sterility of theatres and techniques used within them, i.e. asepsis within an area. Medical is more likely to be the asepsis practised with most techniques, i.e. reducing organisms and their spread individually, but the principles frequently overlap. Asepsis is necessary for every invasive procedure.

### The sterile field

Medical and surgical asepsis both work on the principle that a sterile field is established and additional sterile items are passed without de-sterilising the field. An assistant is therefore required to maintain true asepsis – the midwife once 'scrubbed' can only handle sterile items. The assistant is required to handle/open the external wrappers and pass the sterile contents to the sterile field or directly to the midwife (see Fig. 11.2). If working alone the midwife may adapt the principles by opening the pack, adding the other sterile items, rewashing hands, applying gloves and then continuing with the procedure. This is less efficient, particularly if the woman has to be positioned and exposed before the midwife has established the sterile field (e.g. for urinary catheterisation).

# Principles of asepsis

### Hand hygiene

Hand hygiene is the most important principle of asepsis (for greater detail, see Ch. 10). Briggs et al (1996) state that hand hygiene is one aspect of asepsis that is 'vital, well researched and uncontroversial'. The use of an alcohol-based hand rub is acceptable mid-procedure in many circumstances. It is only acceptable, however, when hand hygiene initially has been thorough and when the items handled subsequently have not been heavily contaminated. Hand hygiene is as important after a procedure as before – microorganisms can grow in gloved hands.

### Use of protective clothing

Microorganisms can also be carried on clothing. The use of a clean plastic apron is indicated; this protects the clothing from bacteria, and thus the spread from one situation to another. Sterile gloves are worn after the hands have been washed and dried, whether sterile instruments or gloved hands are to be used (no-touch technique).

### Use of sterile packs and equipment

Equipment that is sterilised centrally is usually autoclaved. The colour change on the packet indicates sterility but the pack should be inspected to ensure that it has not been damaged or wet in the meantime. Sterile items should be used within their expiry date. Sterile lotions, syringes, cannulas, etc. are all supplied for single use only (unless otherwise stated) and are disposed of after use.

Dressings trolleys should be used purely for aseptic procedures and should be washed daily (using detergent and dried with paper towels) and at any time if visibly contaminated. They should be wiped with an alcohol-impregnated wipe prior to each use.

### Use of no-touch technique
Once a sterile field is established, usually on a dressings trolley, the hands, or any other item, should not de-sterilise it. Equally, contaminated hands should not touch the woman and so gloves or forceps are used to achieve this no-touch principle.

### Arranging the sterile field
The sterile field is arranged on the top shelf of the trolley, the other items 'await' on the bottom shelf. Firstly, the outer wrapper of the sterile pack (whatever sort it is) is opened by the midwife or the assistant. The inner part of the pack is 'dropped' onto the trolley without touching it or the trolley with the hands. This part is sterile and should then only be touched initially with washed hands and then only by sterile gloved hands. The sterile 'inner' is opened out using only the corners or edges of the paper/cloth and flattened out (Fig. 11.1). Sterile gloves are then applied. The other requirements are then added to the field. Ideally, as discussed earlier, an assistant uses a no-touch technique by sliding, holding open for the midwife to take, or 'dropping' them onto the field (Fig. 11.2). The contents of the pack are then arranged according to the procedure or practitioner's preference. However, any items that may be needed quickly (e.g. cord clamps) are arranged towards the edge, within easy reach. Lotions, needles, syringes, etc., whatever is needed, are added by the assistant using the same no-touch technique.

### Retaining sterility
Ideally nothing contaminated is returned to the sterile field. The principle of a 'dirty' and a 'clean' hand can be upheld. This means that the midwife uses one hand (dirty) for initial direct contact with the woman, while the other (clean) is retained over the sterile field, ready to be used for the cleaner part of the procedure. Items are passed from the clean hand to the dirty hand and then disposed of when used, preventing the dirty hand from contaminating anything on the sterile field. The clean hand is often the dominant or examining hand. If undertaking a urinary catheterisation for example, the non-dominant (dirty) hand does the swabbing while the clean hand later inserts the catheter.

**Figure 11.1** Opening a sterile field (Adapted with kind permission from Nicol et al 2000)

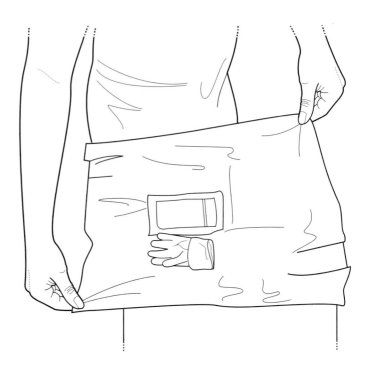

### Managing the sterile field

As the procedure progresses and it is necessary to return items to the sterile field, the field may be divided into clean and dirty areas. Any used items are returned to a designated dirty separate area. This is often at the edge or side of the field, both to prevent the midwife leaning over the sterile field each time to retrieve them but also to prevent them contaminating the larger sterile part of the field.

### Sterility around the woman

A sterile field is also established around the woman that gives the midwife a field to work from, but also encourages the woman to uphold the principles of asepsis by not placing her hands or other items on the sterile drapes. This can be difficult to maintain, and so is often more of a clean field than it is a sterile one! Equipment may be placed on the drapes and returned to the trolley if necessary, if not over-contaminated.

### Environmental contamination

The longer the sterile field is open to the environment the more likely it is to be contaminated. It should be covered over with the sterile wrapper if the procedure is interrupted or delayed. Environmental disturbances such as open windows, curtains wafting, use of fans and doors opening all increase the levels of airborne bacteria.

**Figure 11.2**  Assistant passing items to maintain sterility of sterile field

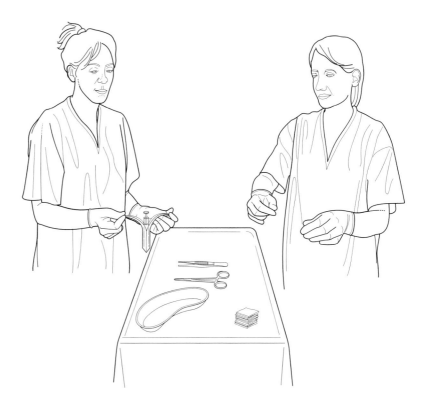

*Correct disposal*

Before leaving a room the sterile field is disposed of by wrapping the remaining contents (if disposable) in the paper and placing them into the refuse sack. Non-disposable items may be covered with the wrapper and taken out of the room into a sluice area. Gloves are removed after used items are disposed of; dirty gloves should not touch anything else, door handles included! Non-disposable equipment is returned to the sterile supplies department in the agreed format. The midwife washes her hands after glove removal, as discussed earlier.

**Role and responsibilities of the midwife**

These can be summarised as:

- undertaking evidence-based care in a consistent manner in order to reduce the transfer of microorganisms
- educating the woman when caring for herself and her baby.

## Summary

- The principles of asepsis should be included (adapted if necessary) for every invasive procedure
- Hand hygiene is essential; a no-touch technique is indicated in which sterile items are transferred on to a sterile field that only the 'scrubbed' midwife may touch
- Further research is indicated.

### Self-assessment exercises

The answers to the following questions may be found in the text:

1. Give four examples of the circumstances in which asepsis is indicated.
2. List the principles of asepsis.
3. Describe how to establish a sterile field, both on a trolley and around the woman, using a no-touch technique.
4. Summarise the role and responsibilities of the midwife when undertaking an aseptic procedure.

### REFERENCES

Briggs M, Wilson S, Fuller A 1996 The principles of aseptic technique in wound care. Professional Nurse 11(12):805–810

Nicol M, Bavin C, Bedford-Turner S et al 2000 Essential nursing skills, 2nd edn. Mosby, Edinburgh

Chapter **12**

# Principles of infection control — obtaining swabs

The midwife may be required to obtain a swab from the woman or the baby when infection is suspected. By culturing the microorganisms obtained by the swab, specific antibiotics can be prescribed to prevent them multiplying and so stop the infection. Swabs may be required even if there is no evidence of infection (e.g. a pregnant woman with a history of vaginal Group B streptococcal infection) to help inform care. This chapter focuses on obtaining swabs from the more common sites of the eye, ear, nose, throat, umbilicus, vagina, wound and placenta.

**Learning outcomes**

Having read this chapter the reader should be able to:

- describe how a swab is obtained from the eye, ear, nose, throat, umbilicus, vagina, wound and placenta
- discuss the role and responsibilities of the midwife in relation to obtaining swabs.

## Obtaining the swab

To increase the likelihood of isolating a microorganism, it is important that the swab is coated all over. This can be achieved by rotating the swab around the area to be swabbed. Different organisms thrive and die in different cultures, thus it is important to use the correct swabstick and transport medium. For the majority of swabs a dry swab and normal transport medium is sufficient.

However, it is important to ensure that alternative swabs and media are used where indicated; for example *Trichomonas, Chlamydia* and *Bordetella pertussis* need charcoal-based swabs and media. Thus the midwife should be aware of which microorganisms are being considered as the causative organism for the presenting symptoms in the woman or baby and, if unsure, the midwife should verify with the doctor in order to use the correct swabs, media and bottles. The woman should also be aware of why several swabs are undertaken.

In some situations the midwife may need to collect pus, exudates, moisture, etc. from the woman or baby (e.g. from the umbilical stump). These may need collecting via a swabstick, although where pus is being collected, a sterile spatula can be used to collect the pus and place it in a specimen container.

Once obtained, the swab should be placed in the transport medium, the lid secured and it should be correctly labelled. This should be placed in a transport bag that is sealed to prevent spillage and contamination. It should be sent for laboratory analysis (culture and sensitivity – C&S – culture of the microorganism and sensitivity to antibiotics that can prevent its growth and replication) as soon as possible. If delay is anticipated, refrigeration is necessary.

In high risk situations, the swab should be double wrapped and labelled accordingly and the midwife should ensure she is wearing gloves and, if appropriate, goggles. Standard precautions should be followed where there is a risk of cross-infection (Ch. 9).

If swabs are required from more than one site (e.g. both eyes, ears, nostrils), a separate swab should be used for each site to minimise the risk of cross-infection from an infected to a non-infected area. Usually only one swab is required; the area that appears most affected is swabbed.

The midwife should record in the notes which swabs have been taken and the time and date. This will ensure that all staff are aware the swabs have been obtained and will serve as a reminder to check the results as soon as they are ready.

### Eye

To obtain a swab from a woman, she should be sat up, with her head supported. If the swab is from a baby, the baby should be supported, with the head held steady. The lower eyelid should be pulled down gently. The swab should be held parallel to the cornea and rubbed very gently against the conjunctiva in the lower eyelid. Usually just one swab is sufficient.

### Ear

To obtain a swab from the ear of a woman, she should be sat up with her head tilting to the unaffected side. If the swab is from a baby, one of the parents or another midwife should hold the baby with the head up and tilted to one side. If the baby is too ill to be moved he can be laid on his side. The external canal is straightened by gently pulling the pinna upwards and backwards and the swab is inserted gently into and rotated around the external canal. It is also important to withhold medication administered via the ears for 3 hours prior to obtaining the swab as the medication can interfere with the growth of the microorganism.

### Nasal

To obtain a nasal swab from a woman, she should be sat up with her head tilting back or lying down with her face forwards. If the swab is from a baby, the baby can be cradled in someone's arms or laid on his back. The procedure may be easier if there is someone to hold the baby's arms; alternatively wrap the baby in a blanket. The end of the swab should be moistened with sterile water. The swab should be inserted gently into the nose, moving it upwards towards the tip of the nose and rotating it.

### Throat

The woman should be sitting or lying facing a strong light source and asked to open her mouth widely. The tongue should be depressed using a disposable spatula and the swab inserted to the back of the throat. The swab is then rotated quickly around the back of the throat, using the faucial tonsils as the boundary, to ensure it is coated (this is likely to make the woman gag). When removing the swab, ensure it does not come into contact with any part of the mouth, tongue or saliva.

### Umbilicus

The baby should be positioned to allow easy access to the umbilicus (e.g. cradled in someone's arms or lying in a cot) and undressed to expose the umbilicus. The swab is moved gently around the umbilicus, rotating it. The baby should be redressed following the procedure.

### High vaginal

This is undertaken following the insertion and opening of a speculum (Ch. 31). The swab should be inserted through the speculum to the top of the vagina and rotated around. When the procedure is completed the speculum should be removed and the woman assisted into a comfortable position.

### Low vaginal

The swab is inserted into the lower vagina for 2–4 cm (a speculum should not be used) and the swab rubbed around the front, side and back walls of the vagina.

### Wound

Donovan (1998) recommends using normal saline (at room temperature) to irrigate the wound prior to swabbing (to remove surface contamination) and to moisten the swab. The swab should be moved across the wound in a zigzag direction, covering the entire wound if small, or 1 cm$^2$ if large.

### Placental

The swab should be moved around the placenta (fetal side) in a zigzag direction and the placenta disposed of appropriately.

| PROCEDURE | obtaining a swab |
|---|---|

- Gain informed consent and gather equipment:
  — disposable gloves
  — sterile swab and appropriate transport medium
  — speculum and lubricating jelly, e.g. KY Jelly (high vaginal swab only)
  — sterile water (nasal swab)
  — sterile normal saline (wound swab only)
- Wash hands and apply gloves
- Position the woman or baby appropriately and obtain the swab specimen
- Remove the swab and insert into the transport medium, sealing securely
- Label the container with the name, hospital number (if applicable) and date of birth of the woman or baby, date and time the swab was obtained, nature of specimen, whether right or left (if applicable) and signature and place into transport bag
- Assist the woman or baby into a comfortable position
- Remove and dispose of gloves
- Wash hands
- Arrange transportation of the specimen to the pathology laboratory
- Document findings and act accordingly.

### Role and responsibilities of the midwife

These can be summarised as:

- recognising the need for a swab to be taken
- ensuring the procedure is undertaken correctly, with minimal discomfort to the mother or baby
- correct documentation.

## Summary

- Obtaining a swab is a significant, simple, but invasive procedure that may be undertaken on either the woman or the baby.

**Self-assessment exercises**

The answers to the following questions may be found in the text:

1. How would the midwife obtain a swab from:
   a. the ear
   b. the eye
   c. the nose
   d. the throat of a woman or baby?
2. How is an umbilical swab obtained?
3. Describe how a wound swab is obtained from a small wound.
4. How would the midwife obtain a high and a low vaginal swab?

## REFERENCE

Donovan S 1998 Wound infection and wound swabbing.
Professional Nurse 13(11):757–759

Chapter **13**

# Principles of hygiene needs — for the woman

This chapter considers the skills required to meet the complete range of hygiene needs of the woman. Cleanliness and attention to physical appearance can be significant in promoting psychological wellbeing, as well as physical health. Bed bathing, assisted washing, vulval toilet and oral toilet are all considered in detail.

**Learning outcomes**

Having read this chapter the reader should be able to:

- discuss the components of safe bed bathing
- describe the techniques for assisted washing, vulval and oral toilets
- describe how a bed is made when occupied or unoccupied
- discuss the midwife's role and responsibilities in relation to each of these aspects of care.

## Bed bathing

Bed bathing aims to meet the complete hygiene needs of a woman if she is confined to bed. The skin gathers perspiration, sebum, dead skin cells and bacteria over a 24-hour period. Pregnant women are often warmer and may sweat more, due to their general rise in body temperature. The extent to which the midwife performs a bed bath will depend upon the woman's level of dependence and is modified according to her needs. Baker et al (1999) indicate that bed bathing is the least effective method of patient hygiene and that therefore the woman should be encouraged and assisted whenever possible to wash by another means.

### Indications

- After surgery
- Immobility, for whatever reason
- Receiving intensive or high dependency care.

Personal preferences play an important role in this aspect of care. It can be difficult and embarrassing to have someone else performing these personal tasks. In providing holistic and individualised care, the midwife will complete other observations or aspects of care while bed bathing. These include:

- observation of consciousness and levels of pain (on both resting and moving)
- observation of the skin, particularly areas of pressure (see Ch. 57), inflammation, infection or allergy
- general health and nourishment, oral intake of diet and fluids
- ante- or postnatal examination
- assessment of vital signs
- wound care
- catheter or bladder care, vulval toilet
- bowel care
- attention to circulation, passive or active exercises, observations for varicosities or oedema, prevention of complications associated with immobility (see Ch. 58)
- care of intravenous infusion and fluid balance
- oral hygiene
- hair washing, pedicure or manicure
- therapeutic touch, communication, education
- attention to a safe and aesthetic environment.

The procedure should be carried out in a warm environment, in which the midwife is not disturbed. Dignity and privacy must be maintained throughout. Ensuring complete safety includes:

- protecting the woman and midwife by using appropriate moving and handling techniques
- ensuring that the woman does not roll out of bed
- adherence to infection control and standard precaution protocols
- adherence to uniform protocol, i.e. not wearing rings or wrist watches that may scratch the woman.

PROCEDURE    bed bathing an adult and making an occupied bed

- Gain informed consent and gather equipment:
  — bowl of hand-hot water
  — woman's own toiletries, etc. (moist flannels colonise bacteria, consider using disposable ones)
  — non-sterile gloves and apron
  — rubbish bag
  — bath towel
  — linen skip

— clean bed linen and clothes
— disposable wipes
— sanitary towels/disposable sheet
— other equipment, e.g. sphygmomanometer, thermometer, etc.

- Wash hands and apply apron. Ideally, find an assistant
- Loosen the bedclothes, retaining the top sheet
- Remove the woman's clothing, ensuring she remains covered with the sheet
- Place the towel across her chest, wash and dry her face (encourage her to do this herself if able)
- Wash the top half of her body (arms, chest, abdomen) doing first the parts away from the midwife, so that the assistant can dry them while the midwife begins washing the nearer parts. Expose as little of the woman as possible
- Ensure that skins folds, e.g. under the breasts, are as dry as possible. Apply deodorant
- Place the leg furthest away lengthways on the towel, wash and dry it, then repeat with other leg
- Change the water if necessary
- Turn the woman onto her side so that her back is facing the midwife (if possible, an assistant should support her in this position)
- Place the towel lengthways beside her, wash and dry her back
- Put on the gloves and cleanse the perineum from front to back using the disposable wipes
- Cleanse her buttocks in the same way
- Dry the whole area with disposable wipes
- Position a sanitary pad (if appropriate)
- Remove the gloves unless the bottom sheet is heavily soiled (in this case they are removed after handling the soiled bottom sheet but before handling the clean bottom sheet)
- Untuck the bottom sheet from the midwife's side, rolling it as small and as close to the woman as possible (Fig. 13.1)
- Tuck in the clean sheet, rolling it with a clean disposable sheet, to the same place
- Assist the woman to roll back onto her other side, over the two sheets so that she is facing the midwife
- The midwife supports her while an assistant removes the soiled sheet, tucks in the clean sheet and ensures there are no creases
- (Depending on the woman's mobility, the sheets may be changed as described, but from the top to the bottom of the bed (rather than side to side) by asking the woman to raise her buttocks to pass the sheets beneath them)
- Assist the woman into a comfortable position and assist her to redress
- Replace the top sheet, removing the soiled sheet

**Figure 13.1**   Making an
occupied bed

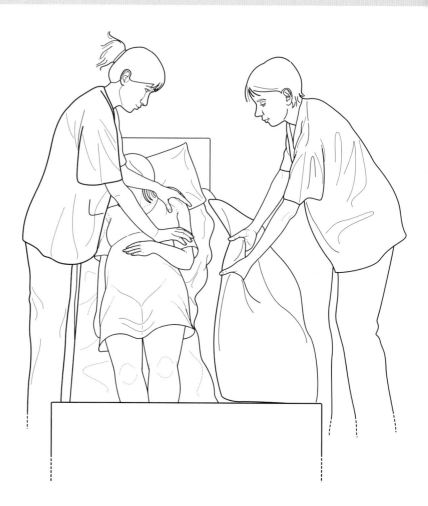

- Remake the bed and dispose of soiled bedding and equipment
- Wash and dry hands
- Comb the woman's hair
- Ensure oral hygiene is completed (p. 117)
- Complete other observations and care as required
- Document findings and act accordingly.

### Partial bed bath

If the woman is seriously ill or too uncomfortable, a partial bed bath may be performed, using the same principles but washing only the hands, face, axillae and genital area.

## Assisted washing

Assisting the woman to wash may be necessary if she is unable to complete this herself; these methods are advantageous in comparison to bed bathing (see above). The plan of care should be individualised to each woman, but may consist of any of the following:

- providing washing equipment and water to a woman on bedrest to allow her to wash all of her body that she can reach, with the midwife washing the remaining parts and changing the sheets
- assisting a woman to sit with a bowl, or at the sink, midwife assisting as necessary
- assisting a woman into a bath or shower, remaining with her or returning after a few minutes to assist as required (supply call bell).

## Making an unoccupied bed

Changing sheets or remaking a bed is indicated if the sheets are soiled, sweaty or dishevelled. The aim is to ensure that the bed is crease-free, protecting skin integrity. It is a difficult and time-consuming procedure to complete alone. Care should be taken that used sheets are disposed of directly, reducing the transfer of microorganisms. Gloves may be worn if the sheets are soiled.

### PROCEDURE   making an unoccupied bed

- Gather equipment:
  — clean sheets and pillow cases
  — blanket and counterpane or duvet with cover
  — gloves if required
  — linen skip
- Work with an assistant, one person on each side of the bed; apply gloves if necessary
- Bring the bed to an appropriate working height, closing the back rest
- Pull out the rack from the foot of the bed, or locate a suitable chair
- Remove the pillows, discarding the dirty pillow cases if necessary, place on the rack
- Loosen the covers, remove the counterpane/duvet, place on the rack ensuring it does not touch the floor (followed by the blanket if used)
- Remove the top sheet, followed by the bottom sheet; either discard or place on rack if to be reused
- Remove gloves
- Place the bottom sheet on the bed with the lengthways crease in the middle of the mattress and sufficient of the sheet at the top to fold under
- Lift the mattress in unison and place the sheet underneath it, return the mattress to the bed
- Mitre the corner (Fig. 13.2)
- Ensuring the sheet is smooth, lift the mattress at the end of the bed, tuck in sheet and mitre the corners in the same way
- Ensure that the sheet is tucked under the mattress lengthways

**Figure 13.2** Mitring the corners of an unoccupied bed (Adapted with kind permission from Lammon et al 1995)

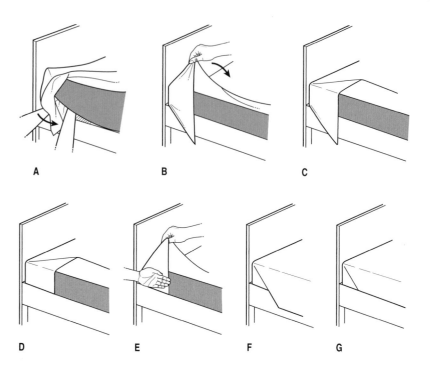

A    B    C

D    E    F    G

- Place the top sheet on the bed, ensure there is sufficient sheet at the head of the bed to fold over, tuck in loosely at the bottom (to avoid compressing the feet) and mitre the corners
- Return the blanket/counterpane in the same way, or place the duvet on
- Return to the head of the bed, straighten the top sheet, fold it over the counterpane or duvet
- Open the back rest to a suitable position and return the pillows, having put clean pillow cases on if necessary
- Return the rack and lower the bed to the correct height
- Dispose of equipment correctly and wash hands.

## Vulval toilet

This is particularly appropriate for women in the early postnatal period, especially after caesarean section or instrumental delivery. While it attends to the hygiene of the perineum, it may also act as a soothing analgesic, and is therefore slightly different from the cleansing of the perineum described when bed bathing. The midwife records this aspect of care and must adhere to infection control policies. The midwife may carry out the procedure or advise the woman how to undertake it herself. Plain water is used; Sleep and Grant (1988) indicated that water was comparable to salt or Savlon in its soothing and healing effects.

There are three methods of vulval toilet:

1. Place the woman on a bedpan, pour warm water over the vulva and perineum, use disposable wipes
2. Sit the woman on the toilet and pour warm water over the vulva and perineum from a jug
3. Sit the woman on the bidet (facing either direction depending upon her mobility and the comfort of her perineum). It is important that:
   — the water is warm, not hot
   — the sprinkle rather than jet is used, gently, so that water does not enter the vagina
   — the perineum is dried carefully afterwards using disposable wipes.

## Oral hygiene

Oral hygiene cleans and freshens the mouth, teeth and gums. It may aid the flow of saliva and prevent dental caries. A healthy woman is likely to require only minimal assistance from the midwife. Poor oral health can cause poor systemic health (e.g. bacterial endocarditis), and the state of the mouth can act as an indicator of general health. Psychological wellbeing is also increased if the mouth, teeth and breath are all clean and fresh (Jones 1998).

### Indications

- Nil by mouth:
  — pre- or post-surgery
  — nasogastric tube in situ
  — unconscious
  — intubated
- Restricted diet or fluids
- Nausea and vomiting
- Oxygen therapy
- Mouth breathing, e.g. labour; use of inhalational analgesia.

### Equipment and preparation

Toothbrush and paste are considered to be the most effective tools for oral hygiene for any woman, conscious or unconscious (Jones 1998). A toothbrush should be of a soft texture and used with a pea-sized amount of fluoride toothpaste (Bowsher et al 1999). The toothbrush should be correctly positioned (bristles pointing towards the roots of the teeth; Fig. 13.3) and moved gently, slightly from side to side, systematically around the top and then the lower jaw, on all surfaces of the teeth (Jones 1998). The mouth should be rinsed thoroughly to prevent any burning sensations from the toothpaste residue (Turner 1996).

**Figure 13.3** Correct position of toothbrush for cleaning teeth (Adapted with kind permission from Jones 1998)

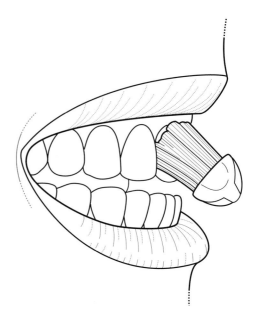

Mouthwashes containing chlorhexidine gluconate notably reduce the bacterial content of the mouth and may be prescribed as mouthwash or gel (Jones 1998). Foam sticks are considered to be less effective than a toothbrush, but may be useful in wiping the gums where the mouth is sore. Vaseline or lip balm may be applied to dried lips (Jones 1998).

The frequency of oral care in a high risk setting is an unresearched aspect of care. It would appear sensible to undertake it twice a day as a minimum.

- For the conscious woman the following are required:
  — toothbrush and paste
  — vomit bowl or receiver
  — cup of water
  — disposable wipe
- For the unconscious woman, the following are required:
  — toothbrush
  — toothpaste
  — disposable wipes
  — 10 mL syringe and water
  — suction apparatus
  — pen torch
  — wooden spatula
  — non-sterile gloves
  — towel, vomit bowl or receiver
  — Vaseline
  — disposal bag.

## PROCEDURE    oral hygiene

### Conscious woman

The conscious, compliant woman will be able to clean her teeth herself if positioned appropriately (sitting upright) and given the necessary equipment.

### Unconscious woman

- Explain the procedure to the woman, and position her so that visibility is good, and secretions can drain from the mouth easily; if necessary, suction can be applied. A lateral position may be the best, but it will depend upon her condition. If intubated with a cuffed endotracheal tube any position may be used, as the secretions will not enter the lungs. Maintain privacy
- Wash hands and apply gloves
- Place the towel and vomit bowl beneath the woman's chin. An assistant may be required to support the lower jaw
- Examine the mouth using the torch and spatula. A swab may be taken for microscopy, culture and sensitivity if infection is suspected
- Clean the teeth, gums and tongue gently, using a toothbrush and toothpaste, as described above
- Inject 10 mL of water gently into the mouth and allow it to drain out; use suction if necessary
- Repeat the rinsing until the fluid is clear
- Dry the area with disposable wipes
- Apply Vaseline to the lips
- Remove gloves and wash hands
- Dispose of equipment
- Document the findings and act accordingly.

## Role and responsibilities of the midwife

These can be summarised as:

- completing the procedures safely with the maintenance of dignity and privacy, using evidence-based care
- undertaking thorough observations (visual, audible, clinical, olfactory)
- maintaining the principles of infection control
- contemporaneous record keeping.

## Summary

- Attention to all types of hygiene benefit the physical and psychological wellbeing of the woman
- The midwife should adapt care according to the individual woman's needs and level of dependence

- Vulval hygiene may be both cleansing and soothing, particularly after a vaginal birth
- Toothbrush and paste are the recommended cleaning agents for oral toilet.

---

**Self-assessment exercises**

The answers to the following questions may be found in the text:

1. List the observations that can be made while completing a bed bath.
2. Discuss the alternative ways to assist a woman to wash when mobility is restricted.
3. Describe the different ways that a vulval toilet may be completed.
4. Demonstrate bed making – occupied and unoccupied.
5. Summarise the midwife's responsibilities in relation to the complete hygiene needs of the woman.
6. Describe how to complete an oral toilet for an unconscious woman.

---

## REFERENCES

Baker F, Smith L, Stead L 1999 Giving a blanket bath – 1. Nursing Times 95(3):40ff

Bowsher J, Boyle S, Griffiths J 1999 Oral care. Nursing Standard 13(37):31

Jones C V 1998 The importance of oral hygiene in nutritional support. British Journal of Nursing 7(2):74–83

Lammon C B, Foote A W, Leli P G et al 1995 Clinical nursing skills. Mosby, St Louis

Sleep J, Grant A 1988 Routine addition of salt or Savlon bath concentrate during bathing in the immediate postpartum period: a randomised controlled trial. Nursing Times 84(21):55–57

Turner G 1996 Oral care. Nursing Standard 10(28):51–54

Chapter **14**

# Principles of hygiene needs — for the baby

This chapter focuses on the hygiene needs of the baby, specifically bathing and washing, and cleaning of the genital area, the cord and the eyes. These are important skills for the midwife when undertaking the tasks and educating the parents. While oral hygiene is important for the baby who is unwell, it is rarely needed for the healthy baby and will not be discussed further.

## Learning outcomes

Having read this chapter the reader should be able to:

- discuss the role and responsibilities of the midwife in meeting the hygiene needs of the baby
- discuss the rationale for not using soap or bath additives
- discuss the principles of bathing and washing the baby
- describe the methods used for applying a non-disposable nappy.

## Baby bathing

The timing of the first bath is dependent upon the condition of the baby. A healthy term baby may be bathed shortly after birth, although in many maternity hospitals this is delayed until the baby and woman are transferred from the delivery suite to the postnatal ward or home. The rationale for the timing of the first bath centres on concerns over the risks of the baby becoming cold and the risk of transferring infection.

Johnston et al (2003) recommend delaying the first full bath until feeding is established to minimise the risks of the baby becoming cold, which they suggest may be towards the end of the first week. However, provided measures are taken to ensure the baby remains warm, this delay is not necessary. Newell et al (1997) suggest that delaying the bath until the baby has acquired his own skin flora may reduce the risk of infection. Equally, early bathing may be advocated to reduce the risk of transmission of blood-borne infection, e.g. human immunodeficiency virus (HIV) (Penny-MacGillivray 1996).

The parents should be involved as much as possible, and be given the opportunity to bath their baby if they choose to, or be shown how to bath their baby if they have not had prior experience. Parents with little or no experience of handling babies may not feel confident to bath them until they are more confident holding them, thus it is important that the midwife considers the needs of the parents and supports them accordingly.

While it is important to minimise the risk of infection, it is not necessary to bath babies every day, nor is it necessary to wash the baby's hair with each bath. Frequent bathing, particularly if alkaline soaps or lotions are used, may predispose the baby to infection. An acidic skin surface – the 'acid mantle' – affords some protection against infection; a pH less than 5.0 has bacteriostatic properties (Blackburn & Loper 1992). At birth the baby's skin is alkaline, with a pH of 6.34, reducing to 4.95 within 4 days (Lund et al 1999). Following a bath where an alkaline soap is used, the skin pH increases, becoming less acidic and it may take up to an hour to regain the acid mantle (Blackburn & Loper 1992) during which time the skin is more vulnerable to microorganisms. It is advisable to undertake a bath using just warm water, as this is usually sufficient to clean the baby. If soap is to be used, it should have a neutral pH, with little or no perfume or dye added. Substances added to the bath may also be absorbed through the skin, which may increase the risk of future allergic sensitisation to topical agents (Blackburn & Loper 1992, Lund et al 1999).

For some parents daily bathing may be an easier and more pleasurable option than washing the baby. There is no right or wrong way to bath a baby, although it is important to adhere to certain principles:

- keep the baby warm
- keep the baby secure and safe
- the water temperature should not be too hot to scald the baby or too cold.

### Keeping the baby warm

The baby can lose heat quickly when undressed or wet. Both the room and water temperature should be warm and the baby bathed quickly, without unnecessary exposure. Additionally, convective heat loss can be minimised by closing windows and switching off fans to stop draughts. Warming clothes, towel and surfaces (e.g. changing mat) minimises conductive heat loss. Drying the baby quickly, particularly the head, reduces evaporative heat loss, and ensuring the baby is not bathed close to cold surfaces such as windows minimises heat loss via radiation.

*Security and safety*

The bath should be filled initially with cold water to prevent the bottom of the bath from becoming too hot. Also, it reduces the risk of other children scalding themselves should they play with the bath water as it is filling. The bath should not be more than half full. The baby should never be left unattended and should always be held to prevent the head from submerging. A woman with epilepsy should place the bath on the floor rather than on a stand and should not be alone. Following a caesarean section, the woman will have difficulty lifting the baby and equipment and will require help.

When washing the face and hair the baby is wrapped securely in a towel and held under the non-dominant arm, secured between the arm and body, with the head and neck supported by the non-dominant hand. To place the baby in the bath, support the baby's head and neck across the forearm and wrist of the non-dominant hand, encircling the forefinger and thumb around the top of the baby's arm. The dominant hand grasps the ankles to lift the baby in and out of the water (Fig. 14.1). Sit the baby up to wash the back, supporting the baby's head across the wrist or forearm of the dominant hand (Fig. 14.2), then return the baby to the original position.

*Water temperature*

The water should feel warm, not hot, no more than 37.8°C (Reeder et al 1997). This can be tested using the inner aspect of the wrist or the elbow. It is inadvisable to use fingers to test the heat of the water, as fingers are able to tolerate quite hot water and so are less sensitive to heat.

## Equipment

- Baby bath – a large bowl will suffice provided it is only used for bathing the baby; the bath or sink can be used, although the latter may be more tiring for the woman's back
- Towel – some towels have an integral hood, useful for drying the baby's head (if using an ordinary towel, fold over about 25 cm of towel lengthways; this can then be pulled up to dry the head)
- Sponge or flannel
- Nappy-changing equipment and nappy
- Baby clothes
- Plastic apron (non-slip)
- Non-sterile gloves, if necessary

## PROCEDURE   bathing a baby

- Gain informed consent from the parents
- Gather equipment and prepare room

Figure 14.1   Positioning of the hands when placing a baby in the bath

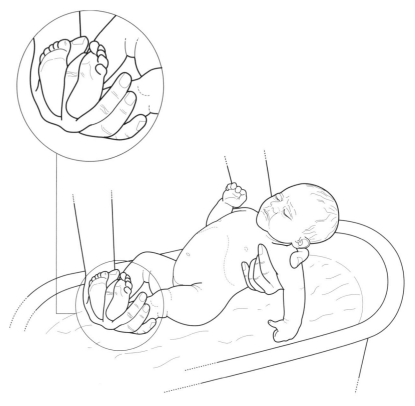

- Wash hands and apply apron (put on gloves if contact with bodily fluids is likely)
- Fill the bath and check the water temperature
- Undress the baby, leaving the nappy on and wrap the baby in the towel

Figure 14.2   Positioning of the hands when washing the back of the baby in the bath

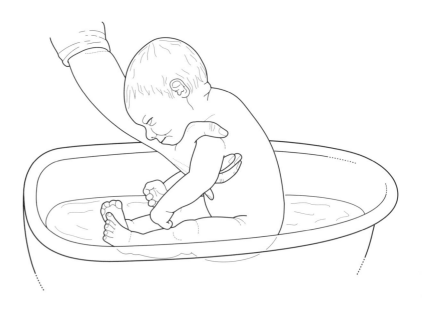

- Wash the baby's face with plain water, using the sponge or flannel to wipe over the face but avoiding the eyes
- Dry the face with the towel, using gentle patting motions
- Wash the hair if required with water, rubbing gently over the baby's hair and dry
- Remove the nappy, cleaning the genitalia if necessary
- Place the baby in the water as discussed, using the dominant hand to gently wash the body and limbs with water
- Wash the baby's back
- Lift the baby out of the water using both hands, taking care as the baby may be slippery
- Wrap the baby in the towel
- Dry the baby quickly using gentle patting motions, with particular attention to skin folds (use either the changing mat or midwife's lap)
- Put on a clean nappy and dress the baby
- Give the baby to one of the parents, or place in the cot
- Empty the bath water and dispose of equipment
- Document the findings and act accordingly.

## Nappy changing

Nappies should be changed as soon as possible following soiling with urine or faeces. The skin should be cleaned at this time with either warm water or a baby wipe to minimise the risk of the skin becoming excoriated and nappy rash occurring. This is likely to happen when urine remains in contact with the skin, particularly if faecal organisms are also present which cause urea to be broken down to ammonia, one cause of nappy rash commonly occurring after the first month (Johnston et al 2003). It is important that the midwife can demonstrate to the parents how to change the baby's nappy, using whichever method the parents will use at home.

## Nappies

Nappies are either reusable or disposable. Reusable nappies are usually made of towelling or cloth, in a variety of styles. The traditional terry towelling nappy is square shaped, requiring folding prior to use. A nappy liner can be placed in the nappy to reduce the amount of urine and faeces coming into contact with the skin. Manufacturers' instructions should be followed when disposing of the nappy liners; they should be used once only and not disposed of down the toilet. Waterproof overpants may be used to prevent urine and faeces seeping onto the baby's clothes. Alternatives are the all-in-one reusables (self-fastening fitted cloth nappies, covered with a waterproof shell), two-piece reusables (cloth nappies that fit into special waterproof pants with self-adhesive fastenings) and wrap-around nappies (cloth nappies with ties, used in conjunction with waterproof overpants). All reusables require laundering. Barrier creams can be used to protect the genitalia and buttocks from the effects of ammonia, but may be contraindicated with some nappy liners.

There are three ways to fold a towelling nappy: the triangle, the kite and the triple-fold method. The triple-fold is useful for boys as it provides extra thickness and absorbency at the front of the nappy where urination is likely to occur.

### The triangle method (Fig. 14.3)
- Place the nappy in a diamond shape, fold in half to make a triangle shape with the longest side at the top and the point at the bottom
- Place the baby on the nappy, bringing up the top layer between the baby's legs
- Wrap one side of the nappy across the baby, then the other side
- Bring up the lower layer of the nappy between the baby's legs and secure with a safety pin.

### The kite method (Fig. 14.4)
- Place the nappy in a diamond shape; fold the outer two points to the centre to make a kite shape
- Fold the top corner down and the bottom corner up towards the centre; the latter fold can be adjusted to suit the length of the baby
- Place the baby on the nappy, bringing up the nappy between the baby's legs
- Wrap one side of the nappy across the baby, then the other side, securing with two safety pins.

### The triple-fold method (Fig. 14.5)
- Place the nappy in a square shape and fold into half lengthways from bottom to top
- Fold in half again, from left to right to make into a four thickness square shape
- Take hold of the bottom right hand corner of the first layer of the nappy and open it to the left
- Turn the nappy over carefully, keeping the layers in position so that the point lies to the left
- Take hold of the next two layers forming the square shape and fold over the outer third towards the centre, then in half, creating a triangle shape with an extra thick pleat in the centre
- Place the baby on the nappy, bringing up the nappy between the baby's legs
- Wrap one side of the nappy across the baby, then the other side, securing with a safety pin.

**Figure 14.3**  Triangle method of nappy folding

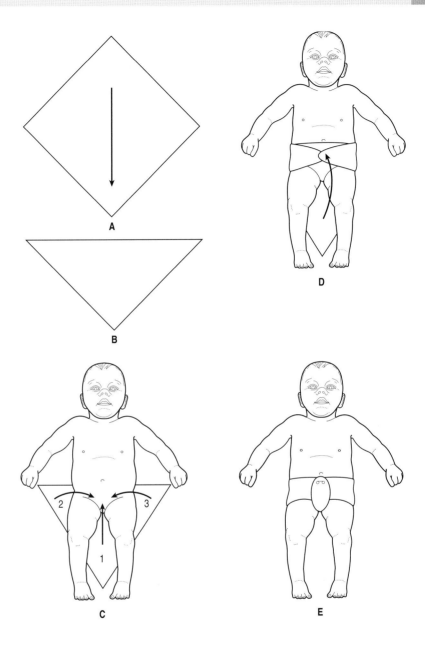

## *Disposable nappies*

Disposables are paper nappies (made from fluffed wood pulp) containing absorbent crystals that form a gel when they become wet from urine. They have an outer plastic layer, fitted elasticated leg bands and sticky tapes at the sides to fasten the nappy. Some disposables also have elasticated waists and some have a hole for the umbilical cord, to allow it to remain dry. They come in a variety of sizes, from newborn to toddler size. Disposables are used once only and should not be disposed of down the toilet.

**Figure 14.4**   Kite method
of nappy folding

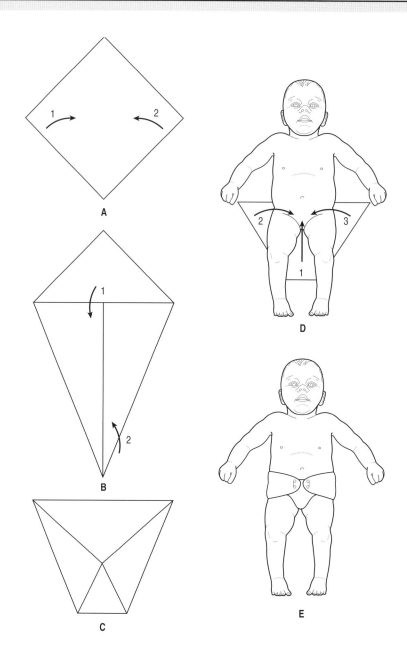

## Use of barrier creams

Barrier creams applied at each nappy change can reduce the effect of friction between the nappy and the skin and minimise contact between the skin and urine or faeces (Atherton & Mills 2004). This, in conjunction with prompt changing and thorough cleansing of the area, can help to reduce the incidence of nappy rash. The cream should allow water vapour to pass through the barrier from the baby but prevent fluid passing the opposite way to the baby's skin. Atherton

Figure 14.5   Triple-fold method of nappy folding

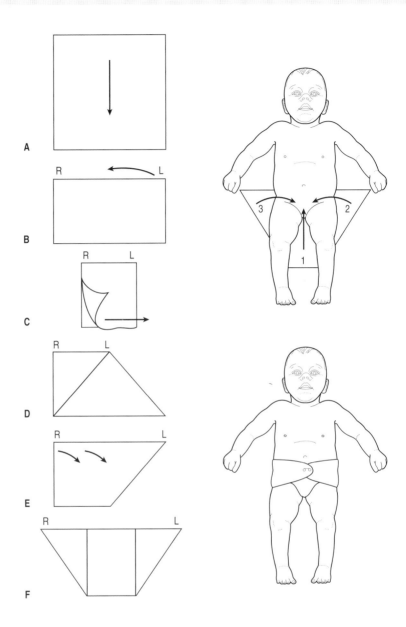

and Mills (2004) suggest that creams containing zinc or titanium oxides should be avoided as they are difficult to remove and white soft paraffin is less effective at allowing transfer from the skin to the nappy. Bacterial preparations are unnecessary as nappy rash is not caused by infection and the cream may interfere with the resident skin flora. Both the Royal College of Midwives and Atherton and Mills (2004) recommend the use of Bepanthen ointment, a mixture containing dexpanthenol and lanolin.

Barrier cream used as a protective layer should meet the following criteria:

- allow the transfer of fluid from the skin to the nappy
- prevent the transfer of fluid from the nappy to the skin
- contain no antibiotics, steroids, perfumes, zinc or titanium oxides
- use lanolin rather than white soft paraffin as the emollient.

Some disposable nappies have a built-in barrier cream that is impregnated into the inner layer or topsheet. The cream is hydrophobic and in response to the warmth of the skin and movement by the baby, the cream should transfer from the nappy to the baby's skin to serve as a protective barrier.

| PROCEDURE | changing a nappy |
|---|---|

- Gain informed consent from the parents
- Gather equipment:
  - non-sterile gloves and apron
  - changing mat or towel
  - small bowl and cotton wool balls or wipes
  - bag or nappy bucket for used nappy
  - clean nappy
  - nappy liner (optional)
  - barrier cream (optional)
- Wash hands, put on gloves and apron
- If using water, put warm water into the bowl
- Lay the baby on a safe, flat surface (e.g. cot mattress, changing mat), with the towel under the baby if required
- Undress the baby sufficiently to gain access to the nappy
- Remove the dirty nappy and put to one side
- Using the non-dominant hand, hold the baby securely around the ankles, enabling the legs to be straightened and the buttocks raised slightly to facilitate cleansing of the genital area
- With the dominant hand, using either a cotton wool ball/wipe moistened with water or a baby wipe, clean the genitalia from front to back before the perianal area to reduce the risk of infection:
  - females: wipe one side of the labia then the other, moving from front to back
  - males: wipe around the penis, towards the scrotum
- Dispose of cotton wool ball/wipe and repeat on the other side until the genitalia are clean
- Clean between the folds of the groin and thigh, then the buttocks
- If water has been used, pat the area dry with the towel
- If a barrier cream is used, apply to the genitalia and buttocks

- Place the nappy under the baby and secure, ensuring a boy's penis points down and the cord is outside the nappy
- Redress the baby
- Dispose of equipment correctly
- Wash hands
- Document the findings and act accordingly.

# Cleaning the eyes

Eyes should not be cleaned unless discharging, in order to minimise the risk of trauma and infection. Sticky eyes are commonly due to blocked tear ducts and are usually not infected. The discharge is a yellowish colour and may be seen as crusting on the eyelid. A profuse or offensive discharge, or a discharge of a different colour, is most likely due to infection and may be accompanied by erythema and localised oedema of the eye. If infection is suspected, a swab may be taken (Ch. 12), referral made and antibiotics commenced. To reduce the risk of cross-infection, each eye is cleaned separately, the cotton wall ball is used to wipe the eye once, then disposed of; the eye should be wiped from the inner part outwards. While sterile water can be used if available, cooled boiled water usually suffices. The midwife should demonstrate this procedure to the parents to enable them to clean the baby's eyes themselves.

PROCEDURE   **cleaning the baby's eyes**

- Gain informed consent from the parents
- Gather equipment:
  — cotton wool balls
  — clean container and cooled boiled water
  — non-sterile gloves if infection suspected
- Wash hands, apply gloves
- Using a cotton wool ball moistened with water, wipe from the inner edge of the eye outwards, using the wipe once only
- Dispose of the wipe and repeat with another cotton wool ball
- Repeat until the eye is clean then undertake for the other eye
- Dispose of the equipment correctly
- Wash hands
- Discuss ongoing care with the parents, e.g. when to repeat the procedure, signs to be aware of
- Document the findings and act accordingly.

# Cord care

The umbilical cord is clamped and cut at birth, leaving 2–5 cm of umbilical cord that has no further function. Following birth, the cord vessels fibrose, the Wharton's jelly dries and the cord separates over the next 5–16 days by a process of dry gangrene. The clamp placed on the cord to prevent haemorrhage is removed on the third or fourth day, once haemostasis is secure. The cord is a potential site of infection, providing ideal conditions for colonisation and replication of organisms. *Staphylococcus aureus* commonly colonises the cord (Newell et al 1997). Current research suggests both cleaning the cord with a spirit-based substance and the application of powder delay the separation time of the cord and may increase the risk of infection by delaying natural colonisation (Zupan & Garner 1998). Current management for the baby not at high risk of infection centres on keeping the cord clean, using water when bathing or nappy changing.

## Role and responsibilities of the midwife

These can be summarised as:

- completing the procedures safely and correctly
- referral, if required
- educating the parents
- correct documentation.

## Summary

- Meeting the hygiene needs of the baby is an important skill for the midwife, who not only undertakes this but also educates the parents
- Bathing the baby can be an enjoyable process for all involved but attention must be paid to keeping the baby warm, safe and secure
- The use of alkaline soaps and bath additives disrupts the acid mantle of the skin, predisposing to infection
- Nappies may be disposable or reusable, with three ways of folding the latter
- The baby's eyes should not be cleaned unless discharging
- The cord should not be cleaned routinely as this can delay separation and increase the risk of infection.

## Self-assessment exercises

The answers to the following questions may be found in the text:

1. How can the midwife ensure the safety of the baby during bathing?
2. Describe how a baby bath is undertaken.
3. Demonstrate the different ways to apply a reusable nappy.
4. When would the midwife clean the baby's eyes and how is this done?
5. What advice can be given regarding cord care?

## REFERENCES

Atherton D, Mills K 2004 What can be done to keep babies' skin healthy? Midwives 7(7):288–290

Blackburn S T, Loper D L 1992 Maternal, fetal and neonatal physiology: a clinical perspective. W B Saunders, Philadelphia

Johnston P G B, Flood K, Spinks K 2003 The newborn child, 9th edn. Churchill Livingstone, Edinburgh

Lund C, Kuller J, Lane A et al 1999 Neonatal skin care: the scientific basis for practice. Journal of Obstetric, Gynaecological and Neonatal Nursing 28(3):241–254

Newell S J, Miller P, Morgan I et al 1997 Management of the newborn baby: midwifery and paediatric perspec-

tives. In: Henderson C, Jones K (eds) Essential midwifery. Mosby, London, p 229–264

Penny-MacGillivray T 1996 A newborn's first bath: when? Journal of Obstetrics, Gynaecological and Neonatal Nursing 25(6):481–487

Reeder S J, Martin L L, Koniak-Griffin D 1997 Maternity nursing family, newborn and women's health care, 18th edn. Lippincott, Philadelphia

Zupan J, Garner P 1998 Routine topical umbilical cord care at birth. (Cochrane Review). Cochrane Library, Issue 3. Update Software, Oxford

# Chapter 15

# Principles of elimination management — micturition

This chapter focuses on micturition, the factors that influence it and how the midwife uses this knowledge. Promoting micturition is an important skill, reducing the need for catheterisation.

**Learning outcomes**

Having read this chapter the reader should be able to:

- define micturition
- describe the physiology of micturition and normal daily urine volumes
- discuss the factors that influence micturition and the changes related to childbearing
- discuss different ways in which micturition can be promoted
- discuss the issues surrounding the use and handling of bedpans
- discuss the role and responsibility of the midwife in relation to elimination.

### Definition

Micturition is the voiding of urine from the bladder via the urethra. It requires coordination between the sympathetic, parasympathetic and somatic nerves and is controlled by higher brain centres contained within the cerebral cortex, thalamus, hypothalamus and brain stem. It is also dependent on normal functioning of the renal system.

### The bladder

The bladder is a hollow, muscular organ, situated in the anterior part of the pelvis, below and in front of the uterus, when empty. When distended with urine, the bladder bulges upwards beyond the pelvic brim and can be palpated above the symphysis pubis. A full bladder can displace the uterus. A baby has a very small pelvis that cannot accommodate the bladder; it lies within the abdominal cavity. Bladder distension compresses the baby's abdomen, increasing pressure on the diaphragm, affecting respiration.

The inner layer of the bladder is composed of transitional epithelium, arranged in folds, accommodating the stretching of the bladder as it fills with urine. The smooth muscle layer beneath this is the detrusor. The ureters are inserted into the upper posterior part of the base of the bladder. The internal sphincter is formed at the junction of the base of the bladder and urethra. The openings of the ureters and internal urethral sphincter form a triangular area – the trigone. Connective tissue separates the base of the bladder from the upper half of the anterior vaginal wall.

Nerve supply to the bladder is via sensory, autonomic and somatic motor fibres, involving the sacral plexus. Somatic motor fibres in the pudendal nerves supply the urethral wall and external sphincter. The spinal micturition centre (between sacral nerves S2 and S4) acts as a relay centre for incoming sensory nervous impulses and outgoing motor impulses, and provides information regarding bladder activity. Information is passed to the higher micturition centres in the pons and cerebral cortex of the brain in response to painful stimuli (e.g. overdistension, spasm or inflammation of the bladder).

## Physiology of micturition

Urine passes from the kidneys into the bladder, where it is stored. As the volume of urine within the bladder increases, the bladder distends and stretches, stimulating stretch receptors within the detrusor. Sensory nerves send impulses to the micturition centre and impulses return causing the bladder to contract rhythmically. A small amount of urine may enter the urethra as the internal sphincter relaxes. When the volume of urine in the bladder reaches 150–250 mL the intensity of the impulses exceeds that of the inhibitory ones, resulting in transmission of impulses to the higher centres. The sensation of filling results in the desire to pass urine. If inappropriate, inhibitory fibres voluntarily delay micturition until convenient. There are 1–2 hours from when the desire to pass urine first arises to the bladder reaching full capacity of 600 mL.

When convenient, impulses from the parasympathetic motor nerves cause the detrusor muscle to contract while the internal urethral sphincter relaxes and opens. As the uterovesical angle changes, urine enters the urethra, stimulating stretch receptors, and the external urethral sphincter relaxes. The presence of urine within the urethra causes further stronger contraction of the detrusor, and urine passes out of the body through the urethral meatus. Contraction of the detrusor muscle continues rhythmically until the bladder is empty.

Micturition is assisted by contraction of the abdominal muscles and forced closed glottis expiration. Contracting the pubococcygeal muscle during voiding can inhibit micturition. The midwife uses this information when assisting the woman to provide a midstream specimen of urine.

### Normal urine volumes

An adult normally voids 1500–6000 mL of urine per day (minimum 30 mL/hour). Disease processes may alter this (e.g. renal disease – oliguria, diabetes mellitus/insipidus polyuria). Oliguria may also accompany shock, hypovolaemia and pregnancy-induced hypertension.

## Factors influencing micturition

These include:

- anxiety/stress
- personal habits: distraction (e.g. reading), privacy, time, etc.
- poor muscle tone due to damage or increasing age
- pain
- position
- disease
- urinary infection
- obstruction: e.g. compression from the enlarging uterus, presenting part, faecal impaction
- damage to the nervous pathway due to trauma, disease or age
- surgery
- stress incontinence
- drugs: anticholinergics (e.g. atropine), antihypertensives (e.g. methyldopa), antihistamines (e.g. pseudoephedrine), beta-adrenergic blockers (e.g. propranolol).

## Changes related to childbirth

### Pregnancy

During pregnancy, a number of structural and functional changes occur within the renal system, some of which continue into the postnatal period.

During the first trimester, the renal calyces, renal pelvis and ureters begin to enlarge, resulting in physiological hydroureter and hydronephrosis becoming more pronounced during the second half of the pregnancy. During the last trimester, the enlarging uterus displaces the ureters laterally; they elongate, becoming more tortuous. The volume of the ureters increases, possibly up to 25 times, resulting in up to 300 mL of urine being stored in the ureters (Blackburn & Loper 1992). This has implications for the accuracy of 24-hour urine collections and increases the risk of urinary tract infection.

Progesterone relaxes the smooth muscle of the bladder, resulting in decreased tone. Hyperplasia of the trigone occurs due to the influence of oestrogen, predisposing to vesicourethral valve incompetence and reflux of urine. Glomerular filtration rate increases by 40–50%

(Blackburn & Loper 1992), resulting in increased urine volume; bladder capacity doubles by term, holding up to 1000 mL. The bladder mucosa becomes more oedematous, predisposing it to trauma or infection. Verralls (1993) suggests 2% of pregnant women develop a urinary tract infection during pregnancy, most usually between 16 and 24 weeks' gestation.

During the first trimester, the enlarging uterus compresses the bladder, increasing the desire to micturate, resulting in urinary frequency. During the second trimester, the bladder is displaced upwards, allowing bladder capacity to return to normal. However, during the third trimester, pressure from the presenting part, particularly following engagement, can once again result in urinary frequency or stress incontinence.

Nocturia may also occur during pregnancy due to increased excretion of sodium and water occurring when the woman lies down (Blackburn & Loper 1992).

### Labour

Pressure may be exerted on the sacral plexus by the presenting part during its descent through the pelvis, resulting in increased frequency or retention of urine; this is also associated with an occipitoposterior position.

Retention of urine occurs when the pressure on the sacral plexus results in inhibition of impulses. The bladder fills but there is no associated desire to void urine, compounded by the distension-inhibiting nerve receptors within the bladder wall. Pressure from the descending presenting part is exerted on the bladder and urethra, particularly at their junction. The resulting compression prevents the passage of urine, even with the desire to void urine. Lack of privacy and poor posture also contribute to retention of urine.

Decreased awareness of the need to void urine occurs if regional anaesthesia is used (e.g. epidural or pudendal block) as the drugs temporarily paralyse the nerves supplying the bladder (Verralls 1993).

Women should be encouraged to void urine every 2 hours during labour to minimise the risk of urinary retention. A full bladder may affect the course of labour in several ways:

- delayed descent of the presenting part, particularly when above the ischial spines (Gee & Glynn 1997, Walsh 2004)
- reduced efficiency of uterine contractions (Morrin 1997, Verralls 1993)
- unnecessary pain (Verralls 1993)
- dribbling of urine during expulsive second stage contractions (Verralls 1993)
- delayed delivery of the placenta (Gee & Glynn 1997)

- predisposes to postpartum haemorrhage by inhibiting uterine contraction (Verralls 1993).

### Postnatal period

During the early postnatal period, a marked diuresis occurs. Between the second and fifth postnatal day, up to 3000 mL of urine may be produced daily, with 500–1000 mL being voided at a time (Blackburn & Loper 1992). Proteinuria may be evident as a result of autolysis (Abbott et al 1997). The structural changes that occurred during pregnancy slowly return to normal during the puerperium, although in some women this may take longer (up to 16 weeks).

Women should pass urine within 6–8 hours following delivery (Blackburn & Loper 1992). However, some women may experience a delayed sensation to void urine. The risk of partial or complete inability to void urine is increased in the presence of:

- trauma to the bladder or urethra
- decreased bladder sensation arising from the use of regional anaesthesia, catheter use or an overdistended bladder
- haematoma formation within the genital tract.

Incomplete emptying of the bladder and urinary stasis increase the risk of urinary tract infection.

Stress incontinence may also occur following delivery as a result of damage to the perineal branches of the pudendal nerves (Abbott et al 1997). If this persists beyond the puerperium medical attention should be sought.

An important part of the midwife's role and responsibilities is record keeping, especially if the woman is experiencing difficulty with micturition (dysuria). Records should show the amount of urine passed and the frequency, with any symptoms associated with dysuria, e.g. stinging (NMC 2004).

### The baby

Micturition is an involuntary process with no control over when and where to void urine. Babies usually pass urine within the first 48 hours of life, with approximately 66% of babies passing urine in the first 12 hours, 93% by 24 hours and 99% by 48 hours (Blackburn & Loper 1992). It is important that the midwife records that the baby has passed urine following birth (NMC 2004). Urinary output is variable, depending on gestational age, fluid and solute intake, the ability of the kidneys to concentrate urine and perinatal events. Urinary output increases during the neonatal period, e.g. breastfed babies pass around 20 mL of urine during the first 24 hours, increasing to 200 mL by the 10th day (Johnston et al 2003). Usually small amounts are passed on a frequent basis, and by the second week of life the baby may produce up to 20 wet nappies a day.

**Summary**

- The desire to micturate begins when the volume of urine approaches 150–250 mL
- If appropriate to void urine, the bladder contracts and urethral sphincters relax
- The adult can inhibit micturition, but it is an involuntary process for the baby. An adult normally voids 1500–6000 mL of urine per day
- Childbirth predisposes the woman to frequency and retention, which may be physiological or pathological in origin
- The bladder should be emptied every 2 hours during labour to minimise the risks of short- and long-term complications
- A marked diuresis occurs following delivery
- Micturition is influenced by a variety of physiological and psychological factors of which the midwife should be aware.

# Promoting micturition

Emptying the bladder minimises the risk of problems such as haemorrhage from a displaced uterus and infection. Knowledge of fluid balance is an integral aspect of elimination management (Ch. 51). This may be of greater importance for some women than others (e.g. women undergoing surgery). The stress of surgery can cause an increased secretion of antidiuretic hormone, resulting in oliguria, compounded by the use of anaesthetic and narcotic drugs, which decrease the glomerular filtration rate and inhibit transmission of nerve impulses. Surgery to the lower abdominal and pelvic structures can result in oedema and inflammation, obstructing the renal tract.

There are three main areas on which the midwife should focus when attempting to promote normal micturition:

1. stimulating the micturition reflex
2. maintaining elimination habits
3. maintaining adequate fluid intake (Ludwick 1999).

## Stimulating the micturition reflex

*Position*
- An upright position, leaning forwards, facilitates contraction of the pelvic and intra-abdominal muscles, forced glottis expiration, bladder contraction and sphincter control
- This is difficult to achieve in bed; use of a bedpan or commode by the bedside or use of the toilet should be encouraged.

*Reduce anxiety*
- Anxiety can cause a sense of urgency and frequency, resulting in voiding small amounts of urine and the bladder may not empty completely as the abdominal and perineal muscles and external urethral sphincter do not relax. Anxiety can result from lack of

privacy, embarrassment, fear of passing urine and the use of cold bedpans

- Staying with a woman while she attempts to pass urine may inhibit micturition; if she feels unsteady she may prefer someone with her; her needs should be ascertained. Warming the bedpan prior to use encourages relaxation
- Use of the toilet can increase the sense of privacy
- Allowing sufficient time to relax and pass urine is also important
- Warm water poured over the perineum may help the woman to relax (measure amount of fluid first if recording fluid balance).

### Use of sensory stimuli

- Ludwick (1999) recommends the sound of running water using the power of suggestion. If the woman is embarrassed by the noise made during micturition, particularly if others are close by, the sound of running water may mask the sound of her passing urine
- Stroking the inner aspect of the woman's thigh, placing her hand in warm water or offering a drink may stimulate the sensory nerves to stimulate the micturition reflex (Ludwick 1999).

### Reduce fear of pain

- Pain, or fear of pain, often has an inhibitory effect on micturition. This is not unusual following delivery with perineal trauma. Concentrated urine may increase pain; additional fluid intake should be encouraged
- Use of the bidet during micturition may reduce discomfort
- Strategies to minimise actual pain should be used, e.g. analgesia.

### Encourage regular emptying of the bladder

- This is important, especially in the absence of the desire to void (caused by prolonged use of an indwelling catheter, damage to the nervous pathways, following surgery, use of drugs, etc.).

### Encourage muscle tone

- Weakness of the pelvic floor muscles (e.g. following vaginal birth), indwelling catheter or severe constipation can affect micturition
- Dolman (1997) recommends undertaking regular pelvic floor exercises to increase muscle volume. This increases the maximum urethral closure pressure, promoting stronger reflex contractions that follow a rise in intra-abdominal pressure
- Prevent severe constipation that can obstruct the flow of urine.

**Maintaining elimination habits**

Supporting the woman to adopt the position and routine (including habits such as reading) that she is used to, assist with micturition.

## Maintaining an adequate fluid intake

Normal renal function requires 2000–2500 mL per day and the midwife should encourage a regular fluid intake.

## Summary

- Stimulating the micturition reflex, maintaining elimination habits and an adequate fluid intake can encourage micturition.

## Bedpans

A bedpan is a container that is sat or laid upon to void urine, used in bed or placed on a chair by the bedside. It is used when a woman is immobile or restricted to bed and is unable to be taken to the toilet. Bedpans are made from plastic or metal, may have disposable liners and come in a variety of shapes and sizes (Fig. 15.1). Slipper bedpans tend to be smaller, being designed to slip under the woman more easily. They may be more comfortable to sit on and do not raise the woman so far from the surface, increasing the feeling of stability.

It can be difficult to void urine while on a bedpan for a number of reasons – feeling of instability, abnormal position adopted, fear of urine overflowing from the bedpan. While the midwife may need to stay with the woman to support her while on the bedpan, this may inhibit micturition. If the bedpan is used on or by the bedside, micturition may also be inhibited due to concern that others may overhear the event.

| PROCEDURE | use of a bedpan |
| --- | --- |

- Gain informed consent and gather equipment:
  — bedpan
  — non-sterile gloves and apron
  — liner (if used)
  — bedpan cover
  — toilet paper
  — sanitary towel disposable bag and clean sanitary towel (if required)
  — handwashing facilities
- Wash hands, apply apron and gloves
- If possible, warm the bedpan prior to administration

Figure 15.1 Different types of bedpan. (A) Non-disposable slipper; (B) bedpan with disposable lining

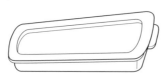

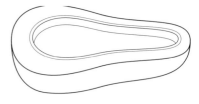

A                                         B

- Take the bedpan to the woman and ensure privacy
- Help the woman to remove her knickers and sanitary towel
- Place the bedpan under the woman, assisting her into a comfortable, preferably upright position
- Stay with the woman if necessary; otherwise supply call bell
- When she has finished, allow time for her to wipe between her legs
- Remove and cover the bedpan
- Assist the woman with replacing her sanitary towel and knickers, ensuring she is comfortable
- Provide facilities for handwashing
- Undertake urinalysis and measure urine if required
- Wash bedpan, if non-disposable, and replace
- Dispose of remaining equipment correctly
- Wash hands
- Document findings and act accordingly.

## Summary

- Bedpans allow the woman to pass urine into an appropriate container on occasions when she is unable to get to a toilet
- Some women find it difficult to use a bedpan; warming the bedpan and ensuring privacy may help
- Standard precautions should be followed (Ch. 9).

### Role and responsibilities of the midwife

These can be summarised as:

- use of the skills that promote micturition
- education of the woman, particularly of the expected physiological changes
- recognition and management of deviations from the norm
- referral as appropriate
- correct documentation.

### Self-assessment exercises

The answers to the following questions may be found in the text:

1. Describe the physiology of micturition.
2. What changes occur during childbirth that can affect micturition?
3. What factors influence micturition?
4. How can the midwife facilitate micturition?
5. Why may bedpans inhibit micturition?

## REFERENCES

Abbott H, Bick D, MacArthur C 1997 Health after birth. In: Henderson C, Jones K (eds) Essential midwifery. Mosby, London, p 285–318

Blackburn S T, Loper D L 1992 Maternal, fetal and neonatal physiology: a clinical perspective. W B Saunders, Philadelphia

Dolman M 1997 Mostly female. In: Getliffe K, Dolman M (eds) Promoting continence: a clinical and research resource. Baillière Tindall, London, ch 3

Gee H, Glynn M 1997 The physiology and clinical management of labour. In: Henderson C, Jones K (eds) Essential midwifery. Mosby, London, p 171–202

Johnston P G B, Flood K, Spinks K 2003 The newborn child, 9th edn. Churchill Livingstone, Edinburgh

Ludwick R 1999 Urinary elimination. In: Potter P A, Perry A (eds) Fundamentals of nursing, 4th edn. Mosby, St Louis, p 972–1008

Morrin N 1997 Midwifery care in the first stage of labour. In: Sweet B R (ed) Mayes midwifery: a textbook for midwifery care, 12th edn. Baillière Tindall, London, ch 29

NMC (Nursing and Midwifery Council) 2004 Guidelines for records and record keeping. NMC, London

Verralls S 1993 Anatomy and physiology applied to obstetrics, 3rd edn. Churchill Livingstone, Edinburgh

Walsh D 2004 Care in the first stage of labour. In: Henderson C, Macdonald S (eds) Mayes midwifery: a textbook for midwives, 13th edn. Baillière Tindall, London, p 428–457

# Chapter 16

# Principles of elimination management — catheterisation

This chapter considers urethral catheterisation of the bladder: what it is, when it is used, aspects of care that the midwife should be familiar with, and the technique itself. Drainage bag emptying and catheter removal are also discussed. Indwelling catheters are rarely required for more than about a week within maternity care; longer term catheterisation requires different clinical management and so other texts should be consulted.

| **Learning outcomes** | Having read this chapter the reader should be able to: |
|---|---|

- define urinary catheterisation, indicating the differences between indwelling and intermittent
- discuss the suitability of equipment available for use
- describe the midwife's role and responsibilities in relation to insertion, care and removal of a urethral catheter
- discuss the management principles involved in the correct use of a urinary drainage system
- describe how a urethral catheter is removed.

## Definition

A sterile catheter is inserted aseptically into the bladder in order to drain it of urine. The most common catheterisation is urethral (via the urethra), for which the catheter may be secured in the bladder (indwelling) or inserted and immediately removed (intermittent).

An indwelling catheter is attached to a drainage system, usually consisting of a urine bag that collects the drained urine and then requires emptying. The bladder can be catheterised through the abdominal wall (suprapubic), but this is seen infrequently within the maternity setting.

**Indications**

- Prior to caesarean section or other abdominal surgery
- During labour if unable to pass urine, especially prior to instrumental delivery
- During the third stage of labour when a full bladder may be impeding normal uterine activity, e.g. during postpartum haemorrhage or retained placenta
- Inability to pass urine, e.g. post-surgery (urinary retention)
- For diagnostic purposes, e.g. postnatal incontinence
- Accurate monitoring of fluid balance when acutely ill or in shock, e.g. pre-eclampsia, major haemorrhage
- Specific urine testing, e.g. to obtain an uncontaminated specimen for protein measurement when pre-eclamptic.

The decision is made as to whether an indwelling or intermittent catheter is required. Jolley (1997) indicates that for postoperative urinary retention, intermittent catheterisation appeared both safe and effective, infection rates were low and the women returned to normal voiding after a relatively short time.

### Considerations for use

Catheterisation is rarely contraindicated, but there are widely recognised side effects and so there should be good clinical indicators prior to its use. Woman-centred care should ensure that the woman is fully conversant with the indications and contraindications before the decision is made and her consent gained. Infection is the most likely complication that can occur (discussed below), but the catheter can also be bypassed or blocked and bladder spasms can be very uncomfortable. There are physical and psychological risk factors associated with catheterisation, particularly as the catheter and the obvious urine bag may affect body image.

# Prevention of infection

There is widespread agreement that urinary tract infection (UTI) occurs with catheter use, particularly with indwelling urethral catheters (Wilson 1997, Winn 1998). The risk is higher for women than for men, due to the close proximity of the urethra to the anus, and the shorter length of the female urethra. Infection is also more likely to occur the longer the catheter is in situ. Crow et al (1986) suggested that bacterial colonisation occurred within 72 hours of catheter insertion.

As a principle, the midwife should consider that bacteria might enter the system in any of the following ways:

- at catheter insertion
- at the port where the catheter and drainage bag meet

- at the port where the drainage bag is emptied
- at the port for obtaining specimens.

Measures can be taken to reduce the risk of infection, including:

- correct aseptic insertion technique
- comprehensive catheter care, including maintaining a closed drainage system that does not allow entry to bacteria (Fig. 16.1). The drainage bag should be maintained at a level lower than the bladder (max. 30 cm) (Evans et al 2001) to allow free drainage and prevent backflow of the urine. Occluding or kinking the catheter (e.g. in the knicker leg) can cause stasis of urine in the bladder and subsequent UTI. The bag should be supported by a catheter stand to avoid contact with the floor. Ongoing catheter care also includes observing the amount, colour, clarity and smell of the urine, in conjunction with the woman's vital signs and clinical signs of illness or UTI
- perineal hygiene, both on insertion of the catheter and on a daily basis. Dance et al (1987) suggested that the use of antiseptic lotions does not reduce urinary tract infection and may be implicated in the development of multiresistance. Soap and water is indicated (Crow et al 1988, Wilson 1997), both on insertion and thereafter. If catheterisation is undertaken at the same time as examination per vaginam in labour it is necessary to swab the perineum using the locally approved solution (often water). The catheter and meatus should be cleaned on a daily basis; showering is preferable
- choice of equipment (discussed below)
- appropriate removal as soon as the condition allows
- general health of the woman. While unresearched, it is traditionally thought that a good daily oral fluid intake is necessary while catheterised (Winder 1999).

**Figure 16.1** Closed drainage system (Adapted with kind permission from Jamieson et al 2002)

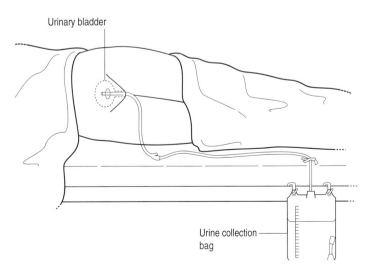

Urinary bladder

Urine collection bag

**Choice of equipment**

Catheter choice should consider reducing:

- tissue inflammation and trauma to the urethra (also improves comfort)
- mineral deposits that may cause the catheter to block
- bacterial growth.

Indwelling catheters were originally made from latex. Caution is recommended with their use because of the danger of latex allergy and the extent to which irritation and urethral strictures have been noted. Consequently, the majority of catheters used are coated latex. A PTFE-coated latex catheter can be used for up to 4 weeks (Colley 1999) and so is often the catheter of choice in the maternity setting. The reader is encouraged to be aware of ongoing new products.

Catheter choice also considers the size of the catheter, both the lumen of the tube and the length. Trauma to the urethra is undesirable because of the increased risk of infection and discomfort. For women, a size 10–12 Ch is recommended; urine is more likely to bypass the catheter if it is too large, and it is in greater danger of being pulled or kinked if too long. A shorter female catheter (23–26 cm long) is available.

Indwelling catheters are retained in the bladder by a balloon inflated with a maximum of 10 mL of water (Foley catheter). Most catheters have a self-inflating balloon; the sterile water is squeezed from the external to the internal balloon (and clamped) when the catheter is in the bladder.

Catheters for intermittent use are generally made from PVC plastic with holes at the tip – there isn't a balloon. A range of sizes and lengths are available; the lumen used for a woman should be 10–12 Ch. Obese women may require a larger size, both in lumen and in length.

All catheters are singly wrapped, sterile and with an expiry date. Correct storage – out of sunlight, heat and humidity in original cardboard and without elastic bands (Winder 1999) – protects the quality of the catheter. Drainage bags are also sterile and sometimes sterile catheterisation packs are supplied, containing a gallipot, receiver and gauze swabs.

### Analgesia

To reduce pain and discomfort on catheter insertion, instillation of anaesthetic gel into the urethra is indicated (Colley 1999). The gel – preprepared 6 mL lidocaine (lignocaine) 2% – acts as a lubricant as well as bringing anaesthesia. It is sterile for single use and needs to be administered 2–5 minutes before the procedure. It can be used for intermittent catheterisation (e.g. during labour) but it is important that the lidocaine (lignocaine) does not enter the bloodstream via any lacerations. Care may therefore be necessary during the third stage of labour if catheterisation is indicated and the gel is being used.

*Documentation*

Details of the catheter – type, length, size, manufacturer and batch number – need to be recorded in the woman's records along with the amount of water in the balloon and the date and time of catheter insertion (Dougherty & Lister 2004).

PROCEDURE    **female catheterisation using an indwelling catheter**

- Gain informed consent and ensure privacy
- Gather equipment:
  — disposable receiver
  — sterile Foley catheter (likely size 10–12 Ch)
  — sterile drainage bag
  — sterile gloves and plastic apron (two pairs of gloves if needing to cleanse the perineum)
  — sterile dressing or catheter pack
  — sterile analgesic gel (likely lidocaine (lignocaine) 6 mL 2%)
  — sterile water (if perineum needs cleansing)
  — catheter bag stand
  — disposable sheet
  — good light source
- Ensure the perineum is cleansed using one of the methods for vulval toilet (p. 117)
- Position the woman (removing sanitary towels and underwear) on a disposable sheet, in a semi-recumbent position, ankles together, knees apart. Keep the woman covered while the remainder of the preparations are made
- Apply apron and wash hands while the assistant opens the pack
- Open the inner wrapper, ask the assistant to slide the gloves, catheter, drainage bag and anaesthetic gel onto the sterile field
- Put on gloves and arrange the contents of the pack while the assistant pours the water into the bowl
- The assistant exposes the woman's genital area
- Establish a sterile field by placing a sterile drape beneath the woman's buttocks and one over her abdomen
- If necessary, cleanse the vulva using the non-dominant hand, ensuring each swab is used once only, cleansing from front to back (pp 247–8). Wash hands and apply new sterile gloves
- Using the non-dominant hand, separate the labia with gauze swabs (this minimises pressure on the labia, increases visibility and makes catheter insertion easier)
- Locate the urethra, insert the anaesthetic gel and wait for this to take effect (2–5 minutes)
- Place the receiver on the sterile field between the woman's thighs

- Using the dominant hand, pass the catheter gently and smoothly in an upwards and backwards direction into the urethra until urine begins to flow. Maintain sterility by pulling back the plastic wrapper as the catheter is advanced. If the urethra is difficult to visualise, ask the woman to take a deep breath in; on expiration the urethra is easier to see (the pelvic floor relaxes)
- Once urine is seen, the catheter should be inserted a further 5 cm to ensure the balloon is in the bladder
- If the woman is very uncomfortable or there is resistance at any stage, stop and seek experienced assistance
- Inflate the balloon by squeezing the fluid from the external balloon and applying the clamp. If there is great discomfort, the balloon may be in the urethra, and the catheter would need to be advanced further into the bladder before the balloon is inflated
- Attach the drainage bag
- Clear the area, assisting the woman to replace her sanitary towel and underwear as required, and to adopt a comfortable position
- Attach the catheter bag to the stand, securing it to the side of the bed
- Discuss ongoing care, e.g. principles of infection control, sufficient mobility, avoiding constipation
- Undertake urinalysis if necessary (using the sample gained when the catheter was inserted)
- Dispose of equipment correctly
- Wash hands
- Document findings and act accordingly.

*Precautions*
- In the event of mistakenly placing the catheter into the vagina, it should be retained while a new one is sought and appropriately placed into the urethra. The vaginal one is then removed. A contaminated catheter should *never* be placed into the urethra
- Excessive loss of fluid from the body quickly in one episode, i.e. up to 1 L, can result in shock. The immediate drainage of urine should be observed and the flow halted with a clamp, if the volume is approaching 1 L.

| **Intermittent catheterisation (female)** | The procedure is exactly the same as inserting an indwelling catheter, except that the catheter is a single-use residual one, which is removed once the urine has been drained. It is an aseptic procedure and the receiver should be large enough to hold the volume expected. |

| **Emptying and changing the drainage bag** | A drainage bag has a life of approximately 5 days (Winder 1999). Getliffe (1996) suggests the drainage bag is emptied before it is two-thirds full to minimise pressure exerted on the urethra and to promote |

continued drainage. It should be emptied into a disinfected or disposable container. The midwife should have clean hands, wear disposable gloves and should wipe the tap with an alcohol-impregnated swab before and after the emptying (Wilson 1998). The urine should be measured and recorded.

# Removing a urethral indwelling catheter

Catheter removal should occur as soon as the woman's condition allows. Depending on local protocol a catheter specimen of urine (CSU) may be obtained before removal to screen for infection. Traditionally catheters are removed early in the morning. However, Kelleher (2002) suggests that removal at midnight allows the woman to rest and begin a normal voiding pattern in the morning. The reader is encouraged to be aware of the evolving research on this issue.

PROCEDURE   **removing an indwelling catheter**

- Gain informed consent and ensure privacy
- Gather equipment:
  — disposable receiver
  — sterile gloves and plastic apron
  — disposable sheet
  — equipment for perineal cleansing (p. 117), depending on chosen method
- Position the woman on the disposable sheet, as for insertion, placing the receiver between her legs; keep covered
- Apply apron, wash hands and apply gloves
- Ask the woman to lift up the sheet that is covering her
- Deflate the balloon by removing the clamp, allowing the fluid to drain into the external balloon
- Ask the woman to take a deep breath, remove the catheter smoothly but quickly as she exhales, placing it into the receiver
- Cleanse the perineum using one of the methods described on page 117 or 247–8
- Assist the woman to replace her sanitary towel and underwear as required and to adopt a comfortable position
- Provide explanations regarding:
  — possible frequency and urgency of micturition due to urethral irritability
  — the need to pass a good volume of urine over the next 6–8 hours
  — possible urinary retention
  — a fluid intake of 2–3 L to wash out any bladder debris
- Measure and record the drained urine
- Dispose of equipment correctly
- Document findings and act accordingly, ensuring the next urine output is measured and recorded.

**Role and responsibilities of the midwife**

These can be summarised as:

- ensuring the woman understands the reason for catheterisation and the ongoing care required
- undertaking the procedures correctly
- correct documentation.

# Summary

- A urethral catheter may be retained (indwelling) or removed (intermittent)
- Infection is one of the greatest risks associated with catheterisation, and the midwife must be aware of all the care that contributes towards reducing the infection risk.

**Self-assessment exercises**

The answers to the following questions may be found in the text:

1. Define catheterisation of the bladder.
2. List the situations in which a midwife is likely to undertake catheterisation for a childbearing woman.
3. Discuss the similarities and differences between indwelling and intermittent catheterisation.
4. List the equipment required for catheterisation using an indwelling catheter.
5. Which is the most likely complication to occur from catheterisation and how may this be prevented?
6. Describe how to empty a drainage bag.
7. Describe how a urethral catheter is removed.

## REFERENCES

Colley W 1999 Female catheterisation. Nursing Times Nursing Homes 14(14):30f

Crow R, Chapman R, Roe B et al 1986 A study of patients with an indwelling urinary catheter and related nursing practice. Nursing Practice Research Unit, University of Surrey

Crow R, Mulhall A, Chapman R 1988 Indwelling catheterisation and related nursing practice. Journal of Advanced Nursing 13(4):489–495

Dance D A, Pearson A D, Seal D V et al 1987 A hospital outbreak caused by chlorhexidine and antibiotic resistant *Proteus mirabilis*. Journal of Hospital Infection 10(1):10–16

Dougherty L, Lister S 2004 The Royal Marsden Hospital manual of clinical nursing procedures, 6th edn. Blackwell Publishing, Oxford

Evans A, Painter D, Feneley R 2001 Blocked urinary catheters: nurses' preventative role. Nursing Times 97(1):37–38

Getliffe K 1996 Care of urinary catheters. Nursing Standard 11(11):47–50

Jamieson E M, McCall J, Whyte L 2002 Clinical nursing practices, 4th edn. Churchill Livingstone, Edinburgh

Jolley S 1997 Intermittent catheterisation for post-operative urine retention. Nursing Times 93(33):46–47

Kelleher M 2002 Removal of urinary catheters: midnight vs. 0600 hours. British Journal of Nursing 11(2):84–90

Wilson J 1997 Control and prevention of infection in catheter care. Nurse Prescriber/Community Nurse June:39–40

Wilson M 1998 Infection control. Professional Nurse Study Supplement 13(5):S10–S13

Winder A 1999 Female urinary catheterisation. Community Nurse 5(10):33–34, 36

Winn C 1998 Complications with urinary catheters. Professional Nurse Study Supplement 13(5):S7–S10

# Chapter 17

# Principles of elimination management — urinalysis

This chapter considers 'normal' urine, changes that may occur during childbirth, the significance of abnormal findings and the procedure for undertaking urinalysis. While pregnancy tests may also be undertaken using a specimen of urine, this is not discussed within this chapter.

**Learning outcomes**

Having read this chapter the reader should be able to:

- discuss the midwife's role and responsibilities in relation to urinalysis, identifying when and how it is undertaken
- recognise 'normal' urine and gain some understanding of the significance of the findings of urinalysis.

## Definition

Urinalysis is the testing of both the physical characteristics and the composition of freshly voided urine. It is undertaken for the purposes of:

- screening – for systemic and renal disease
- diagnosis – of a suspected condition
- management – to monitor the progress of a particular ·condition (Getliffe & Dolman 1997), e.g. pregnancy-induced hypertension.

Urinalysis can be undertaken by laboratory testing, or, for immediate results, by using a chemical reagent strip, in addition to assessing the physical characteristics of colour, clarity and odour of urine.

## Assessing the physical characteristics

- Colour – urine ranges from pale straw to amber colour, depending on its concentration. The colour results from urochrome, a by-product of haemoglobin breakdown. Urine voided in the morning is usually more concentrated and darker than urine voided throughout the day when fluids are taken in.

- Clarity – urine is usually transparent when freshly voided
- Odour – urine has a characteristic inoffensive odour.

### Composition of urine

Urine has a pH of 4.5–8, specific gravity of 1.003–1.030 and is mainly water (96%) with 4% dissolved substances:

- urea (2%)
- uric acid, creatinine, sodium, potassium, phosphates, sulphates, oxalates and chlorides
- cellular components, e.g. epithelial cells, leucocytes
- protein and glucose are present in negligible amounts, normally undetectable by routine testing.

### Normal changes during childbirth

- Pregnancy – glycosuria is more common due to changes in renal function (Blackburn & Loper 1992)
- Labour – proteinuria may occur following rupture of the membranes or as a result of contamination by the vaginal discharge or the operculum
- Ketonuria may occur and, provided it is mild, is insignificant.

---

## Indications for urinalysis

- As part of the antenatal examination
- Throughout labour
- On admission to hospital for any reason as a baseline observation
- Specific maternal disorders or treatment, e.g. hypertensive disease, diabetes mellitus, anticoagulant therapy
- Clinical symptoms, e.g. stinging on micturition
- Altered micturition.

---

## Significance of findings

### Colour

Dark yellow urine is associated with concentrated urine, pale urine with dilute urine. Bilirubinuria colours the urine very dark amber; this should also be suspected if the urine develops yellow foam when shaken. Haematuria also affects the colour: dark red if bleeding is within the kidneys or ureters, bright red if bleeding is from the bladder or urethra. Diet may also influence the colour, with beetroot and rhubarb causing a deep red colour, as can drugs (e.g. sulfasalazine may result in orange-coloured urine).

### Clarity

Urine becomes cloudy (turbid) if left to stand for several minutes due to precipitation of some of the dissolved substances (e.g. uric acid). Proteinuria may cause the urine to appear cloudy or foamy and bacteriuria may cause it to appear cloudy and thick.

## Odour

The odour becomes stronger as the concentration of the urine increases. Stagnant urine smells of ammonia due to the breakdown of urea into ammonium carbonate. A sweet odour could indicate the presence of ketones, a by-product of fat metabolism. Infection may cause the urine to smell offensive. The smell of urine can also be affected by the ingestion of fish, curry and other strongly flavoured food.

## Specific gravity

This reflects the kidneys' ability to concentrate or dilute urine. Low levels are associated with water diuresis, high levels with dehydration.

## pH

A low pH indicates the urine is more acidic than normal and may predispose to the formation of calculi (stones) within the bladder or kidney.

## Protein

This may indicate a contaminated specimen, infection or underlying renal disease. Transient positive tests are usually insignificant, due to the presence of small amounts of albumin and globulin in the urine; to detect larger amounts of protein an early morning specimen is required. To exclude infection, a midstream specimen (MSU) should be obtained, tested and sent for laboratory analysis (if necessary).

## Blood

Blood should not appear in the urine. Its presence might be indicative of infection, trauma, tumour or calculi, or may be due to contamination by blood from another part of the body (e.g. vaginal discharge, haemorrhoids). A positive result warrants further investigation.

## Glucose

Glucose appears in the urine when blood glucose levels rise (hyperglycaemia) or if renal absorption lowers. It may be indicative of diabetes mellitus, stress or, less commonly, acute pancreatitis or Cushing's syndrome.

## Ketones

These may occur due to fasting, vomiting and uncontrolled diabetes mellitus; some drugs may give a false positive result.

## Bilirubin

This is due to hepatic or biliary disease, particularly if the flow of bile into the duodenum is obstructed. A false positive result may occur when certain drugs are taken (e.g. chlorpromazine) and a false negative result if the urine is stale, particularly if the sample is exposed to sunlight.

### Urobilinogen

Normally present in small quantities, larger amounts may be indicative of liver abnormalities or excessive haemolysis.

### Nitrite

Nitrates from the diet are converted to nitrites in the presence of bacteria, particularly Gram-negative bacteria (e.g. *Escherichia coli*). Nitrites in the urine are indicative of a urinary tract infection and an MSU should be sent for laboratory analysis. A false negative result can occur if the bacteria have had insufficient time to convert the nitrates; the urine should be in the bladder for at least 4 hours prior to obtaining a sample.

## Equipment

Urinary reagent strips or 'dipsticks' are the current method used for testing the composition of urine. They are quick and easy to use with good reliability, particularly for detecting proteinuria (Craver & Abermanis 1997). Accuracy for detecting glycosuria increases as the plasma glucose level increases (Li & Huang 1997); glycosuria may not be detected when hyperglycaemia is mild.

The strips can degenerate with time, compounded by storage at temperature extremes or exposure to excessive humidity. Storage should be according to the manufacturer's instructions, in a cool, dry, dark area. The lid should be tight and the desiccant should not be removed from the bottle.

---

**PROCEDURE**    urinalysis

- Obtain a fresh specimen of urine for testing (if refrigerated, allow it to warm to room temperature prior to testing; invert the sample to ensure even distribution of constituents)
- Gather equipment:
  — reagent strips
  — non-sterile gloves
  — apron (if contact with urine is likely)
- Examine the reagent strip to ensure it is not contaminated
- Wash hands, put on gloves and apron
- Observe the colour, clarity and odour of the urine
- Insert the reagent strip into the urine to cover the reagent areas, remove immediately
- Tap the edge of the strip against the side of the urine container to remove excess urine, keeping the strip horizontal to avoid it running down the strip and mixing the colours
- If reading the reagent strip manually, follow the manufacturer's instructions for timing, hold the strip close to the colour charts and read the results in good lighting (alternatively a urine chemistry

analyser may be used in accordance with the manufacturer's instructions)

- Dispose of urine and equipment correctly
- Wash hands
- Discuss the findings with the woman
- Document the findings and act accordingly.

## Role and responsibilities of the midwife

These can be summarised as:

- undertaking the procedure correctly, using an appropriate urine specimen and equipment
- recognising deviations from the norm, referring if necessary
- correct documentation
- education of the woman.

## Summary

- Urinalysis may be undertaken for the purpose of screening, diagnosis or assessment of management
- It is quick and easy to do, with instantaneous results, detecting abnormal constituents in the urine
- False negative and false positive results may occur; these can be minimised if the correct procedure is followed.

## Self-assessment exercises

The answers to the following questions may be found in the text:

1. What are the normal constituents of urine?
2. For what reasons might urinalysis be undertaken?
3. What observations are undertaken on urine prior to urinalysis and why?
4. List the substances that may be found on urinalysis and discuss the significance of each.

## REFERENCES

Blackburn S T, Loper D L 1992 Maternal, fetal and neonatal physiology: a clinical perspective. W B Saunders, Philadelphia

Craver R D, Abermanis J G 1997 Dipstick only urinalysis screen for the pediatric emergency room. Paediatric Nephrology 11(3):331–333

Getliffe K, Dolman M 1997 Normal and abnormal bladder function. In: Getliffe K, Dolman M (eds)

Promoting continence: a clinical and research resource. Baillière Tindall, London, ch 2

Li K, Huang H 1997 Comparing urinary reagent strips for detecting glycosuria in patients with diabetes mellitus. Laboratory Medicine 28(6):397–401

Chapter **18**

# Principles of elimination management — defaecation

This chapter focuses on defaecation, the passage of faeces through the anal sphincter. Relevant physiology, factors influencing defaecation and a discussion on how the midwife promotes defaecation are all included.

Having read this chapter the reader should be able to:

- describe the physiology of defaecation
- discuss the factors that influence defaecation
- discuss the ways in which the midwife can promote defaecation.

## Physiology

Faeces are normally semi-solid in consistency, containing 70% water. The remaining constituents are the end products of digestion, the residue of unabsorbed food, bile pigments, epithelial cells, mucus, bacteria, cellulose and some inorganic material. Faeces are propelled through the large intestine to the sigmoid colon by peristalsis, while water is absorbed from the faeces. The longer the faeces remain in the large intestine, the greater the amount of water absorbed, the harder the faeces become; and the opposite is true. Faeces usually stay in the sigmoid colon until the stimulus for defaecation occurs.

The stimulus to defaecate arises in response to the presence of faeces in the sigmoid colon, causing the faeces to pass from there to the rectum. The rectum is very sensitive to changes in pressure and, as the faeces enter the rectum, the pressure rises by 2–3 mmHg. As the rectal walls distend, the internal anal sphincter relaxes, reducing anal pressure – the inhibitory reflex – creating an awareness of the need to defaecate. The puborectalis muscle contracts, decreasing the anorectal angle – the inflation reflex (Edwards 1997). If appropriate to defaecate, the diaphragm, abdominal and levator ani muscles contract and the glottis closes. This results in a rise in pressure within the rectum and a decrease in pressure exerted by the internal and external sphincters. The pelvic floor lowers as the puborectalis muscle relaxes, increasing the anorectal angle, facilitating the passage of faeces into the anal canal by peristalsis. The posture adopted can assist this process by increasing the action of the abdominal muscles and pushing the walls of the sigmoid colon and rectum inwards. A sharp increase followed by a decrease in blood pressure can occur during defaecation.

This reflex stimulus can be ignored and inhibited; defaecation is, to a limited extent, under conscious control. When ignored, the external anal sphincter contracts, increasing the anal pressure. As a result, the rectal pressure decreases and the puborectalis muscle contracts. The anorectal angle is reduced as the rectum is pulled backwards and the faeces move back to the rectum from the anal canal. The stimulus will disappear and return several hours later. If the stimulus continues to be inhibited, suppression of the reflex occurs and constipation ensues.

If it is inconvenient to defaecate, impulses pass to the cerebral cortex to inhibit defaecation. In babies and young children this ability is absent, and defaecation becomes a reflex response to faeces in the rectum.

---

**Factors that may inhibit defaecation (possibly resulting in constipation)**

- Diet, e.g. inadequate bulk
- Dehydration
- Drugs, e.g. opiates, iron supplements
- Disease, e.g. Hirschsprung's disease, paralysis
- Lack of exercise or immobility
- Psychological – unfavourable conditions (e.g. lack of privacy, bedpans), fear of damaging a sutured perineum
- Pain – may be associated with haemorrhoids
- Psychiatric disorders, e.g. depression
- Pregnancy – progesterone relaxes the smooth muscle of the bowel, slowing down the movement of faeces through the large intestine, allowing more water to be absorbed.

---

**Factors that may increase defaecation (possibly causing diarrhoea)**

- During the onset and early part of labour (this could result in defaecation being delayed in the first 48 hours post-delivery)
- Diet – excessive intake of certain food, e.g. very spicy food
- Drugs, e.g. antibiotics, iron supplements, laxatives
- Disease, e.g. carcinoma, diverticulitis
- Infection

- Damage – lax pelvic floor muscles provide little support for the anal sphincter; as the abdominal pressure rises, faeces will be forced down the anal canal and pass out through the sphincter.

## Principles – promoting defaecation

- Posture – sitting forwards with the forearms supported on the knees allows the diaphragm to move down and facilitates the action of the contracted abdominal muscles; the glottis should be closed, the jaw should be relaxed, lips open and teeth apart. The use of a footstool to raise the legs may facilitate this position
- Diet – a high fibre diet with an adequate fluid intake will stop the stools becoming too firm to pass
- Education – advice on care of the perineum and likelihood of causing damage to a sutured perineum; reassurance of expected changes and return to normal bowel function following birth
- Soft toilet paper – this may help psychologically
- Conditioning – sitting on the toilet following a meal may help bowel habits be relearned
- Mobility – constipation is associated with decreased mobility, so mild exercise will help
- Easy access to toilet facilities – avoid using the bedpan which increases straining and oxygen consumption and causes embarrassment
- Suitable barrier cream to prevent anal excoriation
- Use of laxatives – but these should not be the first course of action
- Suppositories and microenemas may provide immediate but short-term relief of constipation; the cause of constipation should also be treated.

### Role and responsibilities of the midwife

These can be summarised as:

- asking the woman about her bowel habits is part of the daily examination during the postnatal period; this should be undertaken in such a way so as not to embarrass the woman
- any difficulties with defaecation should be discussed and advice given to promote defaecation
- a record of any problems, advice given and evaluation of the advice should be recorded in the woman's case notes
- any drugs given to assist defaecation should be in accordance with the responsibilities of drug administration
- if difficulties with defaecation do not resolve, the midwife should refer the woman for further investigation.

## Summary

- Defaecation is primarily under conscious control (in the adult)
- Inhibition of defaecation can lead to constipation
- Defaecation can be promoted by a number of different factors.

### Self-assessment exercises

The answers to the following questions may be found in the text:

1. Describe the physiology of defaecation.
2. What factors influence the ability to defaecate?
3. How can the midwife promote defaecation?

### REFERENCE

Edwards C 1997 Down and away: an overview of adult constipation and faecal incontinence. In: Getliffe K, Dolman M (eds) Promoting continence: a clinical and research resource. Baillière Tindall, London, ch 6

# Chapter 19

# Principles of elimination management – obtaining urinary and stool specimens

Specimens should be obtained correctly to increase the reliability of the results. The midwife may be best placed to appreciate that a specimen is indicated, but care should be taken to avoid unnecessary specimen collection as it is resource heavy and can be stressful for the woman. This chapter considers how the range of urine and stool specimens is obtained.

---

**Learning outcomes**

Having read this chapter the reader should be able to:

- describe the procedure for obtaining a catheter specimen, a midstream specimen and a neonatal specimen of urine
- describe how a 24-hour urine collection is taken
- describe how a stool specimen is obtained
- summarise the midwife's role and responsibility in relation to specimen collection.

---

## Catheter specimens of urine (CSU)

Urine may be taken from a catheterised woman for the purposes of urinalysis (e.g. infection screening) but occasionally a catheter may be inserted (often residual) to obtain an uncontaminated specimen (e.g. protein urinalysis when pre-eclamptic). This section focuses on obtaining a catheter specimen from an indwelling catheter.

It is important that the following principles are applied:

- sterility, for both accuracy of the result and prevention of infection
- maintaining a closed drainage system, also for prevention of infection (specimens should only be taken when absolutely necessary)
- fresh urine is screened
- correct technique, sample bottle and dispatch to laboratory within the required time for the nature of the test
- recording of the test to avoid duplication.

The type of urinary drainage bag will determine the way in which the specimen is taken:

- a resealing rubber 'window' port in the tubing
- a needleless port in some part of the drainage bag (depending on manufacturer) (Fig. 19.1).

Wilson and Coates (1996) found that using an alcohol-impregnated wipe did not destroy bacteria. Its use is questionable, but recommended at this time.

| PROCEDURE | catheter specimen of urine |

- Gain informed consent and gather equipment:
  — sterile specimen pot (correct one for the nature of the test required)
  — sterile gloves
  — sterile syringe (and needle if it is a resealing port, with sharps box)
  — alcohol-impregnated swab
  — gate clamp
- Ensure privacy

**Figure 19.1** (A) Rubber resealing needle sampling port; (B) needleless sampling port

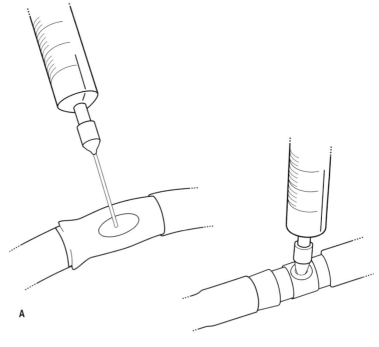

A

B

- Examine the tubing for fresh urine; if none present apply the gate clamp below the level of the port and wait a few minutes for urine to collect (Semple & Elley 1998)
- Wash hands and apply gloves
- Wipe the port (both sorts) with the swab for 30 seconds (Wilson 1998) and allow to dry
- Resealing port: insert the needle into the rubber port
- Needleless port: insert the syringe firmly into the port
- Both: withdraw the required amount of urine and place into the specimen pot. Wipe the port for 30 seconds with the swab. Dispose of needle and syringe into sharps box
- Remove the clamp
- Label the specimen correctly and dispatch to the laboratory, often within 1 hour; this will depend on the nature of the test (if delayed, refrigeration is sometimes acceptable)
- Document the findings and act accordingly.

# Midstream specimens of urine (MSU)

If a urine specimen is to be specifically screened for infection it is important that any bacteria from the vulva or urethra are excluded to enhance the accuracy of the result. Consequently, the middle part of a urine specimen is collected, with the initial voiding clearing the urethra of bacteria. The woman is required to contract her pubococcygeal muscle to 'stop and start' the urine flow, something that may be harder to achieve in late pregnancy.

PROCEDURE  **midstream specimen of urine**

- Explain the procedure to the woman and gain her consent
- Gather equipment:
  — sterile specimen pot (correct for the investigation)
  — sterile receiver – usually a single-use tinfoil bowl or MSU pack that may contain a funnel with the pot and gauze swabs
- Ask the woman to wash her hands and part the labia (perineal cleansing is not necessary unless personal hygiene is poor) (Dougherty & Lister 2004)
- Ask her to void the first part of the urine into the toilet, halt the flow, collect the specimen using either the funnel with the pot, or the foil bowl, then complete the voiding into the toilet. Wash hands
- Transfer the urine from the bowl to the pot, if necessary (wear non-sterile gloves while doing this)
- Dispose of equipment and wash hands
- Label the specimen and dispatch to the laboratory immediately
- Document the findings and act accordingly.

## 24-hour urine collection

The entire amount of urine passed in 24 hours is sent for analysis, usually for protein.

- The collection is started in the morning and is completed and sent the following morning
- Urine is passed and discarded, the exact time noted and the collection begins
- The woman is supplied with a sterile jug and asked to void into the jug then transfer the urine into the correct specimen container. Every single drop of urine passed during the 24 hours needs to be collected. If testing of the urine is required this is done using the specimen in the jug prior to its transfer to the container
- 24 hours later the woman is asked to pass urine as near to finishing time as possible. Once the last collection is added, the container(s) are sent directly to the laboratory with the request card
- Any other specimens required are taken before or after the 24-hour collection.

## Urine specimens from the baby

These are usually obtained from ill babies as part of an infection screen. The urine may be caught in a sterile bowl (clean catch), but this is unpredictable! Sterile specimen bags may be placed over the baby's genitalia and the specimen poured into the pot when collected. Repeated specimen collection can cause the skin to be damaged.

A suprapubic bladder aspiration may be completed by the paediatrician by inserting a sterile needle through the abdominal wall into the bladder and drawing urine off.

## Obtaining a stool specimen

Stool specimens are required to screen for gastrointestinal infection. Parasites such as hookworm can cause anaemia in infected pregnant women. Ease of travel may mean that midwives need to be increasingly aware of this area of care. Stool specimens should be assessed for their colour, consistency, odour and frequency, and the information recorded. Gill (1999) cites the Bristol stool chart (Fig. 19.2), which describes the seven main types of stool classification.

### PROCEDURE stool specimen (adult)

- Explain the procedure to the woman and gain informed consent
- Gather equipment:
  — clean bedpan
  — stool specimen pot with integral scoop or spatula
  — non-sterile gloves

**Figure 19.2** Bristol stool classifications: Type 1, separate hard lumps; Type 2, lumpy sausage; Type 3, sausage but with cracked surface; Type 4, smooth sausage; Type 5, soft blobs; Type 6, mushy/fluffy; Type 7, watery, no solid

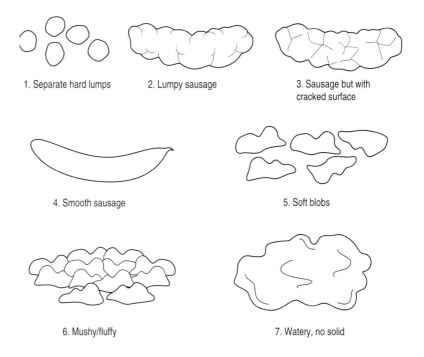

1. Separate hard lumps

2. Lumpy sausage

3. Sausage but with cracked surface

4. Smooth sausage

5. Soft blobs

6. Mushy/fluffy

7. Watery, no solid

- Ask the woman to defaecate into the bedpan, but not to urinate
- Wash hands and apply gloves
- Using the scoop, place the stool sample in the specimen pot, filling approximately one-third of the container, and seal the lid
- If any parasite is visible, aim to place all of it in the pot
- Dispose of equipment, wash hands, label and dispatch specimen, document findings (including stool classification) and act accordingly.

| PROCEDURE | **stool specimen (baby)** |

- Gain parental consent
- Observe the baby for signs of straining (to obtain a fresh specimen)
- Using non-sterile gloves, fill one-third (if possible) of the stool specimen pot with the stool taken from the baby's nappy, seal the lid
- If the stool is too wet and has been absorbed, efforts should be made to catch the sample in a sterile foil bowl on the next evacuation
- Dispose of equipment correctly
- Wash hands
- Label and dispatch specimen (immediately for some screenings), indicating whether contamination with urine is a possibility
- Document findings and act accordingly.

## Role and responsibilities of the midwife

These can be summarised as:

- explaining the procedure and gaining consent
- ensuring correct specimen collection and dispatch
- correct documentation.

## Summary

- Specimens should be obtained, labelled and dispatched correctly
- A catheter specimen is taken from the recognised port, causing minimal disruption to the closed drainage system
- An MSU is the middle part of the voided urine
- Urinary specimens from babies may be obtained using a specimen bag, a clean catch or sterile suprapubic aspiration
- Stool specimens from the woman are obtained from a clean bedpan; from the baby they are obtained from the baby's nappy.

## Self-assessment exercises

The answers to the following questions may be found in the text:

1. Describe how a catheter specimen of urine is obtained.
2. Why is a midstream specimen of urine so named?
3. List the ways a urine specimen may be obtained from a baby.
4. Describe how a stool specimen is obtained from a woman.
5. Summarise the role and responsibilities of the midwife in relation to specimen collection.

### REFERENCES

Dougherty L, Lister S 2004 The Royal Marsden Hospital manual of clinical nursing procedures, 6th edn. Blackwell Publishing, Oxford

Gill D 1999 Stool specimen 1. Assessment. Nursing Times 95(25):40ff

Semple M, Elley K 1998 Catheter specimen of urine. Nursing Times 94(30):33ff

Wilson M 1998 Infection control. Professional Nurse Study Supplement 13(5):S10–S13

Wilson M, Coates D 1996 Infection control and urinary drainage bags. Professional Nurse 11(4):245–252

# Chapter 20

# Principles of drug administration – legal aspects

This chapter considers the legal regulations covering drug administration by the midwife. Errors in drug administration can have serious consequences not only for the person to whom the drug was administered, but also for the midwife who could face charges of professional misconduct and ultimately be removed from the NMC register.

## Learning outcomes

Having read this chapter the reader should be able to:

- discuss the supply, storage, administration, surrender and destruction of controlled drugs
- discuss the responsibilities of the midwife in relation to drug administration.

## Legislation

A number of Statutory Acts and Regulations govern the use of drugs by the midwife, including the Medicines Act 1968 and the Misuse of Drugs Act 1971 (of particular relevance when using controlled drugs). Rule 7 of the Midwives Rules and Standards (NMC 2004a) sets out the responsibilities of the midwife in relation to the administration of medicines, and this should be followed in conjunction with the Guidelines for the Administration of Medicines (NMC 2004b). Drugs are classified according to whether they are non-prescription or prescription drugs (non-controlled and controlled). Midwives can supply and administer non-prescription medicines without a prescription; however for prescription drugs, a prescription chart signed by a medical practitioner is a requirement unless the medicine is covered by a patient group direction. The midwife should ensure that the prescription chart is for the correct woman, the drug is written clearly and correctly with the dose, route of administration, frequency and starting date. The signature should be recognisable as that of the doctor overseeing the woman or baby. It is also important that the midwife is familiar with the drug to be administered, knowing why it is to be given, contraindications and side effects.

## Patient group direction

A patient group direction (PGD) is a specific written instruction covering the supply and administration of a named (prescription only) medicine or vaccine drawn up locally by doctors to cover particular clinical situations (e.g. labour). This allows the midwife working both in hospital and in the community to administer named drugs without a signed prescription chart. Locally agreed policies may be developed to provide guidance surrounding the circumstances when a PGD may be used and administration and dosage for medicines the midwife is able to supply and administer. The consultant obstetricians or paediatricians must sign the PGDs and these should be dated; some may require reviewing each year to ensure they are up to date. They should also be replaced whenever there is a change of consultant. They are usually displayed in a prominent place close to the drugs cupboard.

## Controlled drugs

A controlled drug refers to narcotic drugs and those that cause drug dependence. There are five controlled drug schedules:

Schedule 1: Drugs usually used illegally, e.g. cannabis
Schedule 2: Drugs that are extremely addictive, e.g. pethidine, morphine
Schedule 3: Some barbiturates, e.g. pentazocine
Schedule 4: Includes benzodiazepine tranquillisers, e.g. diazepam, nitrazepam, temazepam
Schedule 5: Medicines containing a small amount of a controlled drug, e.g. cough mixtures, analgesia.

Legislation covers the supply, storage, administration, surrender and destruction of controlled drugs.

### Supply of controlled drugs

For use by the midwife, this relates to pethidine, morphine and diamorphine, listed on Schedule 2. Following notification of their intention to practise, midwives can be supplied with pethidine for use with home confinements using a supply order procedure. This provides details of the midwife's name, the drug, purpose for which it is required and total quantity to be supplied.

**PROCEDURE    obtaining a supply of controlled drugs**

- The supply order is taken to the supervisor of midwives for signing (inspection of the midwife's drug register, record of cases and remaining stock may be undertaken prior to signing)
- The signed supply order is taken to a pharmacist who has a prior agreement to supply the drug and who has a record of the midwife's signature
- On supply of the drug, the name and amount of the drug supplied and name and address of supplier are recorded in the midwife's drugs book (this also contains details of the dates the drug is administered, the woman's name and amount).

The alternative, and usually preferable, option is for the general practitioner to prescribe pethidine directly to the pregnant woman; the woman then becomes responsible for the destruction or return of any unused ampoules. Midwives working in hospital should follow their local policy for obtaining controlled drugs.

### Storage of controlled drugs

Drugs on Schedules 1 and 2 are kept in a locked cupboard within a non-moveable locked cupboard that should only be opened by the midwife. Drugs on Schedules 3, 4 and 5 are not kept in a controlled drug cupboard, but are locked away.

### Administration of controlled drugs

The prescription chart should be written and signed by a medical practitioner unless covered by a PGD. It is important that the prescription chart for any drug is written in ink and is legible. It should contain details of:

- the name of the drug
- dose
- method of administration
- frequency of administration
- date of prescription
- doctor's signature.

When the drug has been administered, the midwife should record the details on the prescription chart, indicating:

- date and time of administration
- dose administered
- route
- midwife's signature.

| PROCEDURE | administration of a controlled drug |
|---|---|

Two people (one of whom is a registered nurse or midwife) are required to check the drug, observe its administration and sign the drug register.

- Obtain the signed prescription chart (if not covered by a PGD)
- Check the stock of the drug in the cupboard with the drug register total
- Record the woman's name, amount of drug to be given, date of administration and amount remaining in the drug register
- Check the name, amount and expiry date of the ampoule
- Draw up the drug, take to the woman
- Confirm her identity (name and date of birth or identity band)
- Administer the drug and dispose of equipment
- Sign the drug register, recording details of the time of administration
- Record the amount and name of the drug, route, time and date of administration in the appropriate documentation, e.g. prescription chart, obstetric notes, partogram.

### Surrender of controlled drugs

Stocks of controlled drugs no longer required are surrendered to an authorised person (e.g. the pharmacist who supplied the drugs). A record of when and to whom the drugs were surrendered is made in the midwife's drugs book.

### Destruction of controlled drugs

Unwanted or expired controlled drugs can be destroyed by the midwife in the presence of an authorised person, and both should sign the midwife's drugs book confirming this. An authorised person includes:

- a supervisor of midwives in England, Wales, Scotland or Northern Ireland
- a regional pharmaceutical officer in England
- a pharmaceutical officer of the Welsh Office
- chief administrative pharmaceutical officers of health boards in Scotland
- in Northern Ireland, an inspector appointed by the Department of Health and Social Services under the Misuse of Drugs Act 1971
- medical officers in England, Scotland or Wales
- an inspector of the Royal Pharmaceutical Society of Great Britain
- a police officer
- an inspector of the Home Office drugs branch.

Unused drugs supplied to a woman on prescription should be destroyed by the woman in the presence of the midwife or the woman can return the drugs to the pharmacist who supplied them (NMC 2004a).

# Prescription only medicines (POM)

Midwives who have notified their intention to practise may be supplied with certain drugs (usually only available on prescription) for use in their practice (NMC 2004a). These may include:

- ergometrine maleate tablets and injection
- pentazocine and pethidine (controlled drugs)
- promazine hydrochloride (Sparine)
- lidocaine (lignocaine) hydrochloride
- phytomenadione (vitamin K)
- naloxone hydrochloride (Narcan)
- oxytocin.

The drugs a community midwife can use are determined locally.

Any non-controlled drugs should have a correctly completed prescription chart (or PGD), which should be completed by the midwife following administration of the drug. It is advisable, wherever possible, for two midwives to check the drug prior to administration to minimise the risk of errors occurring.

## Role and responsibilities of the midwife

In addition to the statutory requirements laid down by Parliament, midwives are also bound by the Midwives Rules and Standards (NMC 2004a). Rule 7 governs the administration of medicines and other forms of pain relief by the midwife. A midwife can only administer medicines following appropriate training in the use, dosage and methods of administration of drugs and equipment. This also encompasses the proper maintenance of equipment and only using equipment approved for use by the NMC (e.g. Entonox apparatus).

The midwife should have a good working knowledge of both the Midwives Rules and Standards (NMC 2004a) and the Guidelines for the Administration of Medicines (NMC 2004b). Local policy relating to drug administration should also be adhered to. Record keeping is an integral part of drug administration. The midwife should also have knowledge of pharmacokinetics (Ch. 21).

## Summary

- Legislation, the NMC and local policy govern the administration of drugs by the midwife; the midwife requires a good working knowledge of how these affect the supply, storage, administration, surrender and destruction of drugs
- All drugs should be written on a prescription chart by a medical practitioner unless covered by a patient group direction

- The midwife should receive appropriate training in the administration of drugs and use of equipment before taking on this responsibility
- Ensuring the drug is administered correctly and knowledge of pharmacokinetics are essential.

## Self-assessment exercises

The answers to the following questions may be found in the text:

1. How does the midwife obtain a supply of pethidine?
2. What is the procedure for the administration of a controlled drug?
3. Identify three people who are authorised to destroy pethidine.
4. Discuss the responsibilities of the midwife in relation to drug administration.

## REFERENCES

NMC (Nursing and Midwifery Council) 2004a Midwives rules and standards. NMC, London
NMC (Nursing and Midwifery Council) 2004b Guidelines for the administration of medicines. NMC, London

# Chapter 21

# Principles of drug administration — pharmacokinetics and anaphylaxis

Pharmacokinetics is the absorption, distribution, metabolism and excretion of drugs. As part of drug administration, an understanding of pharmacokinetics is important and may help the midwife to:

- recognise adverse reactions early
- minimise the risk of unwanted drug interactions occurring
- prevent drugs being used inadvertently during pregnancy and lactation
- educate the woman to help her make an informed choice regarding drug administration.

This chapter discusses pharmacokinetics for both the woman and baby; management of anaphylaxis is also considered. Some drugs in the maternal circulation do not pass through to the fetus during pregnancy and labour, as the placenta acts as a barrier. However, some drugs are able to pass through the placental barrier and can have an effect on the fetus (e.g. pethidine). Drugs may also pass from the maternal circulation to the baby via breast milk. This chapter does not consider fetal pharmacokinetics or drugs and breastfeeding, and the reader is directed towards the growing number of books that look specifically at this topic if further information is required.

## Learning outcomes

Having read this chapter the reader should be able to:

- understand how drugs are absorbed, distributed, metabolised and excreted
- identify factors that influence absorption of drugs via the oral route
- list the factors that can interfere with the metabolism of drugs
- discuss how pharmacokinetics differs for the baby
- recognise the signs and symptoms of anaphylaxis and discuss the management of this condition.

# Adult pharmacokinetics

## Absorption

Drugs administered orally are usually absorbed from the gastrointestinal (GI) tract, entering the bloodstream (some drugs bind to plasma albumin – protein binding) via the portal vein to pass through the liver where metabolism begins. Capsules and tablets must disintegrate prior to absorption; liquid or soluble drugs are absorbed quicker than capsules and tablets. For a rapid response, an oral drug should be administered in a soluble form. Modified release drugs take longer to be absorbed and are also inappropriate if a rapid response is required.

Drug absorption via the oral route is influenced by:

- gut motility and transit time – less drug is absorbed if it passes rapidly; the reverse is also true
- presence of food in the stomach – always follow the recommendations of taking before, with or after food
- acid and enzymes of the GI tract
- lipid solubility (lipid-soluble drugs are easily absorbed and distributed throughout the body water compartments)
- drug formulation.

Certain drugs cannot be administered orally because the acid or enzymes of the GI tract would destroy them and so are administered parenterally (e.g. benzylpenicillin, insulin).

Drugs administered via the sublingual route enter the bloodstream directly and avoid the liver. Drugs administered intravenously enter the bloodstream immediately and can be distributed to the tissues quickly.

Drug plasma concentrations can be measured. Initially the rate of concentration usually declines rapidly, but then slows over several hours. Administering a drug on a regular basis maintains the plasma concentration of the drug at a constant level, although a peak occurs following administration.

## Distribution

The drug is distributed around the body via the circulation until it penetrates the organs or tissues and has an effect. Drugs that distribute into body fluid can be affected by fluid balance (e.g. dehydration, oedema) and those that distribute into fatty tissues are influenced by the amount of fat (e.g. malnutrition, obesity). Different drug dosages may be required depending on the clinical condition of the person.

## Metabolism

This usually occurs within the liver and may be impaired by:

- age
- severe liver disease

- respiratory or cardiac disease affecting hepatic blood flow and oxygenation
- drug interaction
- genetic factors.

### Elimination

The kidneys are responsible for the majority of drug excretion. The half-life of a drug is the time taken for the plasma concentration of the drug to reduce by 50%. A drug that has a short half-life is quickly removed, necessitating frequent doses. A drug with a long half-life requires smaller doses as it remains in the body, having an effect, for longer periods. Loading doses – an initial total dose given to attain high plasma concentrations – may be needed with long half-life drugs to achieve a therapeutic plasma concentration.

### Changes in pregnancy

Physiological changes occurring during pregnancy can affect pharmacokinetics. Decreased absorption in the stomach and increased absorption in the small intestine may occur due to decreased transit time. The latter may increase the time taken to attain optimal plasma concentration. The increase in plasma volume increases the volume of distribution of water-soluble drugs. The increased renal blood flow and liver activity increase drug clearance and elimination, possibly necessitating higher dosages. Different doses may be required during pregnancy; their effect may be slower.

# Neonatal pharmacokinetics

### Absorption

A variety of factors may affect drug absorption via the oral route. At birth, the pH of the term baby's stomach is 7. It becomes more acidic (pH 1.5–3.0) over the first hours of life, followed by a decrease in acid production during the first 10 days of life. Preterm babies have less ability to secrete gastric acid (Jackson 1999).

Drugs remain longer in the baby's stomach as gastric emptying time is slower. The stomach surface is less absorptive than the small intestine (Jackson 1999), and it can take longer to achieve the desired plasma concentration of the drug. Less absorption of fat-soluble drugs occurs as bile output is reduced.

Intramuscular absorption is dependent on blood flow to the muscle, muscle activity, muscle mass and amount of subcutaneous fat. Decreased blood flow to the muscle is common during the first few days of life and absorption is unreliable.

### Distribution

Drugs are more able to affect the brain due to greater membrane permeability of the blood–brain barrier. The baby, particularly preterm, has a higher percentage total body water content, necessitating higher doses (mg/kg) of water-soluble drugs to achieve an effective plasma concentration. However, lower doses of lipid-soluble drugs are required as the proportion of adipose tissue is reduced for both the term and the preterm baby.

Protein binding is decreased in the baby, possibly due to competing substances (e.g. bilirubin) attaching to the plasma albumin. Toxicity may occur as a result of high levels of the unbound drug (e.g. theophylline, diazepam) in the body; lower plasma concentrations are desirable. Drugs such as sulphonamides may displace bilirubin from its protein-bound site, increasing the risk of jaundice.

Metabolism and elimination are both reduced in the baby.

# Anaphylaxis

The administration of a drug is not without risk; many drugs have known side effects and the midwife should be familiar with these. Anaphylaxis is a rare but potentially fatal reaction that can occur following the administration of any drug, as well as food, fluid or topical applications (e.g. plasters, latex gloves), taking anything from several minutes to several hours to appear. Most reactions occur in people with no known risk factors, although it occurs more commonly with drugs such as antibiotics (e.g. penicillin) and whole blood. Early recognition of the signs and symptoms is essential to ensure prompt management of the condition. Mild anaphylaxis occurs more slowly, and symptoms tend to be less serious. Severe anaphylaxis presents with cardiovascular collapse and is more urgent.

## Signs and symptoms
- Urticaria
- Nausea and vomiting
- Tachycardia initially, followed by bradycardia
- Hypotension
- Diarrhoea
- Extreme anxiety
- Cardiovascular collapse
- Pulmonary oedema causing bronchospasm, dyspnoea, stridor, chest pain
- Loss of consciousness.

## Management (Resuscitation Council 2002)
- Position the woman in the left lateral position (inserting an airway if unconscious) and administer 100% oxygen therapy
- Call for medical assistance urgently; do not leave the woman
- If mild anaphylaxis – administer oral antihistamines or subcutaneous adrenaline (epinephrine), closely observing condition for signs of improvement or deterioration, reassuring the woman

- If bronchospasm persists, administration of a bronchodilator may be required, e.g. nebulised salbutamol
- If severe anaphylaxis – administer intramuscular adrenaline (epinephrine) 1:1000 solution (1 mg/mL); repeat twice more at 5–10 minute intervals if needed (adult dose, 0.5–1 mL; baby, 0.05 mL)
- Administer an antihistamine (chlorphenamine) 10–20 mg intramuscularly or by slow intravenous injection
- Resuscitate accordingly
- If the woman is asthmatic, hydrocortisone 100–150 mg should be administered intramuscularly or by slow intravenous injection
- If hypotension persists, 1–2 L crystalloid solution (e.g. normal saline) should be administered rapidly intravenously
- Document the cause and management clearly, informing the woman of this (to avoid recurrence)
- Closely observe the maternal or baby's condition over the next 72 hours as a secondary reaction may occur.

## Role and responsibilities of the midwife

These can be summarised as:

- being familiar with pharmacokinetics and the implications for drug administration
- understanding how pregnancy affects pharmacokinetics
- understanding why pharmacokinetics is different for the baby
- asking about known allergies at the booking interview
- recognising and managing anaphylaxis correctly
- correct documentation.

## Summary

- Pharmacokinetics is the absorption, distribution, metabolism and excretion of drugs
- Pregnancy affects pharmacokinetics and optimal plasma concentrations may take longer to attain
- The differences with neonatal pharmacokinetics result in the oral and intramuscular routes being unreliable
- Anaphylaxis is a rare but potentially fatal reaction that can result from drug administration, occurring from several minutes to several hours following administration.

## Self-assessment exercises

The answers to the following questions may be found in the text:

1. What are the four aspects of pharmacokinetics?
2. How does pregnancy affect pharmacokinetics?
3. How does pharmacokinetics differ for the baby?
4. How would the midwife recognise and manage anaphylaxis?

## REFERENCES

Jackson M P 1999 Impact of age, pregnancy, disease and food on drug action. In: Luker K, Wolfson D (eds) Medicines management for clinical nurses. Blackwell Science, Oxford, ch 4

Resuscitation Council UK 2002 The emergency medical treatment of anaphylactic reactions for first medical responders and community nurses. Online. Available http://www.resus.org.uk (accessed 29 Oct 2004)

# Chapter 22

# Principles of drug administration — oral administration

This chapter considers the different preparations suitable for oral use, the procedure for administering them to an adult and a baby, and the midwife's role and responsibilities.

**Learning outcomes**

Having read this chapter the reader should be able to:

- discuss the different preparations available for oral use, giving an example of each
- describe the procedure for administering a drug orally to a woman and a baby
- summarise the role and responsibilities of the midwife.

Medication taken via the mouth (orally) is absorbed by the gastrointestinal tract. The woman or baby needs to be compliant, alert and able to swallow. If this is not possible or if faster absorption is required then an alternative route should be prescribed. Many preparations can be found in alternative forms. Oral preparations may be affected by other constituents in the stomach, and so the manufacturer's directions should be followed (e.g. before, during or after a meal) for maximum effectiveness. The medication is prescribed as for any other prescription: p.o. (through the mouth) is the agreed abbreviation. Medicine cups with gradations on the side are used; these may be disposable or washed and reused. Some inhalational drugs (e.g. Entonox, oxygen) may be taken via the mouth, but in this chapter only the following oral medications are considered.

- Tablets: these should generally be swallowed whole. If scored they may be divided in half using a tablet cutter, according to the required dosage. Some tablets are coated to protect the stomach lining or to make them more palatable; chewing them would destroy this effect. Examples of tablets include analgesics, antibiotics, iron supplementation

- Granules, powders and soluble tablets: these need to be thoroughly dissolved before administration. This is generally in water, but the manufacturer's guidelines should be followed. Examples include analgesics, e.g. paracetamol
- Capsules: these should always be swallowed whole, never chewed or opened. Examples include antibiotics and analgesics
- Elixir: this may be supplied prepared, or require careful dilution according to the instructions. The bottle needs inverting several times to ensure thorough mixing before administration. Examples include antacids and antibiotics
- Lozenges: these may be used specifically to treat the mouth and are sucked rather than swallowed, or used to coat the tongue. Examples include antifungal preparations
- Sublingual preparations: these are absorbed in the sublingual pocket beneath the tongue. Examples include analgesics and antihypertensives. Preparations for buccal use are required to be placed between the gum and mouth, usually the cheek.

Helping the woman to understand her medication – how to take it correctly, what to expect and what to report – is a significant part of the drug administration process. If a drug is taken incorrectly it can have serious consequences including under- or overdose.

## PROCEDURE    oral administration to a woman

- Ensure that the medication is required and the prescription chart is correct
- With clean hands, check and dispense the drug:
  — Tablets and capsules: tip the required number into the bottle cap, then into a medicine cup. If in foil packaging, check the strip, then push the tablets through the foil into the cup. (Both methods avoid handling the medication)
  — Elixir: invert the bottle several times, hold the bottle with the label to the rear (to avoid obscuring the label with spilt medicine), hold the medicine cup at eye level and pour the liquid into it, ensuring the fluid is accurately on the line
- Approach the woman by name and confirm her identity
- Advise the woman on how to take the medication, providing a glass of water if necessary and observe her swallowing the drug (for sublingual preparations, the medication should be placed beneath the tongue; other directions to suck, chew, etc. should be given as indicated)
- Document administration

- Observe for the effects of the medication and take any necessary action.

### Precautions

- If the woman is unable to take the medication at the time of administration, it is recorded and the late administration checked before being given. A drug dispensed but not administered should be disposed of safely, rather than left in anticipation or returned to the bottle
- Compliance is increased if the woman understands the reason for the medication, likely effects and possible side effects. Refusal to take a drug should be recorded, with the reason and the prescribing medical officer informed
- If the woman vomits soon after administration and only if the tablet is clearly visible, a further dose may be prescribed
- Controlled drugs may also be prescribed in an oral form; administration should be according to local policy. Tablets are counted; elixir should be measured very carefully using a syringe.

# Oral administration to a baby

Depending upon local protocols a healthy baby may be prescribed vitamin K orally. Babies who are unwell or preterm may be administered oral drugs via a nasogastric tube if in intensive care. Standard procedures are undertaken regarding the prescription and dispensing of the drug. Parental consent is necessary for the administration of any medicines. The baby needs to be calmly awake and able to swallow.

Medicine syringes are available for babies and children. An adapter is inserted into the bottle neck, which allows the syringe to be inserted snugly into the opening so that the bottle is then inverted and the medication drawn up with the scale the correct way for viewing. The end on such syringes facilitates this, but also prevents the attachment of a needle. The midwife needs patience when administering medication to babies and children; it can be difficult to assess how much the baby has taken if some is seen to dribble down the chin. If this occurs consultation with the paediatrician is necessary regarding the necessity of a further dose.

## PROCEDURE    oral administration to a baby

- Wash hands, check the drug and prescription
- Gain parental consent and confirm the identity of the baby
- Measure the drug accurately in a sterile syringe, either by drawing it up as for an injection or by using an adapter and medicine syringe with a bottle

- Place the syringe into the baby's mouth towards the cheek, squeeze a small amount (0.5–1 mL maximum) into the mouth and observe the baby swallowing
- Administer the next part of the dose, observe the swallow and continue in this way until the drug is fully administered
- Wash hands
- Document administration
- If appropriate, observe for the effects of the medication and take any necessary action.

### Role and responsibilities of the midwife

These can be summarised as:

- practising within the NMC (2004) guidelines for the safe and effective administration of medicines
- ensuring the drug is dispensed and taken correctly by the woman or baby
- observing the effects and side effects of the drug administered
- education of the woman to aid compliance and effectiveness
- correct record keeping.

## Summary

- Oral drug administration involves all the standards for good practice when checking and administering a drug
- Medication may come in different forms; while the majority of oral preparations are swallowed, some are for sucking, chewing, buccal or sublingual use
- Babies have oral drugs administered in liquid form via a medication syringe where possible.

### Self-assessment exercises

The answers to the following questions may be found in the text:

1. Give an example of each of the different types of preparation available for oral administration.
2. What would the midwife do if the drug was dispensed but the woman was not available to take it?
3. Describe how a midwife would administer a sublingual drug to a woman.
4. Describe how drugs are administered orally to a baby.
5. What would the midwife do if the woman vomited her medication shortly after taking it?

### REFERENCE

NMC (Nursing & Midwifery Council) 2004 Guidelines for the administration of medicines. NMC, London

# Chapter 23

# Principles of drug administration – injection technique

Preparations are administered via an injection if they cannot be absorbed, or are absorbed too slowly, when given via other routes. In this chapter the safe administration of drugs via intradermal (I.D.), intramuscular (I.M.) and subcutaneous (S.C.) injection will be reviewed. Suitable sites in the adult and baby are highlighted and there is discussion about appropriate equipment to use. Intravenous injection is reviewed in Chapter 26.

## Learning outcomes

Having read this chapter the reader should be able to:

- list the situations in which a midwife is likely to administer medication by injection
- describe the suitable sites for I.D., I.M. and S.C. injections in the adult and I.M. in the baby
- demonstrate an injection, giving a rationale for each stage
- summarise the role and responsibilities of the midwife.

## Indications

The midwife administers drugs by injection on a number of occasions; the following is an indicative, but not exhaustive list:

- oxytocic agent (active third stage of labour or postpartum haemorrhage)
- analgesia or antidote, e.g. pethidine, morphine
- anti-D immunoglobulin
- rubella vaccine
- vitamin K (babies)
- subcutaneous heparin (thromboembolic prophylaxis)
- iron therapy
- steroids (fetal lung maturity in preterm labour)
- intradermal local anaesthetics.

### Safety

Giving an injection exposes midwives to potential needlestick injury and contact with blood. Used needles must never be resheathed, unless using a one-handed technique or specific equipment, and sharps must be disposed of correctly in a sharps box. A variety of safety devices are becoming increasingly available to reduce the dangers of percutaneous injury; the reader is encouraged to be aware of their availability and use (Trim 2004). Disposable gloves are indicated to protect the midwife from contact with blood.

# Intradermal injection (I.D.)

A small amount of solution (up to 0.5 mL) is injected locally into the skin using a 25 g (orange) needle at a 10–15° angle (Workman 1999) (Fig. 23.1). The bevel of the needle is inserted upwards so that a small weal forms and is seen on the skin. The same sites as S.C. injection may be used, but frequently midwives inject intradermally prior to cannulation (Ch. 50) and therefore inject over the site of the vein to be cannulated. Local anaesthetic is also injected intradermally when infiltrating for perineal repair (Ch. 37).

# Intramuscular injection (I.M.)

## Choice of site in the adult

As suggested, intramuscular is injection into muscle. A good blood supply ensures the drug is absorbed quickly and the effects are maximised. Choice of site is important; a large muscle is able to support up to 4 mL of fluid. Good knowledge of anatomy is needed in order to avoid nerves, bone and blood vessels at all times. The skin should also be free of bruising and infection; the muscle should not be

**Figure 23.1** Intramuscular, subcutaneous and intradermal injections

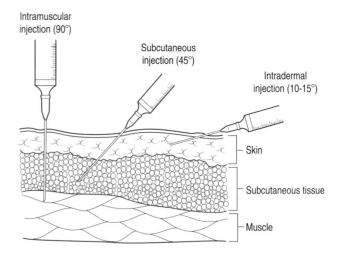

atrophied. There are now five recommended sites for I.M. injection (Workman 1999), the ventrogluteal site having gained popularity in recent years:

- Deltoid muscle of upper arm (maximum 1 mL) (Fig. 23.2A): the site is approximately 2.5 cm below the acromial process on the lateral surface of the arm
- Quadriceps muscle (vastus lateralis): this is found by measuring a hand's breadth down from the greater trochanter, and one up from

**Figure 23.2** Sites for adult intramuscular injection. (A) Deltoid muscle; (B) rectus femoris and vastus lateralis (vastus lateralis is the one suitable site for I.M. injection in neonates also);

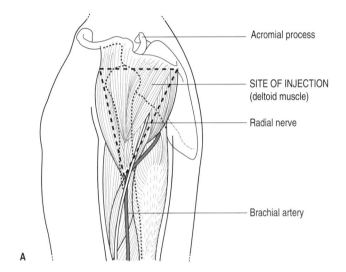

Acromial process

SITE OF INJECTION (deltoid muscle)

Radial nerve

Brachial artery

A

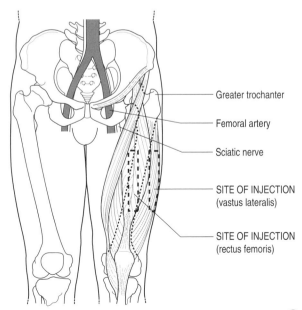

Greater trochanter

Femoral artery

Sciatic nerve

SITE OF INJECTION (vastus lateralis)

SITE OF INJECTION (rectus femoris)

B

*Continues*

**Figure 23.2 cont'd**
(C) gluteus maximus; (Adapted
with kind permission from
Jamieson et al 1997);
(D) ventrogluteal

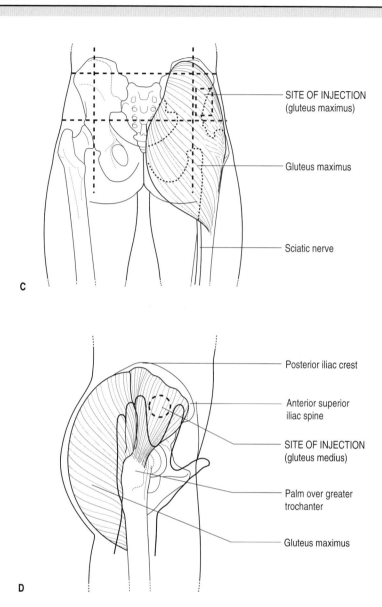

the knee. The remaining middle third of the lateral aspect of the thigh is the correct muscle (Fig. 23.2B). The rectus femoris is adjacent on the anterior aspect of the thigh; it is used less and is not appropriate in children (Fig. 23.2B)

- Gluteus maximus muscle: found on the upper outer quadrant of the buttock (Fig. 23.2C)
- Ventrogluteal site: the palm of the midwife's right hand is placed on the greater trochanter of the woman's left hip or vice versa. The index finger is extended to touch the anterior superior iliac crest while the middle finger stretches as far along the iliac crest as possible. The site is in the 'V' between the index and middle fingers (Fig. 23.2D).

The choice of site often depends on accessibility; the deltoid muscle should be used for anti-D immunoglobulin (Benbow & Wray 1998) and hepatitis B vaccine (Beyea & Nicoll 1996). Beyea and Nicoll (1996) suggest that pain and complications have been documented for all sites except the ventrogluteal.

The muscle should be relaxed for minimal discomfort; the skin does not need to be pinched or held taut, although the site may be supported by the non-injecting hand. Bunching up the muscle in a thin woman may sometimes be necessary (Workman 1999).

### Z track

A Z track technique (Fig. 23.3) ensures the solution does not leak back to the skin. The skin and subcutaneous tissue are moved a couple of centimetres, the needle is inserted into the original site chosen, the solution is injected and after 10 seconds the needle is removed. The skin is then released (Workman 1999). There are advocates in the literature of Z track being the technique of choice for all I.M. injections (Beyea & Nicoll 1996, Rodger & King 2000). The reader will need to consult their local protocol.

### Air bubble

The air bubble technique, when an additional 0.1 mL air is drawn up into the syringe with the solution, is considered to provide a bubble barrier to the outside skin, but its use is not advocated at this time.

## Choice of equipment

In a normal-sized woman a 21 g (green) or 23 g (blue) needle is used at a 90° angle (see Fig. 23.1). This assessment is individualised, and the needle chosen should reach the muscle with approximately one-quarter of it still visible externally. The needle and syringe should be sterile, the syringe being an appropriate size for the amount of fluid to be injected.

**Figure 23.3** Z track injection. The skin and subcutaneous tissue are moved along prior to insertion of the needle and then released once the needle has been removed. The solution is prevented from back tracking to the skin

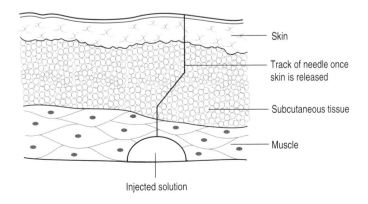

Skin

Track of needle once skin is released

Subcutaneous tissue

Muscle

Injected solution

Skin cleansing is not required for I.M. or S.C. injections but dirty skin should be washed with soap and water beforehand. If an alcohol swab is used, it must be left at least 30 seconds to air dry before injecting. Post-injection, a cotton wool ball is used to cover the puncture site and a plaster applied if necessary.

### Ampoules and vials

Ampoules may be glass or, increasingly, plastic, with a top that 'snaps off'. Vials tend to be glass with a rubber bung beneath the metal top. Preparations may come as solutions or powder for reconstitution. In the event of needing to reconstitute a drug (e.g. diamorphine), sterile water will be required. Ampoules and vials may be completely inverted (without leaking) so that the substance can be removed completely and the scale on the syringe read correctly. A filtered needle should be used when drawing up from a glass ampoule to prevent glass shards entering the woman. Alternatively a new needle can be used to inject with.

## Intramuscular injection for a baby

There is one main site for I.M. injection in the baby: quadriceps muscle (vastus lateralis), lateral mid-third of the thigh (see Fig. 23.2B).

Other sites (e.g. gluteus maximus and ventrogluteal) may be used in older babies, but Hemsworth (2000) suggests that muscular development in these sites is insufficient in neonates. The absolute maximum dose that can be injected is 1 mL. The baby should be in a safe place (e.g. held or in a cot). A 25 g (orange) needle is inserted at a 45° angle.

## Subcutaneous injection (S.C.)

A subcutaneous injection places the medication into the connective tissue and fat beneath the skin. These tissues have a reduced blood supply in comparison to muscle, so drug absorption is slow and steady. Common preparations for S.C. use include insulin and heparin. As a single injection only 1–2 mL can be accommodated, but S.C. infusions can also be established and can add up to 3L of fluid into the circulation over 24 hours.

Generally, a 25g (orange) needle is used at an angle of 45° (see Fig. 23.1) but studies show that S.C. injections can be inadvertently placed into muscle and so it is necessary to grasp the skin and lift the subcutaneous tissue away from the muscle before injecting (Peragallo-Dittko 1997, Workman 1999). Where the medication is prepacked with a shorter needle (1.2 cm or less; Hayes 1998), a 90° angle is used. It has been standard practice to aspirate back with the plunger before injecting to establish that a vein has not been punctured, but this is no longer necessary (Peragallo-Dittko 1997). Chan (2001) also suggests that a slower injection of heparin (over 30 seconds as opposed to 10 seconds) reduces the pain and bruising. It should be noted that this is a small study that only uses heparin, and therefore should be generalised with caution, but nevertheless it is generally accepted that injections should be administered slowly (Dougherty & Lister 2004, Hayes 1998).

The preferred sites are:

- outer surface of the upper arm
- lateral mid-third of the thigh
- umbilical region of the abdomen
- on the back, beneath the scapulae, either side of the spine.

The site should be examined prior to injection for inflammation or hardness, which may indicate poor absorption. For repeated injections, the site is rotated. Safety, skin preparation and sterility issues apply as discussed above.

| PROCEDURE | I.M. and S.C. injections in the adult |
|---|---|

- Ascertain that the prescription is correct
- Gain informed consent and wash hands
- Gather equipment:
  — sterile needle and syringe of correct sizes
  — portable sharps box
  — disposable tray (if sharps box not portable)
  — non-sterile gloves
  — cotton wool ball
  — ampoule
- Assemble the needle and syringe by placing them firmly together
- Loosen the protective sheath over the needle and draw back on the plunger to prepare the syringe
- Ensure all of the solution is in the ampoule (not retained in the top); snap off the top
- Draw up the required amount of solution
- Take the plunger of the syringe back a little further, invert the syringe and examine it for air
- Tap the syringe gently to encourage the air up to the top of the syringe; push the plunger to exclude the air from the syringe and needle, ensuring none of the solution is lost and the dosage in the syringe is correct
- Gently resheath the needle (or change it to a new one) on the tray and take the prescription, sharps box and tray to the woman
- Confirm her identity and expose the injection site
- Apply gloves
- For S.C. injection: identify the site, grasp a fold of skin with the non-injecting hand, decisively inject at the correct angle, release the grasp, but continue to support the skin; administer the injection

slowly, remove the needle quickly and apply pressure with a cotton wool ball

- For I.M. injection: identify the specific site for puncture ensuring the muscle is relaxed, support it with the non-injecting hand. Decisively inject at the correct angle, inserting the needle with approximately one-quarter still visible. Draw back on the plunger (wait for at least 5 seconds); if 'nothing' is seen, push on the plunger smoothly at a rate of 10 seconds per mL to inject the solution. Wait 10 seconds then remove the needle smoothly, pressing gently on the puncture site with the cotton wool ball; avoid massage which may cause irritation
- For Z track injection: following the procedure outlined above, but prior to injecting, move the skin and subcutaneous tissue along 1–2 cm. After injecting, withdraw the needle and then release the traction on the skin
- For all injections: place the syringe and needle directly into the sharps box (or onto the tray) without resheathing the needle
- Assist the woman to a comfortable position; encourage her to gently exercise the muscle of the injection site to encourage drug absorption
- Dispose of equipment correctly
- Document administration and act accordingly; examine the site 2 hours later for any possible reactions.

### Precautions

If blood is seen in the syringe when drawing the plunger back, the needle has punctured a blood vessel and the injection would be intravenous, not intramuscular. The needle and syringe should be withdrawn and discarded. A second injection is prepared and administered.

---

**Role and responsibilities of the midwife**

These can be summarised as:

- correct use of equipment and choice of site to facilitate a correct injection technique
- support of the woman, particularly if anxious
- correct disposal of sharps
- correct record keeping.

---

## Summary

- Intradermal injections inject a small amount of solution just beneath the skin
- Injecting into muscle requires selective use of site and equipment to ensure that the technique chosen is correct

- Subcutaneous injections inject the medication into the tissue beneath the skin and so use a shorter needle and a smaller angle
- The midwife needs to complete the injection decisively, ensuring that a vein has not been punctured
- Used needles should not be resheathed and sharps should be disposed of correctly.

| Self-assessment exercises | The answers to the following questions may be found in the text: |
|---|---|

1. Cite examples of when injections may be necessary for a childbearing woman.
2. List the sites suitable for intramuscular injection for both the woman and the baby.
3. What would the midwife do if blood appeared in the syringe while drawing back?
4. Demonstrate an I.M. injection for a baby.
5. Compare and contrast the similarities and differences between an I.M. and a S.C. injection in the adult, in relation to the equipment, technique and site.
6. Describe how a Z track injection is completed.
7. Summarise the role and responsibilities of the midwife when administering an injection.

## REFERENCES

Benbow A, Wray J 1998 Recommendations for the use of anti-D immunoglobulin for RhD prophylaxis. British Journal of Midwifery 6(3):184–186

Beyea S C, Nicoll L H 1996 Administering IM injections the right way. American Journal of Nursing 96(1):34–35

Chan H 2001 Effects of injection duration on site pain intensity and bruising associated with subcutaneous heparin. Journal of Advanced Nursing 35(6):882–892

Dougherty L, Lister S 2004 The Royal Marsden Hospital manual of clinical nursing procedures, 6th edn. Blackwell Publishing, Oxford

Hayes C 1998 Injection technique: subcutaneous. Nursing Times 94(41):85–86

Hemsworth S 2000 Intramuscular injection technique. Paediatric Nursing 12(9):17–20

Jamieson E M, McCall J M, Blythe R et al 1997 Clinical nursing practices, 3rd edn. Churchill Livingstone, Edinburgh

Peragallo-Dittko V 1997 Rethinking subcutaneous injection technique. American Journal of Nursing 97(5):71–72

Rodger M, King L 2000 Drawing up and administering intramuscular injections: a review of the literature. Journal of Advanced Nursing 31(3):574–582

Trim J 2004 A review of needle-protective devices to prevent sharps injuries. British Journal of Nursing 13(3):144–153

Workman B 1999 Safe injection techniques. Nursing Standard 13(39):47–53

Chapter **24**

# Principles of drug administration – administration of medicines per vaginam

The midwife is actively involved in the administration of medicines per vaginam (P.V.), largely with prostaglandin for the induction of labour. Placing a drug into the vagina is a means of ensuring that the action of the drug can work directly (locally) to produce the desired effect. Other drugs may also be administered P.V. (e.g. antifungal preparations). This chapter considers the midwife's role and responsibilities and the procedure for administration P.V., focusing largely on the administration of prostaglandin $E_2$ ($PGE_2$).

## Learning outcomes

Having read this chapter the reader should be able to:

- describe how a drug is administered P.V.
- discuss the role and responsibilities of the midwife before, during and after administration
- list the factors that are pertinent to the administration of prostaglandin P.V.

## Using prostaglandin

Within its Induction of Labour (IOL) guideline, NICE (2001) is clear about the following points:

- Care should be woman centred with the woman able to make an informed decision
- Where the woman is healthy and has had an uncomplicated pregnancy, vaginal $PGE_2$ may be given on an antenatal ward. Otherwise, prostaglandin should not be given on the ward
- The wellbeing of the fetus should be confirmed prior to $PGE_2$ administration
- Where possible, $PGE_2$ tablets (as opposed to gel) should be prescribed and placed intravaginally, i.e. into the posterior vaginal fornix. The woman should continue to lie down for 30 minutes

following the administration. The prescription is determined according to the presence or otherwise of intact membranes and the favourability of the cervix (determined by Bishop's scoring)

- A continuous cardiotocogram (CTG) should be recorded once contractions have been reported or detected. This may be discontinued once fetal wellbeing is confirmed. Intermittent monitoring is then permitted for healthy women with no other pregnancy complications.

## Role and responsibilities of the midwife

These can be summarised as:

- assessment prior to administration: the midwife must be familiar with the local protocols for the administration of $PGE_2$, most of which are discussed above
- appropriate checking and dispensing of the drug (as for any prescription): the lubricant used with vaginal drugs should be appropriate, e.g. KY Jelly; some interaction can occur with some preparations, e.g. obstetric cream and $PGE_2$
- understanding the action and side effects of the drug, and therefore education and support of the woman to prepare her for the effect: $PGE_2$ can cause hyperstimulation of the uterus, fetal distress and uncomfortable uterine contractions. It may also take time for IOL to occur, something that the woman and her family need to appreciate. Antifungal preparations may be self-administered, for which the midwife can have a significant role in educating the woman in infection prevention and drug administration
- maintenance of dignity and privacy during an embarrassing procedure: survivors of sexual abuse will find the administration of medicine P.V. a traumatic experience. The midwife is well placed to recognise some of the signs and to obtain appropriate help for the woman
- observations made while undertaking the drug administration: e.g. repeated Bishop's scoring, angle of pubic arch, nature of presenting part, other factors that may affect care
- correct administration technique, placing the medication in the correct place: the preparations for vaginal drugs vary, e.g. tablet, pessary (with or without applicator) or gel (similar to a syringe in appearance). The midwife must be competent with vaginal examination before administering $PGE_2$ P.V., as it does need to be placed accurately
- appreciation of care following administration: in all instances the woman will need to adopt a semi-recumbent position following administration, so that the medicine does not dislodge. Antifungal preparations are often administered last thing at night. Observations are made both for the expected action and to exclude deviations from the norm
- contemporaneous record keeping of the care given before, during and after the administration.

PROCEDURE    administration of medicines P.V.

- Gain informed consent and ensure privacy
- Gather equipment:
  — sterile gloves
  — disposable sheet
  — lubricant, e.g. KY Jelly
  — the drug
- Ask the woman to adopt an almost recumbent position (use a wedge to avoid aortocaval occlusion if necessary), with her knees bent, ankles together and knees parted, placing a disposable sheet beneath her buttocks
- Remove any sanitary towels or underwear, keeping the genital area covered
- Open the gloves, place the lubricant and pessary on the sterile side of the paper (a sterile vaginal examination pack may be used)
- Wash hands and apply gloves
- Ask the woman to remove the covers
- For PGE$_2$ administration, part the labia with the thumb and forefinger of the non-examining hand:
  — lubricate the two fingers of the examining hand and gently insert into the vagina, in a downwards and backwards direction along the anterior vaginal wall to locate the cervix, ensuring the thumb does not come into contact with the woman's clitoris or anus
  — when using gel, slide the applicator between the vaginal wall and the examining hand, until it has been guided into the posterior vaginal fornix by the examining hand. The plunger is then depressed by the other hand and the gel administered. Lubricant may be applied to the tip to aid insertion
  — for the application of a tablet or pessary, either insert the examining hand with the pessary secured between the fingers, guiding it into the fornix as before, or slide the pessary into the vagina using the non-examining hand, and guide it into place using the examining hand. Lubricant may be applied to the pessary to aid insertion
- Remove fingers, wipe the vulva
- For administration of a pessary with its own applicator, part the labia with the thumb and forefinger of the non-examining hand (a vaginal examination is unnecessary if the positioning of the pessary is not crucial, i.e. antifungal preparations):
  — slide the applicator along the posterior vaginal wall until the pessary is high in the vagina
  — depress the plunger and withdraw the applicator
- Assist the woman to resume a comfortable semi-recumbent position

- Dispose of equipment correctly and wash hands
- Document administration and findings and act accordingly.

## Summary

- Medicines administered P.V. act locally, but the procedure can be difficult and embarrassing for the woman
- The midwife should ensure that $PGE_2$ is administered correctly following the local protocol
- A semi-recumbent position should be adopted following the procedure.

## Self-assessment exercises

The answers to the following questions may be found in the text:

1. What are the two main types of medicine that are administered P.V.?
2. Describe how the midwife prepares the woman for this administration.
3. Describe how a drug is administered P.V.
4. Discuss the role and responsibilities of the midwife after the administration of a medicine P.V.
5. List the specific considerations when administering $PGE_2$ P.V.

### REFERENCE

NICE (National Institute for Clinical Excellence) 2001 Induction of labour. NICE, London

Chapter **25**

# Principles of drug administration – administration of medicines per rectum

Medicines inserted into the rectum have two predominant actions:

- for laxative purposes
- systemic treatment, e.g. analgesia.

The rectum has a good blood supply and drugs can be absorbed quickly, but the procedure can be embarrassing and it is often not the route of choice. Suppositories or enemas may be administered for constipation; they may also be given for systemic use (e.g. analgesic suppositories postoperatively or steroidal enemas for particular bowel conditions). In this chapter the procedure is reviewed and the role of the midwife is discussed.

| **Learning outcomes** |
| --- |

Having read this chapter the reader should be able to:

- describe the safe administration of suppositories and enemas, making differentiations accordingly
- discuss the role and responsibilities of the midwife in relation to per rectum (P.R.) administration.

## Positioning of the woman

It is easier to insert suppositories and enemas if the woman adopts a left lateral position with one or both of her knees flexed (Fig. 25.1). Insertion then follows the natural anatomy of the colon, permitting the medicine to be placed 2–4 cm into the rectum, beyond the end of the anal canal, thus enhancing retention of the drug. Flexed knees reduce the discomfort of the anus as the suppository is passed through the sphincter (Dougherty & Lister 2004).

**Figure 25.1** Correct positioning for insertion of P.R. medication (Adapted with kind permission from Jamieson et al 2002)

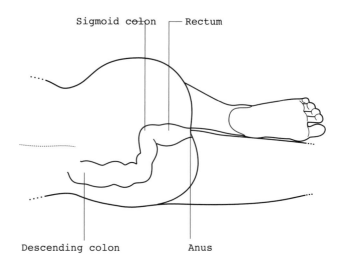

Sigmoid colon — Rectum

Descending colon — Anus

# Suppositories and enemas

### Suppositories for laxative use

Suppositories for laxative use vary in their action; widely used glycerin suppositories are designed to melt in the faeces and so soften it. They are best inserted pointed end first (easier to place into the faeces); this action also aids anal dilatation. Other types of suppository (e.g. Bisacodyl – stimulant laxative) need to be placed between the faeces and rectal wall and so the instructions should be checked prior to administration.

### Suppositories for systemic use

Suppositories for systemic use are often firm in texture. They are tapered, but are easier to retain if inserted blunt end first. Their absorption is enhanced if the rectum is empty and the suppository is placed against the rectal wall.

### Enemas

Enemas for systemic use are often small (microenemas) while laxative ones generally contain more fluid. Both have a nozzle that extends into the rectum (beyond the anal canal), often about 10 cm in length. If a large fluid enema is to be used it should be warmed (40.5–43.3°C) to prevent shock occurring.

Both suppositories and enemas require lubrication (e.g. KY Jelly) on the inserting end so that anal trauma is reduced. Care is always taken not to stimulate the vagus nerve, which may cause bradycardia.

## Role and responsibilities of the midwife

These can be summarised as:

- appropriate checking and dispensing of the drug (as for any pre-scription)
- understanding the action and possible side effects of the drug: the effect/side effect should always be reported and recorded. If given for laxative purposes the quantity, colour and consistency of the faeces should be recorded
- education and support of the woman: she may associate P.R. drugs specifically with laxatives, not appreciating that systemic supposito-ries have no laxative effect. The effect of all P.R. medications will be enhanced if the drug is retained by the woman for the required length of time, often around 20 minutes
- maintenance of dignity and privacy during an embarrassing proce-dure
- correct administration technique, placing the medication in the cor-rect place
- appreciation of care following administration: toilet facilities should be readily available following administration of medicine P.R. for lax-ative purposes
- contemporaneous record keeping of the care given before, during and after the administration.

## PROCEDURE    administration of medicines P.R.

- Gain informed consent and ensure privacy
- Gather equipment:
  - suppository(ies) or (warmed) enema
  - disposable gloves
  - disposable sheet
  - lubricant, e.g. KY Jelly
  - gauze swabs
  - a trolley may be used as a surface to work from
- Position the woman in a left lateral position with one or both of her knees flexed, placing the disposable sheet beneath her buttocks
- Wash hands and apply gloves
- Lubricate the correct end of the suppository(ies)/enema tubing using a gauze swab. Expel the air from the enema tubing by pushing the solution through to the tip
- Ask the woman to take a deep breath (this relaxes the anal sphincter)
- Lift the woman's right buttock with the non-dominant hand, insert the suppository or enema as discussed above (glycerin suppository: tapered end first into faeces; systemic suppository: blunt end first,

place against rectal wall. Check all others before beginning). The fluid of an enema is gradually squeezed in
● Insert a second suppository in the same way if required
● Wipe the perineum and assist the woman into a comfortable position
● Assist later, if needed, to the toilet. Aim for the suppository(ies) to be retained for at least 20 minutes
● Dispose of equipment correctly and wash hands
● Document administration and effect and act accordingly.

## Summary

● Administration of medicines P.R. may be for laxative or systemic purposes
● The midwife should be familiar with the effect of the drug and how to administer it correctly.

**Self-assessment exercises**

The answers to the following questions may be found in the text:

1. Describe how a laxative enema is administered.
2. Discuss the responsibilities of the midwife when administering a systemic suppository.
3. Discuss why the woman is positioned in a left lateral position.

### REFERENCES

Dougherty L, Lister S 2004 The Royal Marsden Hospital manual of clinical nursing procedures, 6th edn. Blackwell Publishing, Oxford

Jamieson E M, McCall J, Whyte L 2002 Clinical nursing practices, 4th edn. Churchill Livingstone, Edinburgh

Chapter **26**

# Principles of drug administration – intravenous drug administration

This chapter considers the administration of medicines intravenously, as bolus or 'push' administration, or intermittent infusion, concluding with continuous administration of drugs using a syringe driver and patient-controlled analgesia. Maximum understanding will be gained from this chapter if it is read in conjunction with Chapters 20, 21, 50 and 51.

| **Learning outcomes** | Having read this chapter the reader should be able to: |

Having read this chapter the reader should be able to:

- describe each of the different ways that drugs can be administered intravenously
- discuss the role and responsibilities of the midwife when undertaking intravenous (I.V.) drug administration
- calculate the infusion rate when using a syringe driver.

Drugs given intravenously act quickly: an advantage if a rapid response is required; a disadvantage if allergy occurs. The midwife should be properly trained to administer drugs intravenously, recognising that in some areas it is an extended role. Updating is often required (according to local protocol) in order to maintain competence. All midwives are able to administer I.V. ergometrine maleate for the treatment of postpartum haemorrhage in an emergency (up to two doses of 500 mcg). Antibiotics are the most common drugs administered intravenously, but many preparations can be administered in this way.

As for the administration of all medicines the woman's details are thoroughly checked, as are the prescription and drug to be administered. Note that the use of medical devices, particularly syringe drivers, features highly in the reported work of the Medical Devices Agency. It is essential that midwives have a thorough working knowledge of the equipment that they use and its correct maintenance (Murray & Glenister 2001).

| PROCEDURE | bolus or 'push' administration |

- A patent cannula should be available with an injection port
- Gather equipment:
  — the drug, including correct solution (often water for injection) if it is to be diluted, and the woman's prescription chart
  — appropriate sized sterile syringe and needle
  — hand rub
  — sterile gloves
  — 20 mL sodium chloride 0.9%, needle and syringe for flushing (or locally approved flushing solution)
  — clean injection tray
  — 70% alcohol-impregnated swab
  — disposable sheet
- Wash hands, prepare and draw up the drug according to the manufacturer's instructions, with a second midwife checking the dosages and expiry dates
- Gently resheath the needle and place the prepared syringe on the tray, retaining the ampoule
- Draw up the normal saline (if unable to differentiate between the syringes, place on a separate tray)
- Confirm the woman's identity, then place her arm on the disposable sheet
- Apply hand rub and gloves
- Inspect the cannulation site and, if present, check the infusion for its smooth running
- Stop the infusion
- Clean the portal for the I.V. drugs with the alcohol-impregnated swab and allow to dry
- Flush the cannula using half of the normal saline, the remainder being kept sterile
- Insert the syringe (or needle, if needle port) (Fig. 26.1) and inject the first 1mL of the drug according to the manufacturer's recommendations, observing the woman's condition throughout (Hayes & Williamson 1998). Restart the infusion. If no problems are noticed, stop the infusion, and continue to administer the rest of the drug at the correct rate
- Repeat the flushing with the remaining normal saline and close the entry portal
- Recommence the infusion at the appropriate rate

**Figure 26.1**  A bolus or 'push' administration of I.V. medication

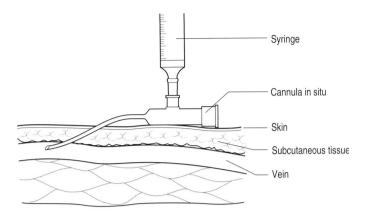

- Syringe
- Cannula in situ
- Skin
- Subcutaneous tissue
- Vein

- Dispose of equipment correctly
- Wash hands
- Document administration and effect and act accordingly.

# Intermittent infusion

Some drugs may be administered as an infusion over 20 minutes to 1 hour. This is done by:

- adding drugs to a burette giving set of an existing infusion, with the existing infusion being stopped until the drugs have been administered, or
- if the drug is already in a prepared infusion (without an existing infusion) it is attached to the cannula with a giving set, or
- if there is an existing infusion, it is 'piggy backed' using a Y giving set, with the existing infusion being stopped until the drugs have been administered.

If the I.V. drugs are the only infusion then the cannula will require flushing before and after administration, as described above. The administration set is often retained for the next dose, but should be renewed after 48 hours. Hand hygiene is essential at each stage of the procedure and it is important that care is taken not to introduce microorganisms into the closed system.

If it is necessary to add drugs to a bag of fluid, it is important that:

- care is taken not to puncture the bag with the needle
- an additive label must be applied with the drug, dose, name and number of the woman and time commenced recorded on it
- the drug and fluid are thoroughly mixed
- the flow rate is correct.

Record keeping should indicate precisely what drug has been administered, over what time and by which method. It should also include whether flushing the cannula was necessary and, if so, with what and should account for any delay of an existing infusion.

### Administration using a syringe driver

Syringe drivers (Fig. 26.2) have the advantage of allowing ambulation while delivering a given dose of drug over a given time. The essential information for the midwife is whether it is a 12- or 24-hour pump. The rate is determined by the distance, i.e. the length of fluid, measured on the ruler, rather than the number of millilitres. The drug is diluted so that the total length is divisible by 12. Instruction booklets will be provided with each driver, but the general rule is:

$$\frac{\text{Length of fluid (mm)}}{\text{Delivery time (hours)}} = \text{rate setting (mm/hour)}$$

Example: If 36 mm of fluid is to be infused over 12 hours then the rate would be 3 mm/hour. The figures often need changing with a screwdriver; they cannot be changed easily.

The setting up of the pump relies on several standard principles:

- calculation of the amount of drug that is required over the given period of time with appropriate solution for dilution
- use of sterile syringe, correct size to fit the driver and inserted so that the plunger is secure
- sterile preparation and dilution of the drug
- use of sterile tubing that will fit the cannula used; the tubing must be primed and attached aseptically, after measurement and calculation of the rate
- the syringe must be labelled correctly
- the driver should be maintained and in full working order; alarms for 'occlusion' and 'infusion complete' must be working and the midwife must make regular observations of the pump to ensure it is running to time.

Figure 26.2 Syringe driver

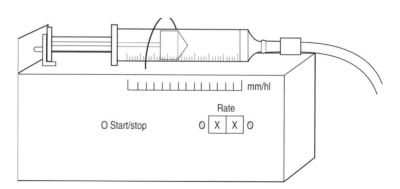

# Patient-controlled analgesia

Syringe drivers sometimes have the facility for the woman to increase the analgesia that she is receiving by use of a 'boost' button. They are valuable for postoperative analgesia because there is control over the overall dosage, but the woman can exercise the boost to receive the analgesia when she needs an increase. The woman has control, improving her pain relief and reducing midwifery staff time in administering analgesia.

A mechanism exists to administer a given dose over a 4-hour period, but the machine also has a facility to 'lock out', i.e. once a dose has been administered, a second dose cannot be given within the next 15 minutes approximately, to ensure that the effect of the first dose is felt before the next one is given. The midwife setting up the infusion must set:

- the lockout interval
- 4-hour dose limit
- limit of the drug that the woman can receive with each boost.

A tamper-proof mechanism is also built in to avoid the woman, visitors or others changing the dose.

## Role and responsibilities of the midwife

These can be summarised as:

- adherence to local protocols for training and updating of skills
- correct administration procedure, as per NMC (2004) and local protocols
- observation of the woman for any unexpected responses
- contemporaneous record keeping.

## Summary

- I.V. drugs have a swift effect
- The midwife needs to be properly trained in their administration and in the correct use of all devices
- I.V. drugs may be given in the following ways:
  — bolus or 'push'
  — intermittent infusion
  — additives to an infusion
  — syringe driver 12- or 24-hour infusion
  — syringe driver with patient control
- Sterility must be maintained and flushing is necessary before and after the drug has been administered.

The answers to the following questions may be found in the text:

1. Describe how a midwife would administer a bolus dose of I.V. antibiotics.
2. Discuss the other ways in which I.V. drugs can be administered.
3. Calculate the rate for a syringe driver: 48 mm of fluid is to be infused over 24 hours.
4. Discuss the advantages of patient-controlled analgesia.
5. Summarise the role and responsibilities of the midwife when administering drugs intravenously.

## REFERENCES

Hayes C, Williamson E 1998 Injection technique: intravenous 2. Nursing Times 94(46):40ff

Murray W, Glenister H 2001 How to use medical devices safely. Nursing Times 97(43):36–38

NMC (Nursing and Midwifery Council) 2004 Guidelines for the administration of medicines. NMC, London

Chapter **27**

# Principles of drug administration — inhalational analgesia: Entonox

Entonox is 50% oxygen and 50% nitrous oxide. In this concentration it acts as an effective analgesic when inhaled. Its use in the maternity setting is, potentially, for all stages of labour, where the analgesic effect is valuable without any known ill effects for the fetus. This chapter reviews its use and the role and responsibilities of the midwife.

## Learning outcomes

Having read this chapter the reader should be able to:

- describe the safe and effective use of Entonox
- discuss briefly its value as an analgesic in labour
- detail the role and responsibilities of the midwife when administering Entonox.

## Principles of Entonox use

- A colourless, odourless gas, supplied piped or in cylinders, the cylinder colouring always being blue with blue and white shoulders. Portable cylinders and administration equipment are available. Care should be taken to store the cylinder horizontally above 10°C; the gases will separate at −6°C and this may pose a problem to community midwives in the winter until the cylinder is brought back to room temperature
- Entonox is self-administered by the woman using a mouthpiece or mask to which an expiratory valve is attached. The mask is held over the nose and mouth with an airtight seal or the mouthpiece is placed in the mouth. As the woman breathes, the Entonox is heard to be released; the apparatus should remain in place during expiration. In this way the woman may breathe through the contraction at a rate that suits her
- Only the woman should hold the apparatus to prevent overdosing; if the woman becomes drowsy she is unable to hold the apparatus to

her face. Other side effects may include poor memory of labour, hyperventilation, tingling in hands, nausea and vomiting

- Taken correctly, Entonox is fully effective within 40 seconds to 1 minute; the effect begins after five deep breaths (approximately 20 seconds) (Street 2000). It is excreted from the body within 2–5 minutes
- The skill for the midwife is to support and assist the woman to gain maximum effectiveness from its use. Entonox needs to be breathed at the onset of the contraction in order for the effect to take the edge off the pain at its peak. The midwife needs to palpate the contractions abdominally and encourage the woman to begin breathing before the woman perceives the contraction pain. Education prior to labour may help the woman to have realistic expectations of the effects of Entonox. Green (1993) indicates that women have good levels of satisfaction with Entonox use in labour
- Entonox may be contraindicated where a respiratory disease exists. Such women may be reviewed individually by an obstetrician if necessary
- Smoking should not occur in the vicinity of any compressed gas; care should be taken in the woman's home environment (Sealey 2002)
- Entonox is believed to be safe for the fetus. Researched evidence is very limited
- Female midwives should be aware that prolonged exposure at work may contribute to congenital abnormality and abortion.

### Role and responsibilities of the midwife

- If appropriately trained in its use, the midwife may, under a patient group direction, administer Entonox to labouring women – all stages of labour are permitted
- All approved apparatus/equipment should be available for inspection when required (NMC 2004)
- The apparatus should be properly maintained and used correctly on each occasion: cylinders have a batch label and a seal on the valve. The midwife should be fully conversant with fitting the head to the cylinder, ensuring that there is no oil or grease present. The mouthpiece and tubing should be cleaned on completion of care
- As a drug, it may only be administered to labouring women, and not to any other group or person 'to try'
- The effect and side effects of the drug are observed; other types of analgesia may be used in conjunction with Entonox if appropriate, e.g. transcutaneous electrical nerve stimulation (TENS), pethidine
- Contemporaneous records are kept.

## Summary

- Entonox is an effective analgesic if taken correctly during childbirth
- The midwife has responsibilities to ensure that it is stored, serviced and used correctly.

**Self-assessment exercises**

The answers to the following questions may be found in the text:

1. Describe how a midwife should support a woman to use Entonox effectively.
2. Discuss the advantages and disadvantages of Entonox as a labour analgesic.
3. Summarise the role and responsibilities of the midwife when caring for a woman using Entonox in labour.
4. Under which regulations can a midwife administer Entonox and to whom?

## REFERENCES

Green J 1993 Expectations and experiences of pain in labour: findings from a large prospective study. Birth 20(2):65–72

NMC (Nursing and Midwifery Council) 2004 Midwives rules and standards. NMC, London

Sealey L 2002 Nurse administration of Entonox to manage pain in ward settings. Nursing Times 98(46):28–29

Street D 2000 A practical guide to giving Entonox. Nursing Times 96(34):47–48

# Chapter 28

# Principles of drug administration — epidural analgesia

A 24-hour epidural service is offered in most consultant delivery units using skilled obstetric anaesthetists. Midwifery skills are required antenatally in the preparation of the woman, during labour (particularly when caring for the woman once the epidural has been sited) and postnatally when additional care is often required. This chapter clarifies the terminology, and details the procedures for epidural insertion, top-up and removal. The indications, contraindications, side effects and midwife's role and responsibilities are all highlighted. The reader is encouraged to be aware that the debates surrounding epidural use and normal birth are greater than this text can examine.

**Learning outcomes**

Having read this chapter the reader should be able to:

- discuss the differences between epidural, spinal and combined spinal epidural analgesia
- list the indications, contraindications and possible side effects from epidural analgesia
- describe how an epidural is sited and a top-up administered
- discuss the role and responsibilities of the midwife throughout the procedures
- describe how to remove an epidural catheter.

## Clarification of terms

### Epidural block

Introduction of local anaesthetic into the epidural space of the lumbar spine provides both analgesia (freedom from pain) and anaesthesia (lack of sensation). The local anaesthetic, often with an opiate analgesic, is injected into the epidural space (Fig. 28.1). A fine catheter is left in situ so that either top-ups (bolus doses) of the local anaesthetic

**Figure 28.1**   Sagittal section of the lumbar spine with tuohy needle in the epidural space

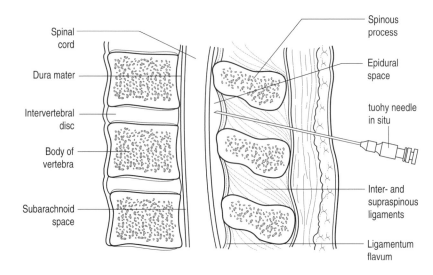

Spinal cord

Dura mater

Intervertebral disc

Body of vertebra

Subarachnoid space

Spinous process

Epidural space

tuohy needle in situ

Inter- and supraspinous ligaments

Ligamentum flavum

can be given once the initial dose has worn off, or continuous infusion can be commenced, often using patient-controlled analgesia (PCA, see Ch. 26). Analgesia and anaesthesia are usually total, but sometimes the pain relief can be patchy. However, the woman is also denied the ability to move her legs, pass urine naturally and experience an urge to push in the second stage of labour. Evidence suggests there is an increased risk of prolonged labour (needing augmentation) and instrumental delivery with epidural analgesia. Fetal heart tracings can have less variability; continuous monitoring is often indicated. Other side effects are discussed below.

### Spinal anaesthetic

A lesser amount of local anaesthetic is injected into the subarachnoid space, below L1 where the spinal cord ends. Analgesia and anaesthesia are usually total; caesarean section is often performed under spinal anaesthetic.

### Combined spinal epidural (CSE)

Usually, opiate analgesic is injected into the subarachnoid space, followed by local anaesthetic into the epidural space, either then or later (a catheter is retained for either bolus or continuous infusion). The advantage of this technique is that analgesia, but not anaesthesia is achieved. The use of opiates provides analgesia of rapid, long-lasting effect, but with retention of sensation. The woman is often able to stand or walk with assistance, pass urine and bear down. The overall doses of opiates given to a woman should be observed; respiratory depression for the woman and the fetus may be a complication of the procedure.

Some evaluation of CSE has taken place, and Hunt (2003) cites the second Comet trial where there was a reduced risk of instrumental vaginal delivery. The midwife's role may be similar when the CSE is being inserted or additional analgesia is being given later.

## Indications for epidural block

- Pain relief/maternal request
- Useful where there is likelihood of instrumental delivery: malposition, malpresentation, multiple pregnancy, prolonged labour
- Hypertension, where the potential side effects of hypotension can be helpful
- Preterm labour, where there may be an early desire to push

### Contraindications

There are contraindications for epidural/spinal analgesia:

- any blood clotting malfunction
- some neurological disorders
- spinal deformity
- local sepsis.

### Side effects of epidural

Some of the side effects are evidence based, others are generally observed. Education of the woman should highlight all the possibilities. These include:

- hypotension (less so with CSE), nausea, faintness, backache, pruritus, tingling and numbness
- dural tap: the epidural needle accidentally punctures the dura mater resulting in reduced intracranial pressure with potential severe headache in the following few days
- total spinal anaesthetic: accidental injection of too much local anaesthetic into the subarachnoid space may cause respiratory arrest
- partial block ('breakthrough' pain): contractions are still felt over one area of the abdomen
- drug toxicity: restlessness, dizziness, tinnitus, metallic taste, drowsiness
- temperature changes: the woman usually experiences the vasodilatory effect of bupivacaine causing her feet to be warm, her temperature to rise but her body to shiver
- urinary retention
- malposition of the presenting part and possibly neonatal hypoglycaemia (Enkin et al 2000).

The technique may be modified if it is a CSE (as discussed above) or if the administration uses continuous infusion.

- Gain informed consent, encourage the woman to empty her bladder, call the anaesthetist and gather the equipment:
  — equipment for intravenous infusion (crystalloid fluid)
  — CTG monitor
  — dressings trolley
  — sterile gown and gloves
  — sterile dressing pack, with fenestrated drape and gauze
  — antiseptic lotion, usually chlorhexidine in 70% isopropyl alcohol
  — epidural pack, usually containing a tuohy needle with stylet, syringe, tubing (catheter) and antibacterial filter
  — local anaesthetics for the skin and epidural, e.g. lidocaine (lignocaine) and bupivacaine
  — opiate analgesia, if required (administered according to controlled drug administration, see Ch. 20)
  — sterile syringes and needles
  — tape/plastic skin dressing
- Site an intravenous infusion; a fluid loading dose to prevent hypotension is less likely to be needed, but seek the anaesthetist's advice
- Position the woman, according to her comfort and the anaesthetist's wishes (usually one of two ways), to promote curvature of the spine so that access can be gained between the vertebrae:
  — in left lateral with knees flexed and chin on chest but with her back very close to the edge of the bed
  — sitting on the edge of the bed with feet supported on a chair, arms resting upon a bed table
- Assist the anaesthetist to 'glove and gown' and to establish a strict aseptic field; pour the lotion, open the needles and syringes, hold ampoules of local anaesthetic for drawing up, etc.
- Encourage the woman to remain still while the epidural is sited by the anaesthetist; all of the activity occurs behind her back, so support and reassurance are needed
  — the woman's back will be cleansed, the drapes put in place and the local anaesthetic inserted into the skin
  — the tuohy needle will be inserted when the woman is contraction free and very still (to avoid advancing too far and causing a dural tap)
  — the stylet will be removed and an epidural syringe will be used (injecting air or saline to assess the resistance) to ensure that the tuohy needle is in the correct place
  — the catheter tubing is then threaded into place and the tuohy needle removed

- If appropriate, spray plastic skin around the puncture site and secure the catheter with tape when the anaesthetist is ready; secure the filter in an accessible place
- A small test dose is given, the first complete dose is given, or a syringe driver attached when the anaesthetist is satisfied that the catheter is correctly inserted
- Assist the woman into the position that the anaesthetist suggests for the initial 20 minutes after administration (often semi-recumbent)
- Assess and record blood pressure and pulse after each 5 minutes for the next 20 minutes, and each 30 minutes thereafter
- Observe the woman's condition, including her level of pain/block, her warmth, safety, intravenous infusion, colour and signs of nausea
- Call the anaesthetist if any observations give cause for concern (hypotension may be corrected by increasing the rate of the intravenous infusion, but the anaesthetist should always be called)
- Dispose of equipment correctly, including sharps
- Monitor the fetal condition and uterine activity, recording the epidural on the CTG tracing
- If after 20 minutes all observations are within normal limits and the level of analgesia has been achieved, reposition the woman according to her choice (avoiding aortocaval compression) or assist to mobilise
- Continue all labour care, including care of the bladder, pressure area care (see Ch. 57) and numb legs (particularly if a total block), maintaining contemporaneous records
- After 2–8 hours observe for signs of recurring sensation; administer a top-up before the woman becomes uncomfortable.

## Epidural top-ups

Epidural top-ups are given if the administration is not continuous. Midwives that have been properly trained and supervised may undertake top-ups, being familiar with local protocol. The anaesthetist prescribes the dose (concentration and volume), the frequency and the position of the woman. Administering the dose in two halves with 5 minutes between them is often prescribed in case the catheter has migrated into the cerebrospinal fluid.

PROCEDURE **epidural top-up**

- Establish the need for the top-up, check the intravenous infusion and gather equipment:
  — the prescribed drug(s)
  — sterile needle and syringe
  — alcohol-impregnated swab

- Position the woman according to the anaesthetist's request, usually lateral during the first stage of labour, sitting for the second
- Wash hands, check the drugs with another midwife and draw up the correct dose
- When the woman is free from contraction, remove the cap from the filter, clean the port with the swab and inject the local anaesthetic at a rate of 5 mL per 30 seconds (half or whole dose according to prescription)
- Observe the woman throughout for adverse reactions such as tinnitus, drowsiness and slurred speech
- Reapply the cap
- Repeat the procedure in 5 minutes (if prescribed in two halves)
- Pulse and blood pressure are undertaken taken as before: every 5 minutes for at least 20 minutes, every 30 minutes thereafter
- Reposition the woman if necessary
- Dispose of equipment correctly
- Document administration and effect and act accordingly
- Continue to observe for the effects or side effects of the block; summon the anaesthetist if required.

## PROCEDURE    removing an epidural cannula

The cannula is removed once the epidural is no longer required, usually once labour is over.

- Gain informed consent and ensure privacy throughout
- Take sterile gloves, waterproof dressing and plastic skin dressing to the woman
- Wash hands, apply sterile gloves
- Remove the tape and ask the woman to arch her back (similar to inserting the epidural); pull the catheter out carefully, but swiftly
- Apply plastic skin and a sterile waterproof dressing
- Examine the tubing for completeness by assessing the gradations and the rounded appearance of the catheter tip; check with a second person if unsure
- Document removal and act accordingly.

# Postnatal care

In the immediate postnatal period the woman may still be numb and may therefore require assistance to care for her baby, to breast feed and help to become mobile again. She will also need observing for signs of urinary retention and headache, two of the most common short-term side effects. Observations for backache may be needed in the longer term.

## Role and responsibilities of the midwife

These can be summarised as:

- education and preparation of the woman, including gaining informed consent
- assessing the suitability of the woman, e.g. progress in labour
- consideration of the delivery suite workload and whether the woman can be given the ideal 'one-to-one' care following its insertion
- correct positioning and support of the woman during the siting of the epidural
- assistance of the anaesthetist during preparation and siting
- ongoing care and observations of the woman and fetus
- recognising deviations from the norm, responding and summoning the anaesthetist
- training and competence for the provision of top-ups or care of continuous infusion
- correct removal of epidural catheter
- appropriate postnatal care
- contemporaneous record keeping throughout.

## Summary

- Epidural, of whichever sort or dose, is generally a very effective form of labour analgesia
- The midwife has a responsible role at the time of siting the epidural, with the ongoing care and with the management of infusion or top-ups, both during labour and postnatally
- The midwife works in conjunction with a skilled obstetric anaesthetist.

## Self-assessment exercises

The answers to the following questions may be found in the text:

1. Discuss the differences between epidural, spinal and combined spinal epidural analgesia.
2. List the indications, contraindications and possible side effects for epidural analgesia.
3. Describe the midwife's role during epidural siting.
4. Describe how an epidural top-up is safely administered by a midwife.
5. Describe how an epidural catheter is correctly removed.

## REFERENCES

Enkin M, Keirse M J, Neilsen J et al 2000 A guide to effective care in pregnancy and childbirth, 3rd edn. Oxford University Press, Oxford

Hunt S 2003 The epidural: a barrier to 'natural' birth? The Practising Midwife 6(7):42–46

# Chapter 29

# Principles of drug administration – transcutaneous electrical nerve stimulation

This chapter considers the midwife's role in the application and use of transcutaneous electrical nerve stimulation (TENS) for the purposes of pain relief in labour and postoperatively. TENS is not a pharmaceutical drug, but its use is widely advocated as a means of analgesia for labour. There are other non-pharmaceutical and complementary therapies available; however, the scope of this text does not permit their discussion.

| Learning outcomes | Having read this chapter the reader should be able to: |

* discuss the principles by which TENS is considered to be effective as an analgesic
* describe how it is applied and used
* summarise the role and responsibilities of the midwife.

## How does TENS work?

The 'gate control' theory of pain suggests that stimulation of larger peripheral nerve fibres inhibits pain signals entering the central pain pathway, reducing perception of pain – TENS provides this stimulation. Additionally, it is believed that the electrical stimulation also activates the release of the body's own endorphins.

TENS is available as a handheld electrical unit. Electrodes are placed onto the skin over specific spinal nerves. The electrodes need to be the correct size to stimulate the nerve fibres at the correct rate and density (Coates 1998). A water-based electrode gel is required to facilitate the current. Tape is used to keep the electrodes securely in the correct place if self-adhesive electrodes are unavailable.

Two frequencies are available: low (pulsed or intermittent) and high (continuous). Low frequency stimulates the release of endorphins, while high frequency closes the pain gate. Most machines are equipped with a boost button, allowing the woman to initiate the high frequency when the contraction occurs, returning to the lower frequency when the uterus is at rest. Pulsation of low frequency occurs throughout. Application in early labour is indicated to promote an increase in the woman's natural endorphin level. The woman experiences the sensation as tingling on the skin; this should be at a comfortable level. If supplied with indicator lights, these are seen to flash intermittently, or to remain on continuously, according to the frequency. Its proven clinical effectiveness is very limited (Robertson 2003), but maternal satisfaction levels are good (Carroll et al 1997).

## Suitability as a labour analgesic

TENS may be described as a non-pharmacological analgesic that allows the woman to mobilise and avoid the side effects of pharmacological analgesia. The woman retains some control, using the boost feature during contractions, increasing the strength and frequency of the pulses as labour progresses. It can be used in conjunction with other analgesics and is often easily accessible for use at home. There are no known side effects for the woman or the fetus, although Mitchell and Kafai (1997) suggest it should not be placed over the uterus in the antenatal period. It should not be used when the woman has a cardiac pacemaker, in water or over areas of damaged skin (Coates 1998). It may interfere electrically with cardiotocography.

## Positioning of TENS

Hawkins (1994) suggests that correct positioning of the electrodes is essential. Bryant and Yerby (2004), Coates (1998) and Hamilton (2003) all indicate the need to place the electrodes over the spinal nerves that supply the uterus and pelvic floor: T10–L1 and S2–S4.

Coates (1998) suggests that if the woman's arms are relaxed and hanging loosely by her sides, then the lower tip of her scapula is at T7. Three spinal vertebrae can then be counted down to locate T10. The top of the upper pad is placed level with T10. S2 is located by identifying the iliac crests and placing the top of the lower electrode one vertebra below this. The pads should be placed centrally either side of the spinal column, with 3 cm between them (Fig. 29.1).

PROCEDURE  **applying a TENS unit**

- Clarify that this is the woman's choice of analgesia; discuss what to expect
- Position the woman so that access can be gained to her back
- Ensure the unit is fully charged with the electrodes connected and all the controls on the lowest possible setting
- Identify the correct positions for the electrodes (see Fig. 29.1) and apply them using tape and electrode gel if required

**Figure 29.1**  Positioning for TENS electrodes (Adapted with kind permission from Coates 1998)

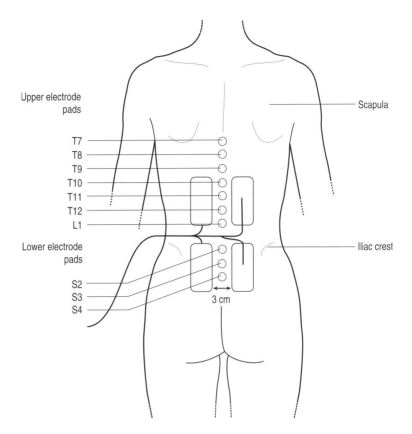

- Switch the unit on, demonstrate the boost and how to increase the intensities according to need
- Ensure that the woman is comfortable
- Replace clothing, securing the unit in a pocket if appropriate, leaving the boost button accessible
- Document application and effect
- Discontinue the use of TENS at the end of labour or according to the woman's wishes (switch the unit off, remove electrodes, clean reusable electrodes, service and maintain the unit according to the manufacturer's instructions).

## Role and responsibilities of the midwife

These can be summarised as:

- education and empowerment of the woman in her choice of analgesia
- appropriate training, updating and application of TENS
- care and maintenance of the TENS unit
- observation of the effectiveness
- contemporaneous record keeping.

## Summary

- TENS works on the 'gate control' theory of pain: electrical impulses of differing frequencies close the gate and encourage the body to release endorphins
- Many women view TENS as being a good non-pharmacological analgesic for labour; research questions its validity
- It has minimal side effects and allows both mobility and control
- The midwife has a role in ensuring that it is applied, used and maintained correctly.

### Self-assessment exercises

The answers to the following questions may be found in the text:

1. How are the effects of TENS achieved?
2. How does a midwife decide where to place the electrodes?
3. Which signs indicate to the woman and the midwife that the TENS unit is working effectively?
4. When should TENS not be used?
5. Summarise the role and responsibilities of the midwife in relation to the use of TENS in labour.

## REFERENCES

Bryant H, Yerby M 2004 Relief of pain during labour. In: Henderson C, Macdonald S (eds) Mayes' midwifery: a textbook for midwives, 13th edn. Baillière Tindall, Edinburgh, p 458–475

Carroll D, Tramer M, McQuay H et al 1997 Transcutaneous electrical nerve stimulation in labour pain: a systematic review. British Journal of Obstetrics and Gynaecology 104(2):169–175

Coates T 1998 Transcutaneous electrical nerve stimulation: TENS. The Practising Midwife 1(11):12–14

Hamilton A 2003 Pain relief and comfort in labour. In: Fraser D M, Cooper M A (eds) Myles textbook for midwives, 14th edn. Churchill Livingstone, Edinburgh, p 471–485

Hawkins J 1994 The use of TENS for pain relief in labour. British Journal of Midwifery 2(10):487–490

Mitchell A, Kafai S 1997 Patient education in TENS pain management. Professional Nurse 12(11):804–807

Robertson A 2003 TENS – a marketing triumph. The Practising Midwife 6(2):20–21

Chapter **30**

# Facilitation of related childbearing skills — optimal fetal positioning

Malposition and malpresentation in labour are associated with an increased risk of intervention during labour, instrumental and/or operative delivery and increased morbidity to the woman and baby. Reducing the incidence of malposition and malpresentation prior to labour could minimise the risks to both the woman and the baby. This chapter focuses on the use of different positions and alternative therapies used by the woman during pregnancy to encourage the fetus into an optimal fetal position.

## Learning outcomes

Having read this chapter the reader should be able to:

- discuss the evidence surrounding the use of optimum fetal positioning
- discuss the different positions and postures a woman can use during pregnancy to encourage the fetal occiput to rotate from a posterior to an anterior position
- discuss the different methods that may change the presentation from breech to cephalic
- identify some of the hazards associated with malpositions and malpresentations for the woman and baby.

## Malposition of the occiput – occipitoposterior position

Approximately 10% of labours at term occur with an occipitoposterior (OP) position. While many of these undergo a long rotation to become an occipitoanterior position during labour, a small number will persist in the posterior position. OP labour and deliveries are associated with a number of possible complications:

- higher presenting part with wider diameters that will take longer to negotiate the pelvis

- early rupture of membranes, increasing the risk of ascending infection
- cord prolapse
- incoordinate uterine action leading to prolonged labour
- urinary retention
- premature urge to push
- increased risk of trauma to vagina and pelvic floor
- increased risk of instrumental and/or operative delivery, which may be associated with an increased blood loss
- abnormal moulding which may result in an unsettled baby and increase the risk of intracranial haemorrhage
- increased perinatal mortality and morbidity.

(Adapted from Lewis 2004)

Sutton and Scott (1996) strongly advocate using different positions and postures to encourage the fetus to rotate to a lateral or anterior position and so facilitate engagement from 34 weeks' gestation onwards. They do caution women to discuss this with the health professional overseeing their pregnancy to ensure there are no contraindications to this.

The assumption behind their recommendations is to provide the fetus with room to rotate within the uterus and adopt a position that is more comfortable and better for delivery. The fetus will be able to adopt a more flexed position if in a lateral or anterior position; as the head flexes the engaging diameters will reduce and hence engagement is likely to occur earlier rather than later. Their advice centres on using upright and forward leaning postures regularly, particularly during Braxton Hicks contractions, as this is believed to assist the fetus to manoeuvre into the optimum position.

### Favourable positions to adopt

- Use upright and forward leaning postures regularly (to create more space for the fetus to turn)
- To read, sit on a dining chair with elbows resting on the table, lean slightly forward and keep the knees apart
- Sit on a dining chair facing the back, stretching and resting arms over the back of the chair
- When sitting generally, make sure the knees are lower than the hips and keep the back straight by placing a small cushion over the small of the back for support
- While watching television, kneel on the floor and lean over a large bean bag or cushion
- When driving, place a wedge cushion under the bottom
- When swimming try to keep the abdomen forward; breast stroke is better for this than back stroke
- When lying on one side, place a pillow between the legs with the top knee resting on the bed.

### Positions to avoid

- Avoid relaxing in semi-reclining positions that cause the knees to be higher than the hips
- If driving using bucket seats, have regular stops to change position and use a wedge cushion under the bottom
- Do not sit with crossed legs
- Do not squat in late pregnancy unless the fetus is no longer in the OP position as the head may be forced into the pelvis in the OP position.

The work of Sutton and Scott (1996) is not research based but they have strong anecdotal evidence to support their claims. This is an area that needs researching but at present does not appear to have any disadvantages for suitable women.

Another method that has been proposed since the 1950s is for the woman to adopt an 'all-fours' position, using knees and hands for support, used in conjunction with pelvic rocking. This method has been recommended over the years and used by many women without being researched as to its effectiveness. Hofmeyr and Kulier's (1998) systematic review of the studies undertaken to evaluate the hands–knees position concluded that although they could not recommend the hands–knees position as an intervention, they would not suggest that the position not be adopted if women found it comfortable. Kariminia et al's (2004) small study compared this intervention (for 10 minutes twice daily) with a control group who had to undertake walking each day from 37 weeks. They concluded that although the hands–knees posture combined with pelvic rocking exercises is a practice commonly used within midwifery to encourage rotation from the posterior to the anterior position, their results did not support this practice and recommended that in the absence of any beneficial effects, the practice should be discontinued. Encouraging rotation of the occiput from a posterior to an anterior position remains an area for further research.

# Malpresentation – breech presentation

The fetus will present by the breech in approximately 3–4% of pregnancies at term; this figure is higher earlier in pregnancy and the majority of breech presentations that turn spontaneously do so by 34 weeks. Midwives need to maintain their skills in undertaking a vaginal breech delivery through simulation, as the number of vaginal breech births is low. Many women with a breech presentation deliver by caesarean section as this is considered to decrease the perinatal morbidity and mortality (Hannah et al 2000).

Breech labour and delivery is associated with a number of complications:

- early rupture of membranes, with increased risk of ascending infection

- incoordinate contractions leading to prolonged labour
- increased risk of cord compression during first and second stage
- cord, foot, leg and arm prolapse
- early urge to push
- increased risk of operative delivery
- no moulding; head undergoes compression and decompression increasing the risk of intracranial haemorrhage during vaginal birth
- increased risk of trauma to vagina and pelvic floor
- increased risk of birth asphyxia
- increased perinatal morbidity and mortality.

A variety of methods can be used to encourage the fetus to turn from the breech to a cephalic presentation, including external cephalic version, adopting a knees–chest position and acupuncture.

### External cephalic version (ECV)

This is undertaken by experienced personnel, usually obstetricians but could include midwives who have undergone further training. It should be offered to all women at or after 37 weeks who have an uncomplicated pregnancy and breech presentation (Hofmeyr & Kulier 2002a). Contraindications include:

- ruptured membranes
- oligohydramnios
- multiple pregnancy
- hydrocephalus
- placenta praevia
- maternal hypertension.

ECV should be undertaken during daylight hours in a unit where emergency facilities are available. Very occasionally the fetus can become compromised during the procedure necessitating immediate delivery as a result of placental abruption or knotting of the umbilical cord.

It is important to ensure the following points are adhered to and the midwife can undertake many of these:

- the location of the placenta should be determined by ultrasonography, as placenta praevia is a contraindication
- an abdominal palpation should be undertaken before the procedure to ensure there has been no spontaneous version and that the breech has not engaged
- cardiotocography should be undertaken before and after the procedure
- the woman should have an empty bladder
- the uterus should not be contracting
- if pain is felt the procedure should be stopped

- anti-D immunoglobulin should be administered to Rhesus negative women within 72 hours of the procedure
- if the membranes rupture during the procedure, exclude cord prolapse
- the procedure is abandoned if the fetus does not turn easily (it can be reattempted after several days).

ECV encourages the fetus to rotate 180° by moving the breech away from the pelvic brim and then with one hand over each fetal pole, the fetal head is turned downwards while the breech is rotated upwards. The fetus is usually rotated face downwards to maintain flexion. However, if this is unsuccessful, an attempt can be made to turn the fetus backwards but it is important to maintain flexion of the head.

### Knees–chest posture

This has been advocated by many health professionals over the years without being properly evaluated. Woman with breech presentations have been encouraged to assume a knees–chest posture for varying amounts of time, either every day or for a set number of days. Although there are variations in the frequency and duration of the posture, one example is the Elkins procedure that requires women to adopt the position for 15 minutes every 2 hours when awake for 5 days (Smith et al 1999). Smith et al (1999) evaluated a modified Elkins procedure (knees–chest position for 15 minutes, three times a day) and found this did not reduce the incidence of breech presentation in labour or increase the success rate of ECV. They conclude that postural management is not an effective management option that should be offered routinely.

Dover (1999) suggests there are unanswered issues resulting from this study and suggests that postural management does not harm and may have some positive effects in relation to maternal emotional well-being. Hofmeyr and Kulier's (2002b) systematic review of the studies found the controlled studies were too small to provide any support or refute the use of postural management with breech presentation. Due to the ease with which postural management could be undertaken they suggest larger randomised trials should be performed to evaluate this further.

## Acupuncture

Acupuncture is a form of traditional Chinese medicine that uses the energy (meridian) lines and acupuncture points believed to run throughout the body. The belief is that a difficulty within one of the energy lines will disrupt the body–mind–spirit relationship, thus correction and rebalancing the energy levels is at the centre of this treatment. Acupuncture can only be administered by a trained acupuncturist who may use conventional acupuncture (insertion of needles into the skin at acupuncture sites), electroacupunture (passing a small electric current through the needles inserted into the skin at acupuncture points) and moxibustion (applying moxa sticks to an acupuncture point on both feet for 15 minutes up to 10 times each day for a set number of days; the sticks are lit and allowed to smoke which applies heat to the acupuncture points).

Several studies report on the efficacy of acupuncture although the study numbers are generally small. One small study of 67 women demonstrated a highly significant effect of acupuncture in altering the presentation (78.7% of the intervention group versus 21.2% of the control group, $p < 0.001$) when undertaken twice a week from 34 to 37 weeks (Habek et al 2003).

Moxibustion has received favourable reports that it increases fetal activity that in turn encourages the fetus to move from a breech to a cephalic presentation (Budd 2000). Budd (2000) suggests that the treatment is cheap, with most women requiring only two moxa sticks, and that with further research to demonstrate the efficacy of moxibustion, midwives could be trained to undertake this.

This is an area of growing interest and the reader is advised to keep abreast of the developments within acupuncture.

## Role and responsibilities of the midwife

These can be summarised as:

- keeping abreast with current changes in optimal fetal positioning to provide good evidence-based care
- assisting at ECV unless trained to undertake the procedure.

## Summary

- Postural management for rotating the occiput from a posterior to an anterior position is mainly anecdotal, with little support for undertaking the hands–knees position during pregnancy
- Postural management for breech appears to bring no benefit but is not considered harmful
- ECV in uncomplicated pregnancies has a high success rate although complications can arise during the procedure
- Acupuncture, particularly moxibustion, increases fetal activity to encourage the breech to change to a cephalic presentation
- Postural intervention requires further research to evaluate its efficacy.

The answers to the following questions may be found in the text:

1. What advice can the midwife offer the woman regarding her posture and positioning that may assist the fetal occiput to rotate from a posterior to an anterior position?
2. What procedures can be used to change the presentation from breech to cephalic?
3. What are the role and responsibilities of the midwife in relation to optimal fetal positioning?
4. List the hazards associated with malpositions and malpresentations for the woman and the baby.

# REFERENCES

Budd S 2000 Acupuncture. In: Tiran D, Mack S (eds) Complementary therapies, 2nd edn. Baillière Tindall, Edinburgh, p 79–104

Dover S 1999 Abstract writers' comments. MIDIRS Midwifery Digest 9(4):450

Habek D, Habek J C, Jagust M 2003 Acupuncture conversion of fetal breech presentation. Fetal Diagnosis and Therapy 18(6):418–421

Hannah M E, Hannah W J, Hewson S A et al 2000 Term Breech Trial Collaborative Group. Planned caesarean section versus planned vaginal birth for breech presentation at term: a randomised multicentre trial. Lancet 356(9239):1375–1383

Hofmeyr G J, Kulier R 1998 Hands/knee posture in late pregnancy or labour for fetal malposition (lateral or posterior). Cochrane Library, Issue 1. Update Software, Oxford

Hofmeyr G J, Kulier R 2002a External cephalic version for breech presentation at term. Cochrane Library, Issue 2. Update Software, Oxford

Hofmeyr G J, Kulier R 2002b Cephalic version by postural management for breech presentation. Cochrane Library, Issue 2. Update Software, Oxford

Kariminia A, Chamberlain M E, Keogh J et al 2004 Randomised controlled trial of effect of hands and knees posturing on incidence of occiput posterior position at birth. British Medical Journal 328(7438):490

Lewis P 2004 Malpositions and malpresentations. In: Henderson C, MacDonald S (eds) Mayes midwifery: a textbook for midwives, 13th edn. Baillière Tindall, Edinburgh

Smith C, Crowther C, Wilkinson C et al 1999 Knee–chest postural management for breech at term: a randomised controlled trial. Birth 26(2):71–75

Sutton J, Scott P 1996 Understanding and teaching optimal foetal positioning, 2nd edn. Bay Print, Tauranga, New Zealand

Chapter **31**

# Facilitation of related childbearing skills — speculum use

This chapter focuses on the use of the Cusco speculum. This is an instrument that is inserted into the vagina to open the vaginal walls and allow access to the top of the vagina and cervix.

## Learning outcomes

Having read this chapter the reader should be able to:

- discuss the indications for using a Cusco speculum
- describe how to insert the speculum
- discuss the role and responsibilities of the midwife in relation to speculum use.

## Indications

The midwife may need to use a speculum:

- during preterm labour to assess the cervix
- to inspect around the top of the vagina and cervix for the presence of amniotic fluid when prelabour rupture of membranes is suspected
- to obtain a high vaginal swab
- to obtain a cervical smear.

## Cusco speculum

The speculum is made of either metal (reusable) or plastic (disposable). It has two short blades that are curved across their width (Fig. 31.1). When the speculum is closed the blades close together, but when it is opened, they separate to press against the vaginal walls. At one end there is a circular opening through which the vagina and cervix can be visualised and swabs inserted when required. Attached to this end are the handles that open and close the speculum by means of a screw mechanism. When the handles are apart the blades are closer together. To open the blades, bring the handles together.

**Figure 31.1** Cusco speculum (Adapted with kind permission from Chilman and Thomas 1987)

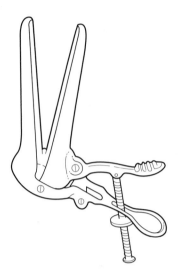

Although insertion of the speculum is not usually painful, it may cause discomfort to the woman, particularly if she has sustained vaginal lacerations. A cold speculum may heighten the discomfort felt. The procedure may also be a source of embarrassment for the woman, provoking anxiety.

### Asepsis

The speculum should be sterile and asepsis maintained throughout as ascending infection can result in uterine and neonatal sepsis. Sterile gloves should be worn in these circumstances; however, when obtaining a high vaginal swab or cervical smear, non-sterile gloves may be worn. A sterile vaginal examination (VE) pack and warm water can be used to clean the area and create a sterile field.

| PROCEDURE | using a speculum |
|---|---|

- Gain informed consent and privacy
- Gather equipment:
    - sterile or non-sterile gloves (depending on the reason for speculum use)
    - speculum and lubricating jelly, e.g. KY Jelly
    - disposable sheet
    - sterile VE pack containing swabs and a bowl
    - warm water
- Encourage the woman to empty her bladder
- Ask the woman to adopt an almost recumbent position (a wedge can be used to avoid aortocaval occlusion if necessary), with her knees bent, ankles together and knees parted

- Remove any sanitary towels or underwear, keeping the genital area covered
- Position the disposable sheet under the woman
- Wash hands and apply gloves
- Clean the genital area by swabbing the perineum from front to back using cotton wool balls or gauze soaked with the warm water, passing the swabs from the examining (clean) hand to the non-examining (dirty) hand; use each swab once and dispose of it
- Lubricate the outer aspect of the blades of the speculum with a water-soluble lubricant, keeping the blades closed
- Part the labia with the non-dominant hand and use the dominant hand to insert the speculum into the vagina (with the width of the blades in the anterior–posterior diameter)
- When in place, turn the speculum 90° so that the handles are uppermost
- Open the blades by unscrewing the handles and bringing them closer together, informing the woman that she may feel pressure as the blades stretch the vagina
- Inspect the vagina and cervix if indicated, using a good light source to obtain the high vaginal swab (Ch. 12) or cervical smear
- To remove the speculum, close the blades, rotate the speculum back to its insertion position and withdraw the speculum
- Remove the disposable sheet and assist the woman to replace her sanitary towel and knickers
- Assist the woman into a comfortable position
- Remove and dispose of gloves and equipment
- Wash hands
- Document findings and act accordingly.

## Role and responsibilities of the midwife

These can be summarised as:

- recognising the need for using a Cusco speculum
- ensuring the procedure is undertaken correctly, with minimal discomfort
- correct documentation.

## Summary

- Speculum use can be an embarrassing and uncomfortable procedure for the woman
- Undertaking the procedure correctly can reduce the discomfort experienced
- Maintenance of asepsis is important to reduce the risk of uterine and neonatal infection.

**Self-assessment exercises**

The answers to the following questions may be found in the text:

1. When might a midwife need to use a Cusco speculum?
2. What are the role and responsibilities of the midwife when using a speculum?

## REFERENCE

Chilman A, Thomas M 1987 Understanding nursing care, 3rd edn. Churchill Livingstone, Edinburgh

# Chapter 32

# Facilitation of related childbearing skills — membrane sweep

This chapter considers the skill of sweeping or 'stripping' the membranes. As the cervical os is gently dilated (stretch) and the amnion is digitally separated from the lower uterine segment (sweep), intrauterine prostaglandin synthesis commences and so labour may be induced. It is generally used prior to formal induction of labour (Enkin et al 2000). However, while the woman may appreciate assistance to commence labour without further intervention, sweeping the membranes is an uncomfortable procedure that may induce per vaginam bleeding and discomfort. Informed consent should include these aspects as well as expected outcome (see Ch. 33 for supporting information).

## Learning outcomes

Having read this chapter the reader should be able to:

- discuss the indications for membrane sweeping
- discuss the current evidence available
- describe how the procedure is performed
- summarise the role and responsibilities of the midwife.

## The evidence

NICE (2001) and RCOG (2001) both indicate that sweeping the membranes increases the likelihood of spontaneous birth within 48 hours and birth within 1 week. It does therefore reduce the incidence of birth after term and formal methods of induction, e.g. prostaglandin ($PGE_2$), both of which have associated risks. The woman and baby would not appear to be at any increased risk of infection, although prelabour rupture of membranes is more likely. Operative delivery figures are unchanged with the use of membrane sweeping. It is noted above that the woman may experience pain and bleeding with the procedure and afterwards and some intermittent uterine activity in the hours and days following. The recommendation is that membrane sweeping should be offered to all women (except placenta praevia and any situation where labour or vaginal birth is not indicated) over 40 weeks' gestation, prior to formal induction of labour (NICE 2001). It is considered that prostaglandin synthesis directly correlates with the surface area of membrane detached. Enkin et al (2000) suggest that where the cervix is closed (and therefore the membranes inaccessible) cervical massage is undertaken. MacKenzie (1999) suggests that the cervix should be favourable, i.e. a Bishop score >8, for a membrane sweep to take place.

The procedure should be completed according to local protocols, but it is likely that the woman already comes into the category of requiring induction of labour, i.e. pregnancy gestation of greater than 40 weeks or pregnancy complication that requires delivery. Care should be taken to avoid membrane rupture when the presenting part is not a well-engaged cephalic presentation, due to the dangers of cord prolapse. The procedure can be carried out in an outpatient setting, the home or hospital; asepsis should be maintained. The woman must be fully informed of what to expect following the procedure. The midwife needs to be trained in this aspect of care before undertaking the procedure. Contemporaneous record keeping should document the findings as well as the action taken.

## PROCEDURE    stretch and sweep of the membranes

- Prepare for and undertake the examination per vaginam as detailed on page 246, as far as 'Locate the cervix…' expecting to find a posterior, largely uneffaced, almost closed cervix (do not rupture the membranes)
- Undertake a Bishop's scoring (or similar) assessment of the cervix
- Insert one or two fingers into the cervix and gently dilate the os
- Insert one or two fingers between the lower uterine segment and the fetal membranes and move the finger(s) with a sweeping circular action through 360° with some inward pressure (Fig. 32.1). Do this fairly decisively as the woman will be uncomfortable and this will be increased if the procedure is unnecessarily prolonged
- Remove the examining hand gently
- Auscultate the fetal heart
- Assist the woman to dress and resume a comfortable position; discuss the findings
- Dispose of equipment appropriately and wash hands
- Document the findings and act accordingly.

Figure 32.1 Sweeping the membranes

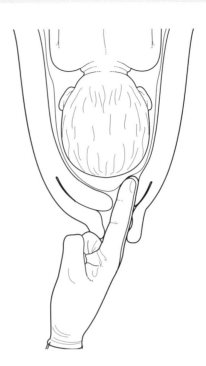

## Role and responsibilities of the midwife

These can be summarised as:

- undertaking evidence-based care with knowledge and professionalism
- correct contemporaneous documentation.

## Summary

- Sweeping the membranes involves dilating the cervical os and separating the membranes from the lower uterine segment prior to induction of labour for women who are to be formally induced
- It is an uncomfortable procedure for the woman but may assist labour to begin naturally.

## Self-assessment exercises

The answers to the following questions may be found in the text:

1. Discuss the indications for membrane sweeping, citing the supporting evidence.
2. What clinical information does the midwife require prior to undertaking the procedure?
3. Describe how a midwife prepares for and carries out a membrane sweep.
4. Summarise the role and responsibilities of the midwife in relation to this procedure.

## REFERENCES

Enkin M, Keirse M J N C, Neilson J et al 2000 A guide to effective care in pregnancy and childbirth. Oxford University Press, Oxford

MacKenzie I 1999 Labor induction including pregnancy termination for fetal anomaly. In: James D, Steer P, Weiner C et al (eds) High risk pregnancy. W B Saunders, London, ch 62

NICE (National Institute for Clinical Excellence) 2001 Induction of labour. NICE, London

RCOG (Royal College of Obstetricians and Gynaecologists) 2001 Induction of labour. RCOG, London

Chapter **33**

# Principles of intrapartum skills – examination per vaginam

This chapter focuses on the principles of examination per vaginam during labour, commonly referred to as a vaginal examination (VE). This is an essential skill for the midwife when caring for a labouring woman, one that should be undertaken sensitively due to the intimate nature of the examination, but efficiently as the information gained will help assess progress and inform care. The procedure is invasive and considered a medical intervention, thus it should only be undertaken when necessary (Mandaza & Nolan 2001). The procedures for performing amniotomy and applying a fetal scalp electrode are described.

## Learning outcomes

Having read this chapter the reader should be able to:

- list the indications for undertaking a VE during labour
- discuss the information that may be obtained from a VE and how this assesses progress
- discuss the role and responsibilities of the midwife when undertaking a VE
- describe the procedures for VE, amniotomy and the application of a fetal scalp electrode.

## Indications

During labour, the midwife may undertake a VE to:

- confirm the onset of labour
- assess progress during labour
- identify the presentation and position
- perform an artificial rupture of membranes
- apply a fetal scalp electrode
- exclude cord prolapse following spontaneous rupture of the membranes where there is an ill-fitting presenting part
- confirm the onset of the second stage of labour, especially with a breech presentation.

### Contraindications

The midwife should not undertake a VE when there is:

- bleeding
- placenta praevia
- preterm rupture of the membranes
- preterm labour (the initial VE should be undertaken by the obstetrician; the midwife may perform subsequent examinations).

# Information gained from undertaking an examination per vaginam

### External genitalia

Any abnormalities such as varicosities, oedema, warts or signs of infection should be noted, as should scarring, particularly if indicative of previous perineal or labial trauma or female genital mutilation. The colour, consistency, amount and odour of any discharge or bleeding from the vagina should be recorded; amniotic fluid may be seen if the membranes have ruptured.

### Vagina

The vagina should feel warm and moist, with soft distensible walls. A hot, dry vagina could be indicative of dehydration, infection or obstructed labour. A vagina that feels tense may be associated with fear or previous scarring. The presence of varicosities, a cystocele or rectocele should be noted. A full rectum may be felt through the posterior vaginal wall.

### Cervix

The cervix is assessed for position, consistency, effacement, dilatation and application to the presenting part. Prior to labour, the cervix is usually in a central or posterior position, firm, non-effaced with the os closed (unripe). In the latter weeks of pregnancy and early labour, the structure and position of the cervix alters as the cervix ripens, resulting in a cervix that feels less rigid and in an anterior position. A ripe cervix that feels soft and stretchy is associated with good dilatation of the os uteri, whereas a tight unyielding unripe cervix at term is more likely to be associated with prolonged labour. An unripe cervix requires three to four times more uterine effort than a ripe cervix (Burnhill et al 1962).

A cervix that is well applied to the presenting part is associated with good uterine activity (Blackburn & Loper 1992). The reverse may be true, that a poorly applied cervix is associated with less efficient uterine activity and slower progress. For example, when the fetus is in an occipitoposterior position, the head is not pushed directly onto the cervix; rather it is directed downwards and forwards against the back of the symphysis pubis, leading to a decrease in the effectiveness of uterine contractility, slower cervical dilatation and prolonged labour

(Chamberlain 1993). The application of the cervix to the presenting part can be assessed by feeling between them.

Effacement usually precedes dilatation with the primigravida; these may appear to occur simultaneously with the multigravida. Effacement is assessed by the length of the cervix and the degree to which it protrudes into the vagina. A non-effaced cervix feels long and tubular, with the os closed or partly dilated. As effacement occurs, the cervix thins out and feels shorter, as the lower uterine segment takes it up (Fig. 33.1). A fully effaced cervix feels continuous with the lower uterine segment and does not protrude into the vagina.

Dilatation of the os uteri is measured in centimetres and is assessed by inserting one or both fingers through the external os and parting the fingers to assess the diameter. In early labour, when the cervix is less than 2 cm dilated, usually only one finger can be inserted. Towards the end of the first stage it may be easier to feel around the remaining rim of cervix to estimate dilatation, e.g. a rim of 1 cm equates to a dilatation of 8 cm, as there is 2 cm of cervix remaining. When the cervix can no longer be felt, full dilatation has occurred, equal to 10 cm. This is the point at which the fetal head can pass through the cervix although for the preterm fetus, this may be less than 10 cm. If the presentation is breech, it is possible for the foot and leg to protrude through the cervix before it is fully dilated (footling breech). Dilatation of the os uteri should occur progressively throughout the first stage of labour and is one factor in determining progress.

The os uteri is usually closed in the primigravida until labour begins, but the os of the multigravida may allow one or two fingers through before labour, commonly referred to as a 'multips os'.

### The membranes

Intact membranes may be felt as a shiny surface over the presenting part. This can be difficult to feel, particularly in early labour or if the forewaters are shallow and the membranes tightly pressed against the

**Figure 33.1** Effacement of the cervix

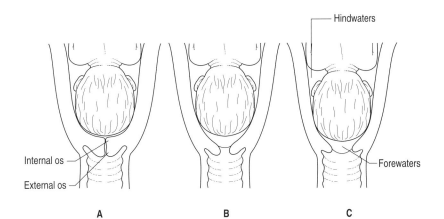

presenting part. If the membranes are difficult to feel, it may be mistaken for ruptured membranes. When the presenting part is poorly applied to the cervix, the membranes contain a greater amount of fluid and may bulge through the cervix. As the pressure increases in the forewaters during contractions, the membranes may become tense and may rupture spontaneously. This usually occurs earlier when the presenting part is ill fitting or poorly applied. If the membranes are felt intact but amniotic fluid is leaking, a hindwater rupture is the likely cause.

### Presentation

In conjunction with information gained from the abdominal examination, the identification of landmarks on the presenting part help to confirm the presentation:

- A cephalic presentation is smooth, round and firm, and sutures or fontanelles may be felt. Moulding can be assessed by the degree of overlapping of the bones of the vault
- Both the breech and face presentation feel soft and irregular. The sacrum may be palpable as a hard bone, with the anus close by. If a finger is inadvertently inserted into the anus, it will be gripped. Fresh meconium is likely to be present also
- With the face presentation, the orbital ridges may be felt and a finger inserted into the mouth will be sucked. If a face presentation is suspected or confirmed, care should be taken to avoid damaging the eyes; application of a fetal scalp electrode is not recommended and obstetric cream should not be used as it could initiate a chemical conjunctivitis
- If the cord presents, the pulsations can be palpated through the membranes – the membranes should not be ruptured due to the danger of cord prolapse.

### Level of the presenting part

This is determined by assessing the distance between the presenting part and the ischial spines in centimetres (Fig. 33.2). The ischial spines are referred to as zero station, with the presenting part being above (−cm) or below (+cm) this. The ischial spines may be difficult to palpate; this becomes a subjective measurement. It is important for the midwife to ensure it is the level of the presenting part being assessed and not caput succedaneum. Descent of the presenting part is one indicator of progress during labour and the assessment should correlate with the findings from the degree of engagement determined during the abdominal examination.

### Position

With a cephalic presentation, identification of sutures and fontanelles will confirm the position and attitude:

**Figure 33.2** Level of presenting part in relation to the ischial spines

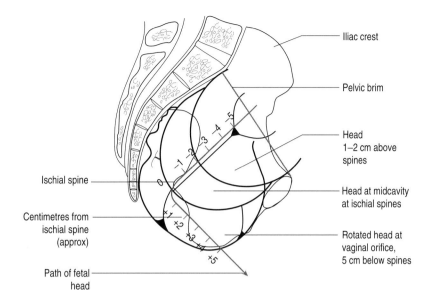

- Iliac crest
- Pelvic brim
- Head 1–2 cm above spines
- Head at midcavity at ischial spines
- Rotated head at vaginal orifice, 5 cm below spines
- Ischial spine
- Centimetres from ischial spine (approx)
- Path of fetal head

- the sagittal suture is easily identified as a long straight suture; its position is taken in relation to the maternal pelvis, moving from back to front
- a sagittal suture in the right oblique is felt moving from the posterior right quadrant of the maternal pelvis obliquely forwards to the left anterior quadrant (Fig. 33.3)
- the posterior fontanelle is felt as a small triangular area, with three sutures running from it; it is indicative of a well-flexed cephalic presentation, usually occipitoanterior position
- the anterior fontanelle is felt as a larger, diamond-shaped area, with four sutures running from it and is associated with a deflexed head, usually with an occipitoposterior position.

Progress is indicated where there is progressive flexion (or extension if a face presentation) and rotation. Comparing the position of the landmarks from all previous VEs should demonstrate this.

### Pelvic outlet

This is assessed by feeling for the ischial spines; if prominent, the transverse diameter of the outlet is reduced and could affect progress, particularly in the second stage of labour. The subpubic angle is assessed by moving the top part of the two examining fingers towards the pubic arch. Two fingers should fit snugly under the pubic arch, indicating an angle of 90° or greater. A reduced subpubic angle is often found with prominent ischial spines and may be associated with an android pelvis. This can result in more pressure being placed on the perineum and increased perineal trauma as well as delay in the second stage of

**Figure 33.3** Rotation of a cephalic presentation felt on examination per vaginam

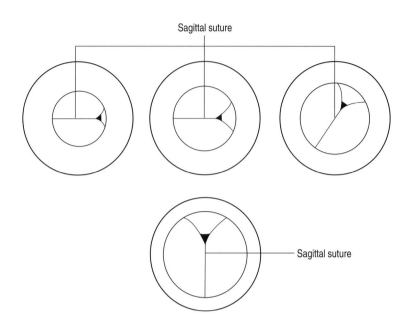

labour. Care should be taken when assessing the subpubic angle to avoid the clitoris; pressure on this structure can be painful.

## PROCEDURE examination per vaginam

The procedure should be carried out using an aseptic technique. While sterile VE packs and lotions to wash the genital area are used in many labour wards, McCormick (2001) has demonstrated that the infection rate is unaffected by their use. She proposes that stringent hand hygiene and using sterile gloves (and avoiding their contamination) is as effective (in minimising the risk of infection) and more cost effective than using VE packs and lotions. The midwife should refer to the hospital policy for local requirements on perineal cleansing. The procedure for perineal cleansing follows this procedure.

- Gain informed consent and ensure privacy
- Gather equipment:
  — apron
  — sterile gloves
  — antiseptic cream, e.g. obstetric cream (except with a face presentation when a water-soluble lubricant should be used, e.g. KY Jelly)
  — disposable sheet
  — other equipment as necessary, e.g. amnihook, fetal scalp electrode
  — Pinard stethoscope or sonicaid

- Encourage the woman to empty her bladder
- Undertake an abdominal palpation to ascertain the lie, presentation, position, degree of engagement and auscultate the fetal heart
- Ask the woman to adopt an almost recumbent position (use a wedge to avoid aortocaval occlusion if necessary), with her knees bent, ankles together and knees parted, placing the disposable sheet beneath her buttocks
- Remove any sanitary towels or underwear, keeping the genital area covered
- Apply apron; wash hands while the assistant opens the gloves
- Dry hands and put on gloves
- The assistant pours antiseptic cream onto the midwife's gloved hand avoiding contact with the gloves and removes the covers from the woman
- Lubricate the first two fingers of the dominant hand with antiseptic cream
- With the thumb and forefinger of the non-examining hand, part the labia, observing the condition of the vulva
- Gently insert the first two fingers of the examining hand into the vagina, in a downwards and backwards direction along the anterior vaginal wall, ensuring the thumb does not come into contact with the woman's clitoris or anus
- Locate the cervix and determine the position, tone, degree of effacement and dilatation and application to the presenting part
- Move the fingers through the cervical os to ascertain the presence of the forewaters and the presentation, position, degree of flexion and level of the presenting part; the presence of caput succedaneum and degree of moulding should be noted
- If necessary, rupture the membranes and/or apply a fetal scalp electrode (pp 249–250)
- Withdraw the fingers gently, assessing the pelvic outlet
- Auscultate the fetal heart
- Assist the woman into a comfortable position and discuss the findings
- Dispose of equipment appropriately and wash hands
- Document the findings and act accordingly.

## PROCEDURE   perineal cleansing

A VE pack and water for cleansing will be required. The midwife should follow the procedure for examination per vaginam up to putting on the apron and washing hands. The assistant will open the VE pack and gloves while the midwife's hands are being washed and slide the gloves on to the sterile field. The midwife is then required to:

- dry hands and put on gloves
- ask the assistant to pour antiseptic cream into the gallipot, warm water into the bowl and remove the covers from the woman
- swab the perineum from front to back using cotton wool balls or gauze soaked with the warm water, passing the swabs from the examining (clean) hand to the non-examining (dirty) hand; use each swab once and dispose of it
- dip the first two fingers of the examining hand into the cream for lubrication.

The procedure then continues as for examination per vaginam from the point 'with the thumb and forefinger . . .'.

## Amniotomy (artificial rupture of membranes, ARM)

Intact membranes provide a cushion that fits appropriately into the cervix during labour, helping to apply an even pressure and giving some protection to the presenting part. When the membranes are not present the presenting part presses more directly onto the cervix; pain is often greater as more prostaglandin is released and so contractions increase in strength and frequency. The UK Amniotomy Group (1994) found that labour was modestly shortened with ARM, but could not justify routine use. Fraser et al (2004) found early amniotomy was associated with both benefits (reduction in length of labour) and risks (reduction in 5-minute Apgar score and an increased risk of caesarean delivery). They concluded that amniotomy should be reserved only for women in whom labour progress was abnormal. Amniotomy is useful for the purposes of augmentation and induction of labour. Many midwives would not rupture membranes unless specifically indicated, believing that spontaneous rupture follows a more natural labour.

Variations of the fetal heart can be seen after ARM (early decelerations) that may lead to further intervention. Amniotic fluid embolism is known to be associated with ARM. The use of standard precautions is indicated and the sharpness of the amnihook means that the midwife must take care to avoid personal injury and must dispose of the hook into a sharps box.

## Indications

- Induction of labour
- Augmentation of labour
- Application of fetal scalp electrode and/or assessment of liquor colour
- Maternal request
- Often prior to birth of second twin.

### Contraindications

- High presenting part (risk of cord prolapse)
- Preterm labour
- Known vaginal infection
- Caution is taken with polyhydramnios or any malposition or malpresentation
- Placenta praevia
- Vasa praevia.

A controlled ARM is sometimes performed when the presenting part is high. An obstetrician performs the ARM while the midwife applies light pressure to the fundus. This encourages the presenting part to engage in the pelvis as the membranes rupture. The obstetrician ensures that the fluid has drained and no cord has prolapsed before removing the hand.

---

PROCEDURE    **artificial rupture of the membranes**

- Discuss the indication with the woman and gain her informed consent
- Gather equipment:
  — equipment as for vaginal examination
  — amnihook
- Undertake a vaginal examination as detailed on page 246, maintaining the sterility of the amnihook
- Locate the cervix using the examining hand; ensure that all factors are favourable for ARM to be undertaken, e.g. descent of presenting part, keeping fingers in the cervix
- Use the non-examining hand to slide the amnihook carefully, with the hook pointing downwards, between the examining hand and anterior vaginal wall
- Guide the amnihook into place with the examining hand, placing the hook against the membranes
- Twist the amnihook slightly using the non-examining hand to tear the membranes
- Withdraw the amnihook gently, retaining the fingers in the cervix as the amniotic fluid drains out (ensuring the amniotic fluid does not come into contact with the midwife's clothing)
- Undertake a reassessment of the cervix, fetal descent and position
- A scalp electrode can be applied if indicated (p. 250)
- Withdraw the hand, auscultate the fetal heart
- Assist the woman re: hygiene, comfort and position
- Discuss the findings with the woman
- Dispose of equipment correctly and wash hands
- Document the indications for ARM with the findings and act accordingly.

Rupturing the membranes with an amnihook is sometimes easier to do if a contraction is present and the membranes are bulging under the pressure. This is not an absolute necessity however. Clearly the membranes do need to be intact; membranes that are tight across the baby's head may be deceptive, causing the midwife to question their presence. Care should be taken to ensure that neither the baby nor the woman is scratched with the hook.

# Application of fetal scalp electrode (FSE)

When continuous cardiotocograph monitoring is indicated a fetal scalp electrode may be applied to ensure continuity of contact. The electrode transfers fetal heart sounds from conductivity in the fetal scalp to a transducer located on the woman's thigh, attached to the ECG port on the monitor. The sound of the fetal heart is continuous regardless of maternal or fetal position. It is not accompanied or confused by sounds of fetal movement or uterine blood flow. It is an invasive procedure for both the woman and the fetus; the electrode is secured under the fetal scalp, with either a clip or spiral connection. It is assumed that the fetus experiences some pain and the transfer of viruses such as HIV from mother to child is more likely. Skin infection or long-term scarring can occur.

Prototype suction electrodes evaluated by Gulmezoglu et al (1996) were found to be difficult to retain. Needs et al (1992) found clip electrodes performed better than other types with regard to attachment. The clip is applied by rotating the end of the electrode: anticlockwise rotation causes the clip to recede into the electrode head; clockwise rotation causes it to emerge from the electrode head and be caught on the scalp. It is often spring loaded and therefore rarely requires an active rotation clockwise. A spiral electrode is rotated in the direction of the spiral, usually clockwise, until caught under the scalp.

Accuracy of scalp electrodes depends upon their correct application. If membrane is between the electrode and the scalp then the tracing is likely to be unreliable, sometimes known as 'artefact'. Interpretation of the trace is impossible. The electrode should not be near or through a fontanelle or suture line, the cervix or vagina – it should be on the skin folds of the scalp. It can be used on the buttocks of a breech presentation, but causes obvious scarring. It should not be used with a face presentation.

## PROCEDURE    application of a fetal scalp electrode

- Discuss the indication with the woman and gain her consent
- Ensure that the monitor has the ECG facility and correct leads
- Gather equipment:

— equipment as for vaginal examination with amnihook if membranes are intact
— fetal scalp electrode
- Undertake a vaginal examination as detailed on page 246
- Perform ARM (p. 248) if membranes intact
- Locate the fetal scalp using the examining hand; ensure that sutures and fontanelles are avoided
- Use the non-examining hand to slide the scalp electrode carefully between the examining hand and vaginal wall
- Guide the electrode into place with the examining hand, supporting the head of the electrode against the scalp
- Turn the end of the electrode anticlockwise, then release to attach to the scalp, using the non-examining hand
- The electrode should be attached to the scalp; a gentle pull will confirm whether or not it is attached
- An assistant may attach the leads to the transducer and the transducer to the monitor while the examining hand remains in place; if the electrode is not working reapplication may be tried
- Check that the electrode is securely placed over an appropriate area of the scalp, withdraw the hand
- Apply conductive gel to the transducer and attach around the woman's thigh using a small belt; ensure that monitoring is satisfactorily taking place
- Assist the woman re: hygiene, comfort and position
- Explain the differences that can be heard
- Dispose of equipment correctly and wash hands
- Document the indications for FSE with other aspects of the examination and act accordingly.

A fetal scalp electrode is usually removed at delivery. To do this the electrode head is held against the scalp while the end is rotated anticlockwise. Care should be taken not to create any trauma while removing it. An obvious scar should be noted on the initial birth examination.

## Role and responsibilities of the midwife

These can be summarised as:

- undertaking a competent examination in which all of the information is gained
- undertaking an amniotomy correctly, if indicated
- appropriate application of a fetal scalp electrode, if indicated
- recognising deviations from the norm and instigating referral
- education, explanations and support of the woman
- appropriate record keeping.

**Summary**

- An examination per vaginam is an invasive procedure but one that can yield valuable information in relation to the assessment of progress in labour
- Amniotomy may be undertaken for induction or augmentation of labour
- Fetal scalp electrodes offer continuity of contact if continuous fetal monitoring is indicated
- The risk of ascending infection is high; an aseptic technique should be used throughout.

**Self-assessment exercises**

The answers to the following questions may be found in the text:

1. For what reasons would the midwife undertake an examination per vaginam during labour?
2. What is the procedure for performing an examination per vaginam?
3. How could the midwife identify a flexed cephalic presentation?
4. How does the information gained help to assess progress?
5. Describe how to perform an amniotomy and application of a fetal scalp electrode.
6. What are the role and responsibilities of the midwife in relation to an examination per vaginam, artificial rupture of the membranes and application of a fetal scalp electrode?

**REFERENCES**

Blackburn S T, Loper D 1992 Maternal, fetal and neonatal physiology: a clinical perspective. W B Saunders, Philadelphia

Burnhill M S, Donezis J, Cohen J 1962 Uterine contractility during labour studied by intra-amniotic fluid pressure recordings. American Journal of Obstetrics and Gynaecology 83:561–571

Chamberlain G V P 1993 Obstetrics by ten teachers, 16th edn. Arnold, London

Fraser W D, Turcot L, Krauss I et al 2004 Amniotomy for shortening spontaneous labour (Cochrane Review). Cochrane Library, Issue 3. Update Software, Oxford

Gulmezoglu A M, Nikodem V C, Hofmeyr G J et al 1996 Randomised evaluation of a prototype suction fetal scalp electrode. British Journal of Obstetrics and Gynaecology 103(6):513–517

McCormick C 2001 Vulval preparations in labour: use of lotions or tap water. British Journal of Midwifery 9(7):453–455

Mandaza P, Nolan M 2001 Clinical file. Case study. Vaginal examinations in labour. The Practising Midwife 4(6):22

Needs L, Grant A, Sleep J et al 1992 A randomised controlled trial to compare three types of fetal scalp electrode. British Journal of Obstetrics and Gynaecology 99(4):302–306

UK Amniotomy Group 1994 A multicentre randomised trial of amniotomy in spontaneous first labour at term. British Journal of Obstetrics and Gynaecology 101(4):307

# Chapter 34

# Principles of intrapartum skills — second stage issues

This chapter will review the current evidence and clinical skills utilised during care in the second stage of labour.

| Learning outcomes | |
|---|---|

Having read this chapter the reader should be able to:

- discuss the evidence and opinions relating to recognition, duration, pushing, positions, nuchal cord and perineal management during the second stage of labour
- discuss the preparation and then describe how a midwife conducts an aseptic delivery
- describe how to infiltrate the perineum and incise an episiotomy
- discuss the role and responsibilities of the midwife throughout.

# Physiology of the second stage of labour

## Recognition

Traditionally, the second stage of labour has been defined by a very clinical description: from full dilatation of the os uteri to the complete birth of the baby. Equally, recognition of the second stage has been classified by signs such as a change in contraction frequency and nature (expulsive), a heavy blood-stained show (as the operculum descends), pouting of the vulva and anus (as the fetal head descends onto the soft tissues), visible fetus at the introitus (always ensure this is not caput succedaneum) or use of vaginal examination which reveals the absence of a locatable cervix. However, skilled, intuitive, observant midwives will be very familiar with situations in which the urge to push is gradual, the urge to push arises before full dilatation, full dilatation is confirmed but there is no urge to push, or there appears to be a resting phase when contractions diminish for a while. Equally, the woman may become particularly vocal or particularly quiet and withdrawn, have a purple line that extends up the anal cleft (Hobbs 1998), display changes in abdominal shape (Burvill 2002) or sacral curve (rhombus of Michaelis; Sutton 2003) or feel that she can't go on, is tired or – in contrast – is renewed with energy. Our researched understanding of these issues remains limited; nevertheless a truly 'tuned in' midwife will support the woman in her intuitive actions and sounds while maintaining good clinical observation and skill.

Latent and perineal stages within the second stage are recognised. It is only when the fetus descends onto the pelvic floor that the Ferguson's reflex is stimulated and the urge to bear down arises. Pushing before this time only exhausts the woman.

## Duration

Placing an arbitrary time limit on the length of the second stage of labour, in view of issues such as latent/perineal phases, is a dubious and discredited activity. Enkin et al (2000) are clear that it is the combination of maternal and fetal wellbeing, and the progress of fetal descent within the contraction pattern, that 'measure' progress in the second stage. Walsh (2002) agrees, stating that for a mobile woman using an upright position and pushing spontaneously, a time restriction is not necessary. This does mean, however, that midwives need to be alert, using skills which can highlight deviations from the norm – e.g. abdominal palpation, observations of fetal heart, liquor, signs of normal mechanism, observance of maternal exhaustion, signs of cephalopelvic disproportion, etc. – which can indicate lack of progress and compromise. Where there are no deviations, Albers (1999) indicates that even with lengthy second stages there is no detriment to mother or fetus.

## Pushing

The physiological dangers to mother and fetus of the breath-holding Valsalva manoeuvre (Brown 1999) have long been recognised. Where a woman is without regional analgesia there is no reason why she should not bear down as her body tells her. This is likely to be with short (4–6 seconds) naturally occurring breath-holding efforts, several times at the height of the contraction.

## Position

Analysis of the studies into maternal position (Gupta & Nikodem 2000) reveals that while the studies are of variable quality and therefore cannot be implemented in their entirety, the trend is in favour of an upright position (standing, squatting, kneeling, all fours, birthing chair or stool, sitting upright), reducing both the length of the second stage and the incidence of instrumental delivery. The incidence of blood loss greater than 500 mL was also noted; care should therefore be taken to assess for anaemia postnatally. Sutton (2003) suggests that pelvic diameters are increased when the woman adopts a lateral position. Midwives can therefore:

- encourage and support women to adopt the positions of their choice in which they are most comfortable, while remembering the advantages of an upright position
- consider the suitability of the environment and accessibility of equipment such as beanbags, birthing balls, rocking chairs, birthing chairs/stools, etc.
- teach women and their birthing partners how to utilise upright positions together
- have confidence in their own ability to facilitate safe deliveries in different positions.

## Asepsis

It is important that delivery is an aseptic procedure for both the woman and the baby to reduce the incidence of postnatal infection. The midwife will use a sterile delivery pack, establishing a sterile field both on the working surface and in the area of the woman's perineum. Adaptations are necessary according to the environment and the position that the woman has adopted. The midwife must attend to scrupulous hand hygiene and the use of all standard precautions including aprons, gowns, sterile gloves and eye protection (eye protection is sometimes interpreted as damaging the relationship with the woman but for certain positions it should be considered). Once the sterile gloves have been applied for delivery they should be kept sterile.

An anal pad may be used to cover or remove any faeces that may escape from the anus. The perineum should be swabbed prior to delivery; tap water is increasingly used but the evidence is sparse and inconsistent (Jessiman 2001) and therefore this may depend upon local protocol.

## Management of the perineum

The HOOP trial (McCandlish et al 1998) provides the means of giving women the choice as to how their perineum is managed. The hands-on approach, i.e. controlling the speed of delivery of the baby's head, guarding of the perineum (placing the hand next to the perineum to support it) and applying traction to deliver the shoulders demonstrated less perineal pain for women at 10 days postnatal. All other outcomes (e.g. perineal trauma) were similar, thus allowing women to make an informed choice. It is possible to achieve control of the speed of delivery with verbal guidance, but equally the woman may wish to deliver the baby herself onto her abdomen; both of these methods are modifications of the hands-on technique. Research into this aspect of care is ongoing and the reader needs to be aware of this.

### The umbilical cord

Another area of discussion is whether or not to feel for the umbilical cord around the fetal neck following delivery of the head, and whether to loop over or cut it if it is found. Evidence is limited and inconclusive (Phillips 2004), but awareness is needed that once the cord is cut the baby's oxygen supply ceases until he is able to breathe. This is significant if shoulder dystocia then occurs.

# Preparation of the environment

As a continuum of labour care it is anticipated that the support, communication, physical care, observations and record keeping that have extended through the first stage of labour will continue. Specifically for the second stage the environment should:

- contain all that is required for management of an aseptic delivery
- be warm and ready to receive the baby
- be calm and relaxed
- have a midwife present throughout, with an assistant for delivery (depending on local protocol, but ideally a second midwife)
- have a mechanism to call for emergency assistance
- be equipped to begin emergency management for mother or baby. All equipment must have been checked and the midwife must be competent in its use.

### PROCEDURE    normal delivery

Adaptations are made according to the birth environment and position of the woman. Note should be taken of the discussions above.

- Prepare the environment and gather equipment:
  — delivery trolley or surface to work from
  — sterile delivery pack, including towels to dry/wrap the baby
  — sterile gloves, gown, etc.
  — disposable sheets, gloves and sanitary towels
  — water/lotion for perineal cleansing
  — obstetric cream/water-based lubricant (depending on local protocol)
  — extras: urinary catheter, amnihook, lidocaine (lignocaine), needles and syringes, oxytocic agent
  — a refuse bag should be available, usually a floor bin
- Ensure that the room temperature is correct (21–24°C) and draughts are excluded

- Give ongoing reassurance and explanations to the woman, support her in her choice of position and analgesia and maintain maternal and fetal observations (utilise assistant once sterility is established)
- Place the disposable sheets strategically in the area of the perineum, while wearing disposable gloves
- When delivery is imminent, put on apron and eye protection, wash hands while the assistant opens the outer covering of the delivery pack
- Open the pack and dry hands while the assistant slides the sterile gloves onto the sterile field
- Apply sterile gloves and gown
- Check the swabs and instruments in the delivery pack while the assistant adds water, lubricant and any other requirements to the sterile field
- Arrange the trolley in a way that suits, having cord clamps and the receiver for the placenta accessible
- Continue to observe the advancing fetus while carrying out these procedures (some women experience short second stages of labour)
- Swab the perineum using gauze and lotion, front to back, using each swab once using a 'clean and dirty' hand technique (p. 101)
- Place sterile drapes appropriately to provide a sterile field
- Position the anal pad, have a towel on hand, e.g. on mother's abdomen, ready to receive the baby
- As the fetus reaches the perineum, the perineum is seen to stretch
- As the head crowns, consider applying gentle pressure to it with one hand to slow the delivery, guard the perineum with the other hand (encourage the woman to breathe and give gentle pushes as the head extends and emerges)
- As the head restitutes, consider feeling below the occiput for the presence of the cord around the neck – if felt, it may be pulled gently to loop over the head, or if very tight two clamps may be securely applied and the cord cut between the clamps and unwound from the neck
- External rotation of the head is seen as the shoulders rotate internally
- As the next contraction occurs and the woman has urges to push again, apply traction to the anterior shoulder (in a direction away from the symphysis pubis) to deliver it, followed by traction in the opposite direction to deliver the posterior one
- Deliver the body and limbs of the baby by lateral flexion, following the curve of the birth canal, in an upward direction towards the woman's abdomen; the woman may assist
- Note the time of delivery
- The baby is placed ideally skin to skin with his mother and is dried completely; parents or midwife will check the gender

- Drying acts as stimulation, during which time the baby will take its first breath and cry; complete Apgar score (Ch. 40) at 1 minute. Act swiftly (before 1 minute) if resuscitation is required (Ch. 60)
- Clamping and cutting of the cord will be undertaken according to the parents' wishes and chosen management of the third stage of labour. Breastfeeding may be facilitated
- Share in the joy of the moment, but stay alert to the clinical situation
- Care moves into management of the third stage of labour; this may have included the administration of an intramuscular oxytocic agent following delivery of the anterior shoulder.

# Episiotomy

Episiotomy is the surgical incision into the perineum to widen the vulval outlet. The work of Sleep et al (1984) indicates that a protocol of restricted episiotomy can be safely applied so that it is performed solely for fetal or maternal distress or with lack of progress and instrumental delivery. Its incidence is less in current practice. Usually a right mediolateral episiotomy is performed; this is less likely to extend to a third degree tear but can be more difficult to repair. A midwife may perform an episiotomy if it is indicated, with the woman's consent, and if properly trained. The timing of gaining informed consent is a more difficult issue; parenthood education during the antenatal period may assist the woman to understand what it is and why it may be necessary; her birth plan may include her wishes. The urgency of the need to undertake one at the time prevents detailed explanations, but consent is still required.

Infiltration of the perineum with an anaesthetic is necessary prior to the incision. The timing of the episiotomy is important; the presenting part needs to descend sufficiently onto the perineum to displace the levator ani (deep muscles). The incision is then only likely to affect the skin, posterior vaginal wall and superficial pelvic floor muscles (Fig. 37.1, p. 284, indicates the muscles of the pelvic floor). If performed too early the deep pelvic floor muscles may be incised and haemorrhage is likely to occur from the wound. The delivery of the presenting part usually follows immediately, the midwife being required to remove the scissors from the vulva, control the delivery of the head and support the perineum so that the episiotomy does not extend, almost simultaneously. The procedure and repair (Ch. 37) are both aseptic events.

PROCEDURE    **infiltration of the perineum and episiotomy**

- Gain informed consent
- Between contractions, draw up the correct dose of anaesthetic agent, e.g. lidocaine (lignocaine) using a sterile needle (21 g green) and syringe

- Swab the perineum as described above
- Insert two fingers into the vagina behind the perineum to protect the presenting part
- Insert the full depth of the needle centrally at the introitus, draw back; if not in a blood vessel inject one-third of the anaesthetic as the needle is withdrawn. Avoid taking the needle completely out of the tissue, but as the introitus is reached reposition the needle and reinsert it in a mediolateral direction. Instil the anaesthetic as described and then repeat for a third time (Fig. 34.1A) to infiltrate a fan-shaped area of the perineum
- Allow the agent time to work, two or three contractions if possible
- Reinsert two fingers to protect the presenting part again. Using the straight scissors supplied in the delivery pack, make one decisive right mediolateral incision of approximately 4–5 cm long at the height of the contraction at which the delivery is anticipated (Fig. 34.1B)
- Immediately apply control to the fetal head, removing the scissors onto the trolley; guard the perineum if able and facilitate the slow delivery of the head
- Continue with the delivery as described above
- Ensure that after examination of the genital tract (Ch. 35) the episiotomy is repaired appropriately (Ch. 37)
- Records should specifically include details of the indication, infiltration and incision.

**Figure 34.1** (A) Infiltration of the perineum; (B) incision of episiotomy

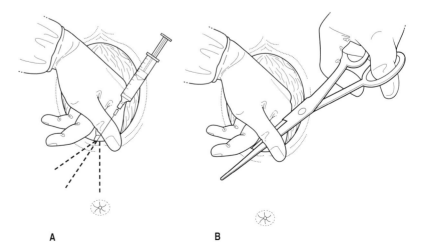

A        B

## Role and responsibilities of the midwife

These can be summarised as:

- thorough preparation of the environment and equipment
- care and observations throughout the second stage
- safe, evidence-based management of the birth for woman and baby
- respect and appropriate facilitation of the woman's wishes
- recognition of any deviation from the norm; referral as necessary
- contemporaneous record keeping.

## Summary

- Many factors contribute to satisfying, safe and evidence-based care in the second stage of labour
- Midwives should have confidence to allow women to push spontaneously in whichever is the position of their choice, preferably upright
- Restricting the length of the second stage is inappropriate providing that there is progress and maternal and fetal wellbeing
- Delivery is an aseptic procedure in which standard precautions are also used
- Controlling the speed of delivery of the head, support of the perineum and lateral flexion to the shoulders are all desirable for perineal integrity
- Episiotomy should be restricted to instances of maternal and fetal distress. It is an aseptic procedure, incising the perineum to increase the vulval outlet. Anaesthetic is used, consent is essential and timing vital
- The midwife has an autonomous and highly responsible role during the second stage of labour.

## Self-assessment exercises

The answers to the following questions may be found in the text:

1. How may the midwife recognise the second stage of labour?
2. Describe how the environment is prepared for birth.
3. Discuss the evidence relating to management of the second stage of labour, including length, pushing and delivery positions.
4. Demonstrate how a normal birth is conducted including management of the equipment and positioning of the hands.
5. Describe how to infiltrate the perineum and incise an episiotomy.
6. Summarise the role and responsibilities of the midwife when providing complete care during the second stage of labour.

## REFERENCES

Albers L 1999 The duration of labour in healthy women. Journal of Perinatology 19(2):114–119

Brown K 1999 Push! Or is that shove? Nursing Times 95(15):58, 60

Burvill S 2002 Midwifery diagnosis of labour onset. British Journal of Midwifery 10(10):600–605

Enkin M, Keirse M, Neilson J et al 2000 A guide to effective care in pregnancy and childbirth, 3rd edn. Oxford University Press, Oxford

Gupta J, Nikodem V 2000 Women's position during second stage of labour (Cochrane Review) Cochrane Library, Issue 1. Update Software, Oxford

Hobbs L 1998 Assessing cervical dilatation without VEs – watching the purple line. The Practising Midwife 1(11):34–35

Jessiman W 2001 Lotions and lubricants. The Practising Midwife 4(3):23–28

McCandlish R, Bowler U, van Asten H et al 1998 A randomised controlled trial of care of the perineum during second stage of normal labour. British Journal of Obstetrics and Gynaecology 105(12):1262–1272

Phillips S 2004 To cut or not to cut? The Practising Midwife 7(7):26–27

Sleep J M, Grant A, Garcia J et al 1984 West Berkshire perineal management trial. British Medical Journal 289:587–590

Sutton J 2003 Birth without active pushing. In: Wickham S (ed) Midwifery best practice. Elsevier Science, Edinburgh, p 90–92

Walsh D 2002 Part six: Limits on pushing and time in the second stage. British Journal of Midwifery 8(10):604–608

Chapter **35**

# Principles of intrapartum skills — third stage issues

The third stage of labour is a dangerous stage for the woman as primary postpartum haemorrhage (PPH) is a cause of maternal mortality (CEMD 2004) and mismanagement of the third stage increases the risk. Following the delivery of the baby, the midwife has a responsibility to deliver the placenta and membranes safely and competently. This chapter focuses on the principles of the management of the third stage of labour, discussing both physiological and active management, examination of the genital tract following delivery of the placenta and estimation of blood loss; relevant anatomy and physiology are included.

**Learning outcomes**

Having read this chapter the reader should be able to:

- describe the physiology of the third stage of labour
- discuss the different methods of managing the third stage
- discuss how blood loss is estimated
- describe how the genital tract is examined following delivery.

# Physiology of the third stage of labour

The third stage is from the birth of the baby to the complete expulsion of the placenta and membranes, involving the separation, descent and expulsion of the placenta and membranes and the control of haemorrhage from the placental site. It also encompasses examination of the genital tract following delivery and, if necessary, perineal repair.

Placental separation has previously been thought to result from the placenta being squeezed following the reduction in the size of the uterus at the beginning of the third stage. This was thought to result in an increased pressure within the blood vessels of the spongy layer of the decidua, causing them to rupture. The escaping blood between the placental surface and the thin septa of the spongy layer resulted in the placenta shearing from the decidua. However, following ultrasound visualisation of placental separation, a different understanding of the physiology has emerged (Herman 2000, Herman et al 2002, Krapp et al 2000) with three phases identified – latent, contraction/detachment and expulsion.

With the delivery of the baby, the intrauterine volume reduces drastically (from 4 L before labour to 0.5 L) as the uterus becomes smaller. Intrauterine pressure increases from 100 mmHg in the second stage to 140 mmHg in the third stage.

### Phase 1 – latent phase

Contraction and retraction of the myometrium continues as with the first and second stages of labour causing extensive thickening of most of the myometrium. However, the area of myometrium beneath the placental site is unable to thicken to the same extent.

### Phase 2 – contraction/detachment phase

With further contraction and retraction, the myometrium under the lower pole of the placenta begins to contract with a reduction in the surface area. Consequently the shearing forces cause the placenta to tear away from the spongy layer of the decidua. With the onset of placental detachment the wave of separation passes upwards and the remaining placenta detaches, with the uppermost part of the placenta detaching last. At this point the maternal sinuses within the decidua are exposed. The oblique muscle fibres surrounding the blood vessels contract, sealing off the torn ends of the maternal vessels, helping to prevent haemorrhage.

### Phase 3 – expulsion phase

The placenta descends into the lower uterine segment, causing the membranes (which had begun to detach from the uterine wall as the internal cervical os dilated) to peel away from the walls of the uterus. As the uterus contracts, the placenta descends into the vagina, assisted by gravity, with the membranes following.

The placenta and membranes are then expelled by maternal effort. The fetal surface appears first at the vulva, with the membranes behind, and any blood loss is contained within this – the 'Schultze' method of expulsion (Fig. 35.1A). Sometimes the lower edge of the placenta descends first, so that the maternal surface appears at the vulva, sliding out lengthways with membranes (Fig. 35.1B). This is a slower process, with increased blood loss (the mechanisms to control haemorrhage are less effective when the placenta is still partially attached) – also known as the 'Matthews Duncan' method of expulsion.

**Figure 35.1** Methods of placental expulsion. (A) Schultze; (B) Matthews Duncan

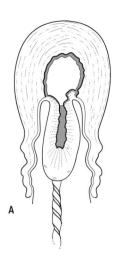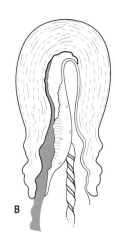

Brandt (1933) demonstrated by radiographic studies that the placenta usually separates within 3 minutes of the birth of the baby. Herman (2000) suggests that the duration of the third stage is dependent on the length of the latent phase; however, the time taken for the descent and expulsion of the placenta and membranes can also vary individually, influenced by factors such as posture and whether the third stage is managed actively or expectantly.

### Signs of separation and descent

These are not absolute and may occur for other reasons:

- Bleeding: 30–60 mL of blood may trickle from the vagina (this may also occur with a partially separated placenta, although bleeding is often heavier, or from a laceration)
- Lengthening of the cord: this occurs as the placenta descends, but may also occur if the cord is coiled and then straightens out
- Uterus becomes globular, hard, high, mobile and ballottable: this is assessed by palpating the fundus and should be undertaken with caution as it may cause irregular contractions, resulting in partially separated placenta and membranes, and excessive bleeding. The fundus is palpable below the umbilicus, and is broad, until placental separation and descent into the lower uterine segment. The fundal height increases, usually above the umbilicus, with the fundus narrowing (Fig. 35.2).

### Control of haemorrhage

Bleeding from the placental site can be profuse and rapid, as the placental circulation is approximately 500–800 mL/minute at term. It is imperative that haemorrhage is controlled. The body attempts to do this in three ways:

**Figure 35.2** Position of the uterus before and after placental separation

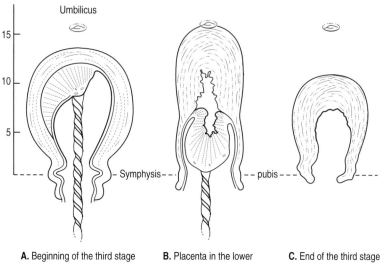

Umbilicus

— Symphysis — — — pubis — — —

**A.** Beginning of the third stage  **B.** Placenta in the lower segment  **C.** End of the third stage

1. The middle oblique fibres of the uterus contract and retract, constricting the blood vessels running through them. This causes the vessels to kink, slowing down and stopping the blood flow, allowing for clot formation at the placental site
2. The walls of the uterus become in apposition to each other, exerting pressure on the placental site
3. The blood clotting mechanism begins to work at the placental site, within the sinuses and torn vessels. The damaged tissue releases thrombokinase, converting prothrombin to thrombin. This combines with fibrinogen to form fibrin, which then combines with platelets to form a clot. Vitamin K, calcium and the other clotting factors are required for this process to happen efficiently.

## Clamping of the umbilical cord

The custom of cutting the cord was introduced in the 17th century, coinciding with the practice of giving birth in bed. Consequently, the bedding would become soaked and the practice of clamping the cord became widespread to reduce this.

Placental separation relies on the ability of the uterus to contract and retract. If the cord is clamped, a counter-resistance is set up in the placenta, preventing the transfer of blood to the baby. The size of the placenta does not reduce as much and this can inhibit contraction and retraction, resulting in a slower separation process. The effect of this is twofold:

1. the delay in complete separation means there is delay in sealing off the torn maternal vessels, resulting in a retroplacental clot and increasing the risk of haemorrhage

2. the cervix may retract before the placenta is expelled, resulting in a retained placenta, which often necessitates a manual removal of the placenta and membranes under an epidural, spinal or general anaesthetic.

### Clamping the cord and Rhesus isoimmunisation

When the cord is clamped, more fetal blood remains in the placenta, increasing the pressure within the placenta. As the uterus contracts, the pressure increases further and the surface placental vessels rupture. Fetal blood cells are released into the uterine cavity and may pass into the maternal circulation. Thus active management can increase the risk of feto-maternal transfusion (Enkin et al 2000). If the baby is Rhesus positive and the woman is Rhesus negative, she will produce antibodies against the Rhesus positive blood cells. Rhesus isoimmunisation can affect future pregnancies, as the antibodies are small enough to pass through to the placenta and will haemolyse fetal cells if the fetus is Rhesus positive. All Rhesus negative women should receive anti-D immunoglobulin at birth if the baby is Rhesus positive to reduce the risk of isoimmunisation occurring.

### Clamping the cord and the effect on the baby

During the third stage 75–125 mL of blood can be transferred from the placenta to the baby while the cord is still pulsating. This extra blood may be required for the newly established pulmonary circulation. Early cord clamping reduces the amount of blood transferred to the baby, with resulting hypovolaemia. This may be a factor in the development and severity of respiratory distress syndrome. Early cord clamping may also compromise the baby who is born with low haemoglobin. Kinmond et al (1993) found that delayed cord clamping, allowing the transfer of blood to the baby, improved the outcome for preterm babies.

If an oxytocic drug is given and the cord is not clamped, there is a risk of overtransfusion, as blood is forced from the placenta to the baby who can receive half of his entire blood volume again. This increases the risk of jaundice developing and, if already compromised, may create circulatory overload. It is important that the cord is clamped early if an oxytocic drug is given to avoid this.

If the baby is placed 40 cm below the introitus, placental transfusion is completed physiologically within 30 seconds; if the baby is above this level, the process is delayed. If an oxytocic drug is required, the baby could be kept below the level of the introitus for 30 seconds (ideal if the woman is upright, on all fours or squatting; difficult if she is semi-recumbent or in left lateral). The oxytocic drug can then be given and the cord clamped. The maternal end could remain unclamped to reduce interference with the physiological process.

# Management of the third stage

## Expectant management

This is either expectant (physiological, passive) or active.

This is delivery of the placenta without intervention – no oxytocic drug, no cord clamping unless it has stopped pulsating, no controlled traction, no palpation of the abdomen. The placenta is delivered by maternal effort, assisted by gravity and the baby suckling at the breast. Signs of separation and descent are seen.

Expectant management is associated with a higher blood loss (Prendiville et al 2004), partly because blood loss measurement is more accurate. Provided this is not excessive and the woman is not compromised, it may be a physiological loss with which the body can cope. Wickham (1999) suggests that the blood loss in the postnatal period is less when the third stage is managed expectantly compared with active management.

Expectant management can take longer to complete than one that is actively managed – up to 1 hour. Provided the woman's condition remains stable, with no excessive bleeding, there is no cause for concern. This may be a time when breastfeeding is initiated, with the added benefit of increased oxytocin release to promote uterine contraction.

## Principles of expectant management

- The midwife continues to wear the gloves worn for delivery of the baby and ensures the woman's bladder is empty
- Note the time of delivery of the baby
- Encourage the woman to adopt an upright position
- Place a bedpan or suitable receptacle under the woman, for the placenta to be expelled into
- Observe the condition of the woman throughout, particularly any blood loss per vaginam, recording the maternal pulse every 15 minutes or more frequently if indicated
- Do not touch the cord, allowing it to stop pulsating naturally
- Encourage and assist the woman to breast feed
- Do not palpate the uterus unless blood loss becomes excessive
- Encourage the woman to deliver the placenta by her own efforts, bearing down to expel the placenta
- Note the time the placenta and membranes are expelled (usually within 1 hour of the birth)
- The cord can be clamped and cut when it has stopped pulsating, applying the clamp 3–4 cm from the abdominal wall (longer if the baby is preterm, as catheterisation of the umbilical vein may be required; this is more successful when the cord is longer)
- Assess the condition of the woman, noting the condition of the uterus, amount of blood loss, pulse and blood pressure following completion of the third stage; the condition of the genital tract

should also be determined, suturing can be undertaken when appropriate
- Assist the woman into a comfortable position, removing any soiled linen; if all her observations are within the expected parameters, leave the woman and her baby together (with her partner or labour supporter), ensuring the call bell is close at hand
- Examine the placenta (Ch. 36) and record total blood loss
- Dispose of the placenta and equipment correctly
- Document findings and act accordingly.

If the woman wishes to have an expectant third stage but the umbilical cord has been severed, the maternal end of the cord should be cut 2–3 cm above the clamp and the cord placed in a sterile receiver. This will allow a limited amount of blood to drain from the placenta, helping to reduce its overall size. The principles of management are the same. However, this is not as effective and may inhibit the physiological process. In the presence of any signs of haemorrhage, an oxytocic drug may be required and the third stage actively managed. Blood drained from the placenta should not be included in the total estimate of blood loss following delivery, being placental and not maternal blood.

## Active management

This involves the administration of an oxytocic drug, early cord clamping and delivery of the placenta using controlled cord traction (CCT). It is often quicker than a physiological third stage, with a reduced blood loss; however, the oxytocic drugs can have unpleasant side effects and there is a higher incidence of retained placenta (Prendiville et al 2004). Prendiville et al (2004) suggest active management should be the management of choice for deliveries in maternity hospitals. Traditionally, active management does not require signs of separation to be seen prior to undertaking CCT (Spencer 1962). Levy (1990), however, recommends awaiting these signs, suggesting that when CCT is attempted before signs of separation are seen and is unsuccessful, blood loss is increased. Further research is required as to whether or not to wait for signs of separation as the results are inconclusive.

The use of oxytocic drugs has been a major contributor in the reduction in maternal deaths from PPH (DoH 1996); active management is recommended for women considered to be at high risk of PPH. These include:

- previous PPH
- grande multiparity
- fibroids
- multiple pregnancy
- polyhydramnios

- anaemia
- pre-eclampsia
- antepartum haemorrhage, both placental abruption and placenta praevia
- tocolytic drugs given for preterm labour
- induced labour
- augmented labour
- prolonged labour
- precipitate labour
- general anaesthesia.

## Oxytocic drugs

These are drugs that stimulate the uterus to contract and consist of oxytocin, in the form of Syntocinon, ergometrine or a combination of the two. They are administered prophylactically during active management to reduce the risk of PPH or as part of the emergency management of PPH to arrest bleeding.

### Syntocinon

Syntocinon causes the uterus to contract rhythmically and strongly, mainly the upper uterine segment, mimicking the body's actions. Given intravenously (I.V.) it takes effect within 40 seconds; with intramuscular (I.M.) use, it takes around 2–3 minutes to take effect. Its main side effect is fluid retention due to its antidiuretic nature. The usual dose is 5 or 10 units.

### Ergometrine

Ergometrine causes a non-physiological continuous spasm of the uterus and cervix, lasting for up to 2 hours; it is therefore a useful drug to give when a PPH is due to uterine atony. It also causes vasospasm, which can increase blood pressure and should not be administered routinely to hypertensive women. Constriction of the smooth muscle of the bronchioles may also occur, which may be problematic for women with asthma. Given I.V., it takes effect within 40 seconds; with I.M. use, it takes around 5–7 minutes. The usual dose is 0.25–0.5 mg. The side effects are mainly related to the effects of smooth muscle contraction and include tinnitus, headache, chest pain and palpitations, cramp-like pains in the back and legs, nausea and vomiting, a sharp rise in blood pressure, and a decreased prolactin level; if the woman has had a general anaesthetic, ergometrine increases the risk of acute pulmonary or cerebral oedema post-delivery.

### Syntometrine

This is composed of ergometrine 0.5 mg and Syntocinon 5 units in 1 mL. It combines the effects of the two drugs and is commonly the drug of choice when the third stage is being actively managed; unfortunately it also combines the side effects of the two drugs. Compared with Syntocinon alone, it significantly reduces the risk of PPH when the blood loss is less than 1000 mL (McDonald et al 1998).

When an oxytocic drug is to be administered prophylactically, it is usually given I.M. as the anterior shoulder is being delivered, as this provides sufficient time for the drug to take effect before delivering the placenta. If there is more than one baby to be delivered, the oxytocic drug should be administered as the anterior shoulder of the final baby is delivered.

## Principles of active management

- As the anterior shoulder of the baby is born, an oxytocic drug is given
- Clamp and cut the cord at birth, ensuring both ends are secure, placing the maternal end (often clamped with artery forceps) in a sterile receiver, positioned close to the vulva
- Place a sterile towel over the woman's abdomen and place the non-dominant hand over the fundus and await a contraction, keeping the hand still, during which time signs of placental separation and descent may be seen
- When the uterus is contracted, place the non-dominant hand above the symphysis pubis, with the thumb and fingers stretched across the abdomen and palm facing inwards (Fig. 35.3)
- Grasp the cord with the dominant hand and apply steady downward traction (controlled cord traction); at the same time, push the uterus upwards towards the umbilicus with the non-dominant hand (to reduce the risk of uterine inversion)
- Controlled cord traction is best achieved if the midwife is able to keep the hand applying traction close to the vulva. The grip should be secure by holding the artery forceps on the cord close to the vulva, as the cord lengthens the clamp should be moved up to remain near to the vulva. Alternatively, wrap the cord around the fingers of the dominant hand, moving them nearer the vulva; as necessary
- If resistance is felt, stop, relieve the pressure from the dominant then the non-dominant hand (the placenta may not have separated) and wait for a minute before attempting again, ensuring the uterus is contracted
- When the placenta appears at the vulva, traction should be applied in an upward direction to follow the curve of the birth canal
- The non-dominant hand is moved down to help ease the placenta into the receiver, allowing the membranes to be expelled slowly
- If there is any difficulty delivering the membranes, they should be 'teased out' either by moving them gently up and down (artery forceps can be positioned on the membranes to help with this) or by

**Figure 35.3** Position of hand to 'guard' the uterus during controlled cord traction

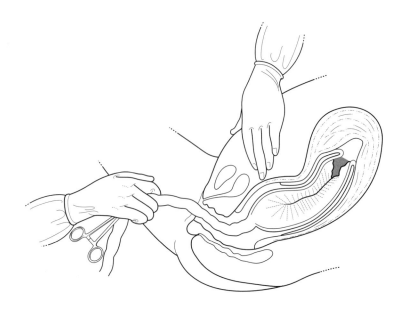

twisting the placenta round to make the membranes into a rope-like structure, either way encouraging the membranes to separate and be expelled

- Observe the condition of the woman throughout, particularly any blood loss per vaginam
- Note the time the placenta and membranes are expelled (often within 5–10 minutes)
- Assess the condition of the woman, noting the condition of the uterus, amount of blood loss, pulse and blood pressure following completion of the third stage; the condition of the genital tract should also be determined, suturing can be undertaken when appropriate
- Assist the woman into a comfortable position, removing soiled sheets; if all her observations are within the expected parameters, leave the woman and her baby together (with her partner or labour supporter), ensuring the call bell is close at hand
- Examine the placenta (Ch. 36) and record total blood loss
- Dispose of the placenta and equipment correctly
- Document findings and act accordingly.

Once third stage management is complete the delivery records are completed in detail, including the birth notification. The new family are given time together, vital sign observations are checked, as is the woman's uterus and lochial loss. Refreshments are given and the baby care is attended to; infant feeding should begin.

# Estimation of blood loss

Estimating blood loss is notoriously inaccurate, with estimates usually lower than the actual amount of blood lost. Brant (1967) demonstrated that although blood loss up to 300 mL was accurately assessed, blood loss in excess of this was generally underestimated. Haswell (1981) used a pouch situated under the woman's buttocks to 'catch' the blood loss and suggested that blood loss over 500 mL was usually underestimated by half. Levy and Moore (1985) conducted a small study to assess midwives' ability to assess blood loss accurately. They set up four trolleys with blood, mixed with fluid to simulate amniotic fluid, spread around on drapes and jugs. As the actual amount of blood increased, the accuracy of the estimation reduced, e.g. 100 mL blood loss was estimated as 111 mL (mean), 300 mL blood loss was estimated as 197 mL (mean), with 500 mL the mean estimate was 307 mL and, when the blood loss was 1200 mL, the mean estimated blood loss was 718 mL.

Blood loss should be estimated as accurately as possible. This includes blood loss on disposable sheets, linen and collected within receivers during and after the third stage. It is important to retrieve as much blood from the sheets as possible into a container for measurement. Obvious blood loss can be measured in a jug, but when the blood has seeped onto the sheets, it becomes harder to estimate blood loss.

The woman who has an expectant third stage often delivers the placenta into a bedpan, or container, enabling blood loss to be collected more easily. The increased blood loss with an expectant third stage may be due (in some instances) to the more efficient collection of blood.

The estimated amount of blood loss should be documented appropriately and referral should be made if this is excessive or the woman is compromised.

# Examination of the genital tract following delivery

Trauma to the cervix, vagina, labia and perineum can increase blood loss, cause increased pain for the woman or result in infection. The midwife should examine the woman's genital tract following birth to ascertain the degree of trauma and whether suturing is indicated. Bruising and oedema may be evident, which can affect the examination. The area is likely to be extremely tender, and the examination should be undertaken sensitively; the woman may use Entonox. It is important that there is a good light source to visualise the genital tract clearly.

| PROCEDURE | examination of the genital tract |
|---|---|

- Explain the procedure to the woman and gain informed consent
- The midwife continues to wear the gloves that have been used for the delivery of the placenta and membranes
- Ask the woman to adopt an almost recumbent position, with her knees bent, ankles together and knees parted
- Wash down the external genitalia gently with a sterile swab, wiping from front to back, using the swab once only to remove any blood or debris
- Examine the vulva, noting any trauma, particularly to the labia
- Wrap a sterile swab around the first two fingers of the examining hand, fingers slightly parted
- Separate the labia gently with the fingers of the non-examining hand and insert the swabbed fingers carefully into the vagina, directing the fingers in a downwards and backwards direction
- Gently press down to examine the anterior and side walls of the vagina and cervix (if the cervix cannot be seen, the woman may need to lie flat) for trauma, replacing the gauze as necessary
- Slowly begin to remove the swabbed fingers from the vagina, examining the posterior vaginal wall
- When the fingers have been removed, examine the perineum for trauma
- Assist the woman into a comfortable position and discuss the findings
- Suturing may be undertaken when appropriate (Ch. 37)
- Dispose of equipment appropriately
- Document findings and act accordingly.

## Summary

- The third stage of labour is concerned with the delivery of the placenta and membranes and the control of haemorrhage
- During this stage, the woman is at increased risk of morbidity and mortality from haemorrhage
- The placenta and membranes may be delivered expectantly (by the woman) or actively (by the midwife)
- Active management decreases the length of the third stage and the blood loss, but is associated with increased side effects from the oxytocic drugs and retained placenta

## Role and responsibilities of the midwife

These can be summarised as:

- undertaking the procedures correctly
- recognising deviations from the norm and instigating referral
- appropriate record keeping.

- Estimation of blood loss is often inaccurate and under-assessed; as the blood loss increases, this inaccuracy also increases
- The genital tract should be examined following delivery of the placenta and membranes for signs of trauma.

---

**Self-assessment exercises**

The answers to the following questions may be found in the text:

1. Describe the physiology of the third stage of labour.
2. What is the midwife's role when the third stage is to be expectant?
3. What are the side effects of Syntocinon and ergometrine?
4. How is controlled cord traction applied?
5. How is blood loss estimated?
6. How does the midwife assess the genital tract for trauma following delivery of the placenta and membranes?

---

## REFERENCES

Brandt M 1933 The mechanism and management of the third stage of labour. American Journal of Obstetrics and Gynecology 23:662–667

Brant H A 1967 Precise estimation of postpartum haemorrhage: difficulties and importance. British Medical Journal 1:398–400

CEMD 2004 Why mothers die. The Confidential Enquiries into Maternal Deaths in the United Kingdom 2000–2002. RCOG Press, London

DoH (Department of Health) 1996 Report on confidential enquiries into maternal deaths in the United Kingdom 1991–1993. HMSO, London

Enkin M, Keirse M J N C, Neilson J et al (eds) 2000 The third stage of labour. In: A guide to effective care in pregnancy and childbirth, 3rd edn. Oxford University Press, Oxford, ch 33

Haswell J N 1981 Measured blood loss at delivery. Journal of Indiana State Medical Association 74(1):34–36

Herman A 2000 Complicated third stage of labor: time to switch on the scanner. Ultrasound in Obstetrics and Gynecology 15:89–95

Herman A, Zimerman A, Arieli S et al 2002 Down–up sequential separation of the placenta. Ultrasound in Obstetrics and Gynecology 19:278–281

Kinmond S, Aitchison T C, Holland B M 1993 Umbilical cord clamping and preterm infants: a randomised trial. British Medical Journal 306:172–175

Krapp M, Baschat A A, Hankeln M et al 2000 Greyscale and color Doppler sonography in the third stage of labor for early detection of failed placental separation. Ultrasound in Obstetrics and Gynecology 15(2):138–142

Levy V 1990 The midwife's management of the third stage of labour. In: Alexander J, Levy V, Roch S (eds) Intrapartum care: a research-based approach. Macmillan, London, ch 7

Levy V, Moore J 1985 The midwife's management of the third stage of labour. Nursing Times 1(5): 47–50

McDonald S, Prendiville W J, Elbourne D 1998 Prophylactic syntometrine vs oxytocin in the third stage of labour (Cochrane Review). Cochrane Library, Issue 3. Update Software, Oxford

Prendiville W J, Elbourne D, McDonald S 2004 Active versus expectant management in the third stage of labour (Cochrane Review). Cochrane Library, Issue 3. Update Software, Oxford

Spencer P M 1962 Controlled cord traction in the management of the third stage of labour. British Medical Journal 1:1728–1732

Wickham S 1999 Further thoughts on the third stage of labour. The Practising Midwife 2(10):14–15

# Chapter 36

# Principles of intrapartum skills — examination of the placenta

Examination of the placenta following delivery is an important skill undertaken by the midwife to reduce the occurrence of both postpartum haemorrhage and infection. This chapter describes the structure and appearance of the placenta, discussing the significance of deviations, and concluding with the procedure for undertaking examination of the placenta.

**Learning outcomes**

Having read this chapter the reader should be able to:

- describe the structure and appearance of the placenta at term
- describe how the placenta is examined
- discuss the significance of the information obtained from the examination
- discuss the role and responsibilities of the midwife in relation to examining the placenta.

## Structure and appearance

The placenta is a disc-shaped structure that has both maternal and fetal surfaces. At term, the placenta weighs approximately 500–600 g (about one-sixth of the baby's weight), has a diameter of 15–20 cm and is 2–3 cm thick. Early cord clamping may result in the placenta being proportionally heavier, whereas late cord clamping can produce a placenta that is proportionally lighter, due to the amount of blood transfused from the placenta to the baby at delivery. A larger placenta may be associated with maternal diabetes and multiple pregnancy, a smaller placenta with chronic intrauterine growth restriction.

Occasionally the placenta may develop with an abnormal structure and appearance such as a circumvallate placenta. The placenta enlarges beneath the endometrial surface and the embryonic sac enlarges above it; the endometrium between the two is compressed and obliterated resulting in an acellular membrane, which may affect the attachment of the placenta to the decidua, increasing the risk of placental abruption. The placenta has a thick, grey/white raised ring around the central part of the fetal surface, caused by the fetal membranes folding back on themselves (Blackburn & Loper 1992).

### Fetal surfaces of the placenta

The fetal side has a white shiny appearance due to the chorionic plate (a thin membrane continuous with the chorion) and the amnion that cover the surface. The fetal side is composed of 50–60 lobes or cotyledons, which are further divided into 1–5 lobules. Occasionally, the placenta may be divided into two (bipartite) or three (tripartite) separate, distinct lobes, each with an umbilical cord inserted into it. The cord presents as one cord until it is near the placental surface when it divides into two or three to supply each lobe (Fig. 36.1).

Blood vessels, branches of the umbilical vein and arteries are clearly visible, spreading outwards from the point of cord insertion, usually centrally or slightly off centre (Fig. 36.2A,B). A cord inserted at the edge of the placenta – a 'battledore' insertion (Fig. 36.2C) – is usually insignificant, although the attachment may be fragile, increasing the risk of detachment during controlled cord traction. Rarely the cord is inserted into the membranes – a 'velamentous' insertion (Fig. 36.2D) – with vessels running through the membranes to the placenta. The attachment can be very fragile, resulting in detachment during controlled cord traction. The vessels may overlie the cervix ('vasa praevia') and if ruptured during spontaneous or artificial rupturing of the membranes will result in massive fetal haemorrhage.

The umbilical cord contains the two umbilical arteries and the umbilical vein, surrounded by Wharton's jelly, and is covered by the amnion. A cord with fewer than three vessels may indicate a congenital abnormality; the baby should be referred to the paediatrician and a sample of the cord may be required for analysis. The cord is 50 cm long (range 30–90 cm), 1–2 cm wide and is twisted spirally to provide

**Figure 36.1**  Bipartite placenta

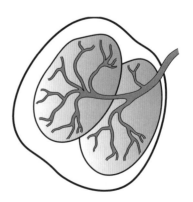

**Figure 36.2** Cord insertions. (A) central; (B) eccentric; (C) battledore; (D) velamentous

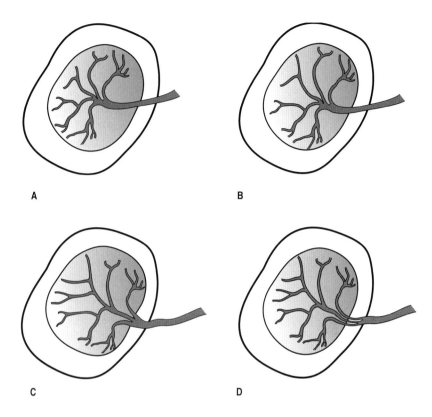

A

B

C

D

some protection to the vessels from pressure. A short cord is one measuring less than 40 cm and is usually insignificant unless very short when descent of the fetus through the pelvis will cause the cord to be pulled taut and apply traction on the placenta. A long cord may become wrapped around the fetus or knotted, resulting in occlusion of the vessels. The risk of cord presentation and prolapse increases with a long cord, particularly if the presenting part is poorly applied to the cervix. False knots can occur when the blood vessels are longer than the cord and form a loop in the Wharton's jelly; these are of little significance. A thick or thin cord may be difficult to clamp securely following delivery.

The amnion and chorion comprise the fetal membranes, which appear fused but are not. Stripping one from the other can separate them; the amnion can be pulled back to the cord. The amnion is smooth, translucent and tough, whereas the chorion is thick, opaque and friable. The chorion begins at the edge of the placenta and extends around the decidua. Following delivery, the membranes will have a hole in them through which the baby has been born. If the membranes appear ragged, a piece of membrane may be retained in utero. This can affect uterine contractility and predispose to postpartum haemorrhage. It also provides a site for microorganisms to grow, predisposing to infection. The passage of any clots postpartum should be examined for membranes.

### Maternal surfaces of the placenta

The dark red maternal side is composed of 15–20 cotyledons (divided by septa) which have arisen from two or more main stem villi and their branches. During the second and third trimesters, fibrin deposition may occur around the villi resulting in isolated villi infarction. This is usually insignificant unless excessive, affecting the exchange of nutrients and waste products between the maternal and fetal circulation, resulting in intrauterine growth restriction. Calcification due to lime salt deposition on the surface can make it feel gritty; this is insignificant. Occasionally, a cotyledon may be present in the membranes, separated from the placenta but connected by a blood vessel – a 'succenturiate' lobe (Fig. 36.3). If this is retained in utero, it predisposes to postpartum haemorrhage and infection as for the retained membrane. The membranes should be carefully examined for evidence of missing lobes, suspected if an unexplained hole appears in the chorion, particularly if blood vessels run towards the hole and stop abruptly.

A pale placenta may reflect delayed clamping of the cord, where less blood is retained in the placenta; it could also indicate intrauterine anaemia. Meconium may also be seen on the fetal surface, as may signs of infection and hyperbilirubinaemia. An offensive smelling placenta is often indicative of intrauterine infection.

---

PROCEDURE    **examination of the placenta**

- Explain the procedure to the parents and ascertain if they wish to observe the examination
- Gather equipment:
  — gloves and apron
  — disposable protective cover
  — disposal bag for placenta
  — placenta

**Figure 36.3**  Succenturiate lobe

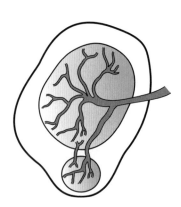

- Wash hands, apply gloves and apron
- Lay the placenta, fetal surface uppermost, onto the cover (placed on a flat surface) noting the size, shape, smell and colour
- Examine the cord, noting the length, insertion point and presence of knots
- Count the number of vessels in the cut end of the cord (if the end has been obliterated, cut off a small portion of the cord and count the vessels in the portion remaining)
- Observe the fetal surface for irregularities
- Taking hold of the cord with the non-dominant hand, lift the placenta from the surface and examine the hole in the membranes and replace on surface
- Spread the membranes outwards, looking for extra vessel or lobes, or unexplained holes
- Separate the amnion and chorion, pulling the amnion back over the base of the umbilical cord
- Turn the placenta over, maternal side uppermost
- Examine the cotyledons, ensuring all are present, noting the size and amount of areas of infarction or blood clots
- Weigh or swab the placenta if indicated
- Dispose of the placenta and equipment correctly
- Wash hands
- Discuss the findings with the parents
- Document findings and act accordingly.

If cord blood is required (e.g. when the mother is rhesus negative), McDonald (2003) suggests this should be obtained from the fetal surface of the placenta as the blood vessels are congested and visible. Sampling should be undertaking quickly before the blood clots and is usually undertaken before the placenta is examined.

In some maternity units the placentae are collected and frozen for research purposes; this may entail either the placenta or cord. Cord blood can be donated to the London Cord Blood Bank and used for a variety of haematological conditions, e.g. leukaemia (Fursland 1998). Histological investigation may be required in certain situations, e.g. multiple deliveries, preterm deliveries, stillbirths, suspected infection.

## Role and responsibilities of the midwife

These can be summarised as:

- undertaking the examination correctly
- recognising deviations from the norm and instigating referral
- appropriate use of standard precautions
- appropriate record keeping.

## Summary

- The placenta has fetal and maternal components; both sides should be examined carefully
- The placenta should be examined to ensure it is complete; retained products predispose to postpartum haemorrhage and infection
- Deviations from the norm can indicate underlying problems for the baby, e.g. infection, congenital abnormality
- Standard precautions should always be followed when handling and disposing of the placenta.

## Self-assessment exercises

The answers to the following questions may be found in the text:

1. Describe the general appearance of the placenta at term.
2. What are the differences between the fetal and maternal placental surfaces?
3. Describe the procedure for examining the placenta.
4. List the deviations that can be detected and discuss the significance of each.
5. What are the role and responsibilities of the midwife in relation to the examination of the placenta?

## REFERENCES

Blackburn S T, Loper D 1992 Maternal, fetal and neonatal physiology: a clinical perspective. W B Saunders, Philadelphia

Fursland E 1998 Blood mothers. Nursing Times 94(33):42–43

McDonald S 2003 Physiology and management of the third stage of labour. In: Fraser D M, Cooper M A (eds) Myles textbook for midwives, 14th edn. Churchill Livingstone, Edinburgh, p 507–530

Chapter **37**

# Principles of intrapartum skills — perineal repair

This chapter examines the procedure, technique and materials used for perineal repair. The anatomy of the pelvic floor is reviewed and the significance of correct perineal repair is highlighted. The reader is encouraged to read widely in other literary sources to appreciate the associated issues (e.g. prevention of perineal trauma, postnatal perineal care).

**Learning outcomes**

Having read this chapter the reader should be able to:

- discuss the role and responsibilities of the midwife when completing perineal repair
- discuss the current evidence for the choice of materials and the technique used
- state the aims of perineal repair
- describe how to infiltrate the perineum
- demonstrate tying a knot, continuous locked, non-locked and subcuticular sutures
- list the factors that should be included with record keeping.

## The pelvic floor

As a hammock-shaped arrangement of muscles and fascia, the pelvic floor is the supportive structure in the woman's pelvis. The muscles are arranged in two layers, deep and superficial (Fig. 37.1). They extend to and from landmarks in the pelvis, encircling other structures (e.g. the vagina) and forming the perineal body. The perineal body is triangular in shape, consisting of skin, two superficial muscles (bulbocavernosus and transverse perineal) and one deep muscle (pubococcygeus). It lies between the anus and vagina and is flattened and displaced as the baby is born. The pelvic floor prevents all of the pelvic organs from

**Figure 37.1** (A) Deep muscle layer of the pelvic floor; (B) superficial muscle layer of the pelvic floor

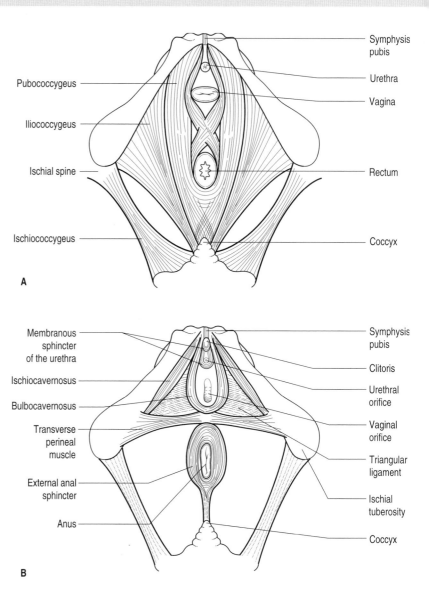

prolapsing and is clearly significant for the correct functioning of the vagina, bladder, uterus and rectum. A pelvic floor that is damaged or weakened may cause long-term urinary, faecal or sexual morbidity.

## Aims of perineal repair

Repairing perineal trauma aims to ensure that the tissues are correctly realigned, haemorrhage is stemmed and dead space (into which bleeding may occur) is reduced. The overall aim is to maintain the integrity of the woman's pelvic floor.

On examining the genital tract immediately post-delivery the extent of any perineal damage is noted and decisions are made as to:

1. whether or not the damage requires repair
2. if so, using which materials
3. by whom
4. in which environment.

Definitions of perineal trauma are based around the structures involved; note that no classification is currently made as to the size of the injury. It may have occurred naturally or be a result of incision (episiotomy). The accepted definitions are:

- first degree: affects skin only
- second degree (tear or episiotomy): affects the skin, posterior vaginal wall and superficial muscle (occasionally deep muscle is affected)
- third degree: affects the same structures as a second degree as well as the anal sphincter
- fourth degree: affects all of the above as well as the rectal mucosa.

However, the damage may be to any part of the pelvic floor, perineal body or vulval tissue.

Suturing is the most likely means of repair, but there is some speculative research into the use of tissue adhesive (Adoni & Anteby 1991). It is the skill of the operator that is important; midwives can provide good continuity of care for the woman, but care needs to be evidence based, with training and updating and within one's capabilities. Hesitations about the task in hand, for whatever reason, should cause the midwife to refer to an obstetrician. The health and wellbeing of the woman may be seriously affected in both the short and long term if the repair is poorly completed (Sleep et al 1984). Extensive perineal damage or third or fourth degree injury requires repair by a senior obstetrician in theatre with additional analgesia (general or regional anaesthesia). Bilateral labial grazes that would be in apposition when standing or sitting should also be sutured so that the labia do not heal together. Arkin and Chern-Hughes (2001) cite a case study in which the labia needed surgically parting some months following abrasions in childbirth. Perineal repair can be undertaken in the home if adaptations are made to accommodate suitable positioning of the woman and midwife (with good light). If the repair is extensive, however, the midwife may consider transfer to a hospital environment.

## Current evidence

Draper and Newell (1996) suggest that failure to adhere to evidence-based practice with perineal repair may have wide-ranging consequences in women's lives. The body of research is now extensive (but still increasing) and therefore there is little excuse for diversity in practice. Kenyon and Ford (2004) discuss the process and implementation of an evidence-based accepted protocol in their maternity unit.

### Choice of material

Absorbable suture material not only reduces the need for suture removal but also has good tensile strength for up to 14 days. Kettle et al (2002) confirm that Vicryl Rapide reduces perineal pain and has less need to be removed when uncomfortable. Size 2/0 is indicated for perineal tissue.

### Instruments

There is little mention of instruments except that Bott (1999) recommends that midwives should learn to suture with instruments (needle holder and tissue forceps) rather than fingers, to reduce the risk of injury to the midwife and possible transfer of HIV. The DoH (1998) also recommends the use of blunt-ended needles for suturing to reduce these risks further.

### Technique

Perineal repair is often completed in three stages:

1. posterior vaginal wall
2. perineal muscle layer
3. perineal skin.

The vaginal wall is sutured using a loose continuous locked (blanket stitch) or non-locked suture. While Kettle et al (2002) recommend non-locked, Enkin et al (2000) note that concertinaing of the vaginal wall is less where the suture is locked. A two-stage procedure is advocated, i.e. the muscle layer is repaired in one or two layers using a continuous suture (Kettle et al 2002). While there are questions about the need to suture the muscle layers, Fleming et al (2003) suggested that healing at 6 weeks post-delivery was poorer where the muscles had not been sutured. Kenyon and Ford (2004) agree, indicating that the existing studies are small and therefore unreliable and that, at this time, suturing of the vaginal wall and muscle layers is indicated. McCandlish (2001) also suggests that it is time to seek the evidence, but not to change practice until reliable evidence exists.

The skin, following the Ipswich trial (Gordon et al 1998), may be left unsutured providing that the skin edges are in apposition with a gap no greater than 0.5 cm. This is considered to reduce dyspareunia at 3 months postpartum, but with no differences in short- or long-term perineal pain. However, if suturing is required (poor apposition or obvious haemorrhage), Kettle (1999) indicates that it should be a continuous subcuticular suture beginning at the distal end and working towards the vagina.

The current evidence may be summarised as:

- if indicated, a perineal wound should be sutured throughout using Vicryl Rapide, with a loose continuous locked or unlocked suture to the posterior vaginal wall and a continuous suture to the muscle layer, bringing the skin into good apposition

- if skin closure is indicated then a continuous subcuticular technique should be used
- for good practice (not evidence based) the midwife should consider standard precautions and use instruments to suture with and if possible blunt-ended needles.

# Perineal suturing

A successful perineal repair incorporates all of the following principles:

## Effective analgesia for the woman

Sanders et al (2002) indicate that pain while being sutured is greater than midwives may realise for women who do not have regional analgesia. The perineum should be infiltrated using lidocaine (lignocaine) according to an approved patient group direction; analgesics such as Entonox are also useful. Following repair Kenyon and Ford (2004) recommend rectal diclofenac 100 mg stat.

## Asepsis and standard precautions

A sterile suturing pack is used and the midwife wears gloves, apron and any other necessary items for infection control and protection purposes that local protocols suggest. Research into suitable fluids for perineal swabbing remains limited; water is widely used, but not proven (Jessiman 2001). Lubricant may also vary according to local protocols between water soluble (e.g. KY Jelly) and chlorhexidine Hibitane cream.

## Alignment of the tissues to encourage granulation and healing

The midwife should be very familiar with the pelvic floor anatomy and therefore be quite certain of the alignment of the tissues. The distinction in colour between the tissues is often very helpful. A good light source and access to the perineum (lithotomy position) is important in order for the repair to be completed properly. Occasionally the midwife may discover on examining the woman in lithotomy position that the tear is more extensive than originally thought. This allows decisions to be reviewed; if necessary an obstetrician is called. Equally, beginning in lithotomy position is better than having to move to lithotomy part way through the procedure. At home suitable alternatives can be found (e.g. sitting on the edge of the bed with legs supported on chairs). When aligned properly the process of wound healing begins (Ch. 55); sutures that are too tight or too loose may impede this process.

## Cessation of all haemorrhage

Suturing must achieve this in each part of the repair, otherwise haemorrhage can continue between the layers resulting in a haematoma or postpartum haemorrhage.

### Reduction of any dead space

Haemorrhage may occur into areas of dead space resulting in a haematoma as described above.

### Minimal amount of suture material

Any foreign material in tissue results in a reaction. Fewer knots and less suture material will result in improved healing.

## Infiltration of the perineum for repair

Using an aseptic technique, anaesthetic – usually lidocaine (lignocaine) – is infiltrated into the four aspects of the tear, along the left- and right-hand sides of the vaginal wall and perineum. The tissue is held with tissue forceps while the needle is inserted at point A (Fig. 37.2). The anaesthetic is instilled as the needle is withdrawn along line B to A, then the needle is reversed rather than removed so that the distance C to A is also infiltrated. It is then inserted into point D and the process repeated B to D, C to D.

### Using a needle holder

In appearance, the needle holder appears very similar to artery forceps, except that the grooves are designed to retain a better grip of the needle. The suture is placed in the packet in such a way that, as the packet is torn at the right-hand side, the needle is exposed in the correct position to attach the needle to the needle holder without having to remove the suture from the packet at that time. The suture is attached to the needle, the needle being appropriately shaped to reduce tissue trauma and also levelled off approximately one-third of the way along the needle to allow the needle holder to grasp it securely.

**Figure 37.2** Infiltration prior to suturing (Adapted with kind permission from Nisbet & Rouse 1992)

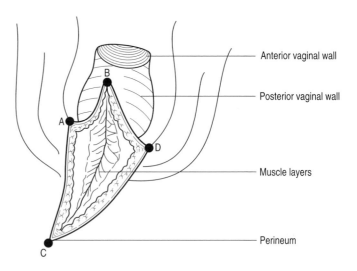

**Suturing techniques**

Described below are some of the basic suturing techniques. They are described for a right-handed midwife; a left-handed person will need to adapt these principles. Note that where there is any possible exposure to the needle, tissue forceps should be used to hold the tissue, rather than fingers (Bott 1999).

### Tying a knot

The knot is tied three times, to the right with two throws, to the left (one throw) and back to the right (one throw) so that it will not slip and will lie flat.

If it is a knot to anchor the suture then the short end is cut short and the stitching continues using the long end (Fig. 37.3).

### Continuous locked suture

This is suitable for use on the posterior vaginal wall. In order to ensure that the tear is repaired completely the apex of the tear must be located and clearly visualised:

1. The first stitch enters the tissue above the apex, where a knot is tied to anchor it
2. The short end is cut
3. The next stitch is placed below and parallel to the first one; the left hand applies slight tension to the thread on the left so that the needle emerges to the right of the thread that is held. This is the action of locking the suture (Fig. 37.4)
4. It is continued at approximately 1 cm intervals down the vaginal wall to the fourchette
5. The suture is tied by not locking the last stitch (emerging to the left of the held thread) and retaining a loop to act as the short end
6. The knot is then tied in the same way and may be buried for comfort.

Burying a knot is achieved by cutting the short end then passing the needle under the suture line to take the knot into the tissue. The long end is then cut (Fig. 37.5).

### Continuous non-locked suture

This is the same as a locked suture (above) except that the needle emerges each time to the left of the held thread (Fig. 37.6) and therefore follows the needle each time.

### Subcuticular suture to perineal skin

As the name suggests, the suture is beneath the skin. Beginning at the anal end, a knot is tied beneath the skin. To do this the needle is inserted deeply on the left-hand side of the tear, emerging (still on the left) superficially just below the skin. A knot is tied (Fig. 37.7). The needle is then reversed on the needle holder (the point of the needle

**Figure 37.3** Instrument tied knot: consisting of three throws to 'lock' and prevent slippage. Key: white thread, left side of suture material; black thread, right side of suture material (Adapted with kind permission from Nisbet & Rouse 1992)
(A–C) Holding the tissue with tissue forceps, use the needle holder to pass through tissue from right to left, leaving 8–10 cm on the right hand side; (D) hold needle holder in right hand parallel to tissue, grasp left thread between thumb and index finger of left hand, pass thread in front of and over needle holder;

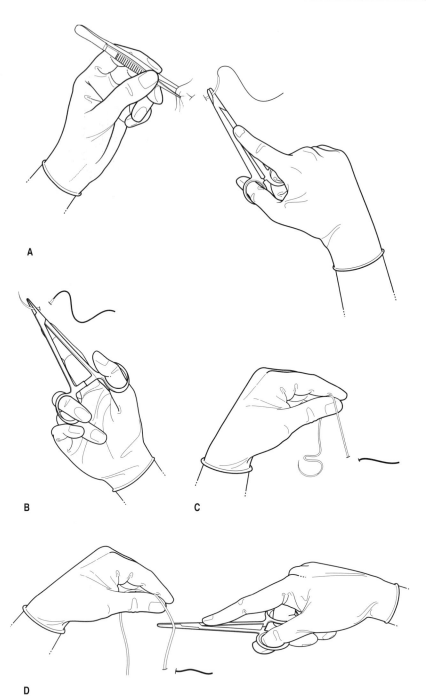

A

B

C

D

*Continues*

**Figure 37.3 cont'd** (E, F) wind two loops of left suture over needle holder, rotate needle holder from 9 o'clock to 11 o'clock position; (G) continue rotating needle holder until 1 o'clock position (right hand should be palm up at this stage), grasp right thread with needle holder as close to the end as possible; (H) pull right thread through loops of left thread;

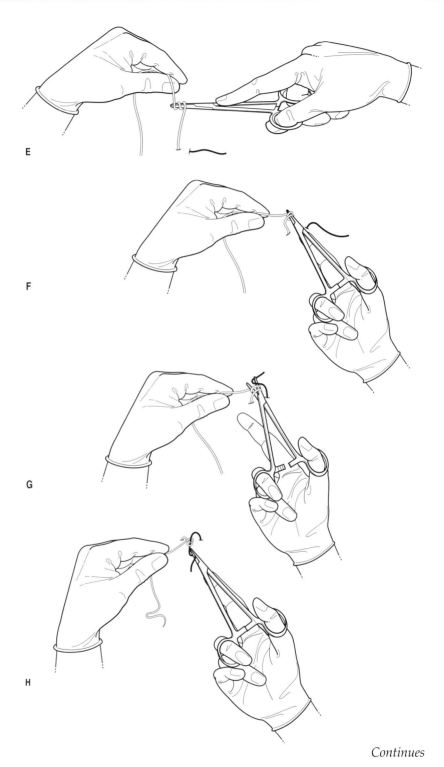

E

F

G

H

*Continues*

**Figure 37.3 cont'd** (I) pull right thread towards the left until the first knot forms, do not pull too tight: this completes the first throw; (J) second throw: hold needle holder in right hand parallel to tissue, grasp thread between thumb and index finger of left hand; (K) pass left thread behind and over needle holder just once; (L) grasp right thread with needle holder;

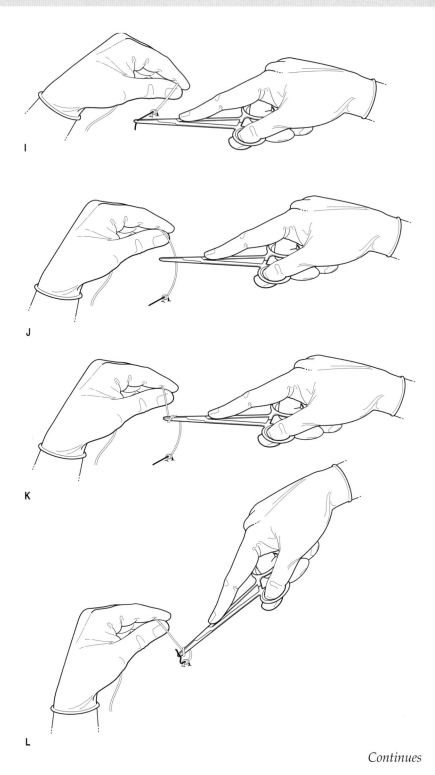

*Continues*

**Figure 37.3 cont'd** (M) pull right thread through loops of left thread; (N) continue pulling until knot is firm. Repeat the first throw (Fig. 37.3D–I) to 'lock' the suture, winding only one loop over the needle holder

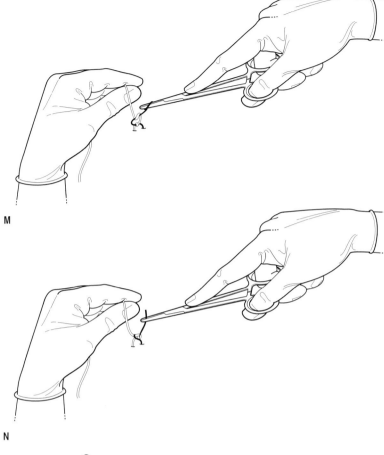

M

N

**Figure 37.4** Continuous locked suture (Adapted with kind permission from Nisbet & Rouse 1992)

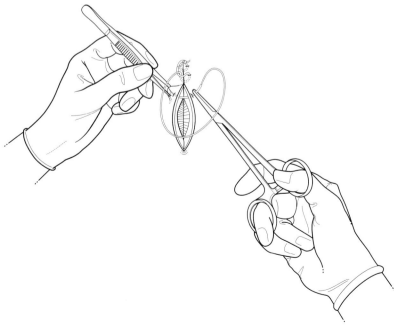

**Figure 37.5** Burying a knot

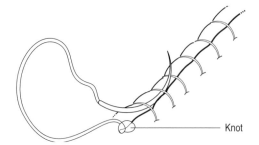

Knot

**Figure 37.6** Continuous non-locked suture (Adapted with kind permission from Nicol et al 2000)

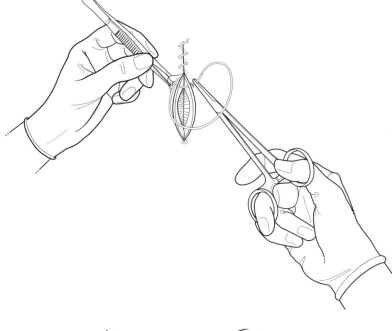

**Figure 37.7** Tying a subcutaneous knot

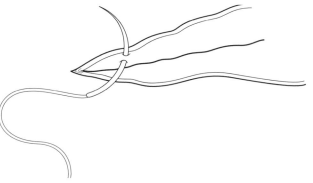

emerging to the right of the needle holder), and on the right-hand side of the tear the needle is entered superficially beneath the skin opposite the knot on the left. The needle emerges superficially (still on the right) at approximately the length of the needle. The next bite is taken along the left side of the incision, entering opposite where the last suture emerged on the right. The process is repeated until the fourchette is reached. A loop is retained with the last suture to tie off a knot. Both ends are cut. There should not be any suture material apparent on the outside of the perineum (Fig. 37.8).

## PROCEDURE perineal repair

- Obtain informed consent
- Gather equipment and place on a dressings trolley or suitable working surface:
  — sterile repair pack with sterile gown
  — water/lotion
  — plastic apron
  — sterile gloves
  — sterile sutures
  — lidocaine (lignocaine) with sterile needle (21 g green) and syringe
  — lubricant
- Correctly assist the woman into the lithotomy position. Keep covered. A stool should be available for the midwife to sit on and the light is positioned appropriately
- Put on apron and wash hands while the assistant opens the outer covering of the repair pack
- Open the pack and dry hands while the assistant slides the sterile gloves onto the sterile field
- Apply gloves and gown
- Check the swabs and instruments in the repair pack while the assistant adds lotion and lubricant to the bowl and gallipot, sutures, needle and syringe on to the sterile field
- Arrange the trolley in a way that suits
- Draw up the anaesthetic

Figure 37.8 (A–C)
Subcuticular suture to the skin
(Adapted with kind permission
from Nisbet & Rouse 1992)

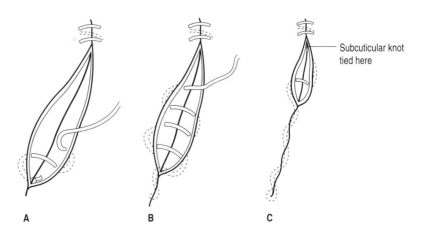

A          B          C

Subcuticular knot tied here

- Ask the assistant to remove the woman's sheet. Cleanse the vulva using the sponge holding forceps, working from top to bottom, using each swab only once
- Establish a sterile field beneath the woman's buttocks, over her legs and abdomen using the sterile towels and fenestrated drape
- Re-examine the genital tract to establish the extent of the trauma; refer if necessary
- Infiltrate the perineum as described above; time is given for anaesthesia to be achieved
- Insert a lubricated vaginal tampon to absorb the lochial loss so that visibility while suturing is good, attaching the tail to the sterile drapes using artery forceps
- Locate the apex, insert the first suture just above it and anchor with a knot
- Complete a continuous loose locked or non-locked suture (local protocol) down the vaginal wall. Secure it with a buried knot at the fourchette
- Locate the deep muscles and suture with a continuous non-locked suture. Repeat for the superficial muscles, securing with a buried knot if the skin is in good apposition (0.5 cm maximum gap)
- If the skin is not in good apposition, complete a subcuticular suture, beginning at the anal end and ending at the fourchette with a subcuticular knot
- Examine the vagina to establish that the tissue is in good alignment and that all haemorrhage has stopped
- Remove the tampon, examine the repair gently and insert one finger into the anus to establish that sutures have not gone through the rectal mucosa. Administer rectal analgesia if required
- Remove the drapes and assist the woman correctly from the lithotomy position, ensuring her comfort and dignity. Advise her re: ongoing perineal care
- Check the swabs, instruments and needles and dispose of sharps correctly
- Dispose of the equipment and wash hands
- Document the repair and act accordingly.

## Record keeping

The following should be included:

- date and time of the procedure
- nature and extent of the tear
- position of the woman
- drugs used
- tampon inserted *and* removed
- suture material used
- order of repair

- techniques used to which area
- examinations per vaginam and per rectum following the repair
- indication that all swabs, needles and instruments are correct
- legible signature of suturing midwife.

## Role and responsibilities of the midwife

These can be summarised as:

- appropriate assessment of the wound to establish who should suture, where, with which analgesic
- use of appropriate materials, technique, asepsis and standard precautions
- education and support of the woman before, during and following the procedure
- contemporaneous records.

## Summary

- Perineal repair is a very important procedure for which the midwife should be correctly trained and updated and able to acknowledge any limitations, thus referring. Undertaking audit is also good practice
- Evidence-based practice should be used with regard to the materials and techniques used
- The repair is a sterile procedure carried out in the lithotomy position, in which the aims include alignment of the tissue, stemming of all haemorrhage and reduction of dead space.

## Self-assessment exercises

The answers to the following questions may be found in the text:

1. What is the function of the pelvic floor?
2. When might a midwife ask a senior obstetrician to complete a perineal repair?
3. Describe how to successfully infiltrate the perineum prior to perineal repair.
4. List the aims of successful perineal repair.
5. What is the current material of choice for perineal repair?
6. Give a rationale for the technique used when suturing the posterior vaginal wall and the muscle layer.
7. What kind of technique should be used for the perineal skin if suturing is indicated?
8. Summarise the role and responsibilities of the midwife in relation to perineal repair.
9. List all the aspects of the repair that should be included in the records.
10. Find some suitable suturing equipment and demonstrate tying a knot, continuous locked, non-locked and subcuticular suturing.

## REFERENCES

Adoni A, Anteby E 1991 The use of Histoacryl for epi-siotomy repair. British Journal of Obstetrics and Gynaecology 98:476–478

Arkin A, Chern-Hughes B 2001 Case report: labial fusion postpartum and clinical management of labial lacera-tions. Journal of Midwifery and Women's Health 47(4):290–292

Bott J 1999 HIV risk reduction and the use of universal precautions. British Journal of Midwifery 7(11):671–675

DoH (Department of Health) 1998 Guidance for clinical health care workers. Protection against infection with blood borne viruses. The Stationery Office, London

Draper J, Newell R 1996 A discussion of some of the lit-erature relating to history, repair and consequences of perineal trauma. Midwifery 12:140–145

Enkin M, Keirse M J, Neilson J et al 2000 A guide to effective care in pregnancy and childbirth. Oxford University Press, Oxford

Fleming E, Hagen S, Niven C 2003 Does perineal sutur-ing make a difference? The SUNS trial. British Journal of Obstetrics and Gynaecology 110:684–689

Gordon B, Mackrodt C, Fern E et al 1998 The Ipswich Childbirth Study: 1. A randomised evaluation of two stage postpartum perineal repair leaving the skin unsutured. British Journal of Obstetrics and Gynaecology 105:435–440

Jessiman W 2001 Lotions and lubricants. The Practising Midwife 4(3):23–28

Kenyon S, Ford F 2004 How can we improve women's postbirth perineal health? MIDIRS Midwifery Digest 14(1):7–12

Kettle C 1999 Perineal care following in Jennifer Sleep's footsteps. British Journal of Midwifery 7(12): 760–762

Kettle C, Hills R, Jones P et al 2002 Continuous versus interrupted perineal repair with standard or rapidly absorbed sutures after spontaneous vaginal birth: a randomised controlled trial. Lancet 359(9325):2217–2223

McCandlish R 2001 Routine perineal suturing: is it time to stop? MIDIRS Midwifery Digest 11(3):296–300

Nicol M, Bavin C, Bedford-Turner S et al 2000 Essential nursing skills, 2nd edn. Mosby, Edinburgh

Nisbet M D, Rouse B A 1992 Perineal repair. Davis & Geck, Cyanamid Australia Pty. Ltd, Australia

Sanders J, Campbell R, Peters T 2002 Effectiveness of pain relief during perineal suturing. British Journal of Obstetrics and Gynaecology 109:1066–1068

Sleep J M, Grant A, Garcia J et al 1984 West Berkshire perineal management trial. British Journal of Medicine 289:587–590

# Chapter 38

# Principles of intrapartum skills — management of birth at home

This chapter focuses on the midwife's role and management of labour and delivery in the home setting. It highlights the considerations for care at home that are different from care in hospital; the reader will need to refer throughout to other relevant chapters (e.g. Chs 34, 35 and 36). For example, the physiology and management of the third stage of labour is not described here, but the considerations for managing it at home are discussed.

## Learning outcomes

Having read this chapter the reader should be able to:

- highlight the researched-based evidence that relates to safe delivery at home
- discuss the differences in skills and attitudes that the midwife utilises when managing birth at home
- discuss the value and principles of good preparation for all the parties concerned
- list the equipment and information that the midwife needs available
- discuss the overall role and responsibilities of the midwife when caring for labouring women at home.

## Safety

The current national average in the UK for births at home is approximately 2% (Hagelskamp et al 2003). Despite this there is evidence which suggests that for a healthy woman with a normal pregnancy and planned home birth:

- birth at home is safer than in hospital (Olsen & Jewell 2002), with no increase in maternal or infant mortality rates
- there are fewer interventions at home, e.g. episiotomies, with fewer low Apgar scores and severe lacerations (Olsen 1997)
- there is good psychological wellbeing (Hodnett 1989).

Safety is naturally enhanced by good preparation (see below), part of which includes low risk criteria to identify women suitable for home birth. The 5th Annual CESDI report (MCHRC 1998) gives a comprehensive list. Broadly it categorises women as being healthy, of normal height and weight, and between 16 and 35 years of age with a normal singleton pregnancy now and without risk factors from previous pregnancies that can affect labour. Parity should not be greater than four. Ongoing assessment throughout the pregnancy and labour will be necessary to ensure that the woman remains within the low risk criteria.

## Midwifery skills

There are many articles of opinion that share highly positive experiences for midwives and their practice as well as the women and families in their care (Cook 2003, Jones 2003, Kitzinger 2001). While midwives may have limited experiences of home birth, those that do often regard it as a professionally enhancing experience. Different skills are needed than when caring for women in hospital including issues such as:

- Needing a full understanding and confidence in labour physiology and a woman's ability to give birth naturally
- Fundamental midwifery skills using limited equipment, e.g. Pinard stethoscope or Doppler sonicaid use rather than cardiotocography monitor, delivery in alternative positions, management of pain with limited availability of pharmacological preparations
- 'Active inactivity': women who have planned their birth at home often assume a greater level of control. A midwife may feel a little superfluous but has in fact to remain 'with woman', to keep alert, being active in, for example, observing for signs of the labour progressing, while appearing to be relatively inactive. As a guest in the woman's home the midwife is obliged to be relaxed, tactful, blending in to the circumstances and events, while still exercising the full range of professional labour care and support
- Flexibility and adaptability are required, e.g. continuing to maintain standard precautions, following aseptic guidelines or maintaining health and safety protocols while working in an unfamiliar environment. Midwives also find that their decision-making skills and professional autonomy are increased
- Management of unexpected situations or emergencies for mothers or babies when assistance may be some miles or minutes away.

It is clear, however, that as well as being professionally well prepared for birth at home, the midwife's personal feelings are significant in the woman's success. Floyd (1995) suggests that a woman has greater success if the midwife has a positive attitude, confidence, competence and willingness. Supervisors of midwives can assist midwives who feel that they are lacking the necessary skills and experience to gain this as part of their annual professional development review. Student midwives should aim to get as much experience as possible while training.

## Preparation

Good preparation is necessary for several agencies involved.

### Maternity services

Each service needs to have considered home birth provision within its service as a whole, including the training and updating of midwives, budgetary provision for items such as mobile phones and birthing equipment, and issues such as midwife availability, referral and transport systems. It is likely that risk management assessments are made frequently in relation to the service. Provision should be made for women who fall outside of the low risk criteria, but continue to choose the home birth option. The supervisor of midwives will provide advice and support in this situation (Jones 2003). Protocols should include whether midwives are expected, for example, to site intravenous cannulae in an emergency.

### The midwife

It can be helpful if the midwife knows the geography and socioeconomic demography of the area. This can highlight potential risk factors to personal safety. Equally, good working relationships with others in the health care team can make the management of problems smoother and enhance the communication that facilitates the woman's care. Knowing which second midwife to call and how to access the supervisor of midwives is essential information which should be easily to hand. The Royal College of Midwives (RCM 2002) rightly point out that midwives are fully equipped to manage normal birth; the essence is to manage it confidently at home with good judgements and actions in the event of abnormality. Updating in emergency drills (including community management) and resuscitation skills are essential. Cannulation and suturing skills are also advisable.

Equipment (e.g. sphygmomanometer, Entonox, suction apparatus, etc.) should all be stored, used and serviced correctly (see Chs 6, 27 and 59/60 respectively), with the midwife ensuring that she is very familiar with the equipment carried and its location. Keeping items together (e.g. equipment for primary postpartum haemorrhage management or resuscitation) means that they are easily accessible and easily moved around the home with the woman. Pethidine is rarely used, but may be supplied from the NHS Trust, via a GP, or via a midwife's private prescription following authorisation by a supervisor of midwives (see Ch. 20). Other medicines that the midwife carries, such as oxytocic agents, naloxone, lidocaine (lignocaine), may be administered according to the agreed patient group direction as for any other woman. Other equipment for the birth should include the items suggested in Box 38.1. Further details can be obtained from RCM (2003). Items such as the delivery pack may be kept at the woman's home in advance, but this may depend on local protocols and the midwife's discretion. The midwife will need to supply her own food and drinks.

---

**Box 38.1  Equipment suggested for managing labour and birth at home**

- Antenatal equipment including Pinard stethoscope and/or sonicaid and gel, sphygmomanometer, thermometer, venepuncture equipment, sharps box, swabs and medium, reagent sticks, MSU bottles, pen torch, scissors, tape measure, gloves (sterile and non-sterile), documentation such as continuation sheets, blood forms
- Labour equipment including sterile delivery and vaginal examination packs, urinary catheters, cannulation equipment and fluids, suturing equipment, gloves, incontinence pads, drugs (including spare Entonox), container for placenta, rubbish bags, water thermometer, documentation for labour care including birth notification and emergency management cards
- Resuscitation equipment for woman and baby including oxygen (with tubings, airways, bags and masks), suction with neonatal and maternal suckers, stethoscope, stop watch, heat source and possibly endotracheal tubes and laryngoscope depending on local protocol, blood glucose sticks
- Postnatal equipment including weighing scales, equipment for neonatal examination and documentation such as neonatal examination forms, child health record, postnatal exercises and advice, transfer of care documentation

---

### The woman and her family

Clearly for a planned home birth the woman is likely to be well prepared. RCM (2003) recommends obtaining items such as plastic sheeting, towels, rubbish bags, light foods and drinks, alternative sources of heating and lighting, massaging equipment, appropriate clothing for mother and baby, pillows and pethidine, amongst other things. However, family poverty should not be a hindrance to home birth and as such the midwife may need to assist with some of these items. The woman should be fully aware of how and when to get hold of the midwife. Reed (2002) provides helpful guidance for mothers, for example: 'Call during the day if waters break and are clear, call anytime if they break and they're brown or green'. One of the most helpful preparations for both the woman and the midwife is a pre-birth home visit that looks at all the practicalities: proposed room for birth, unobtrusive space for equipment, resuscitation area, location of telephone or presence of mobile phone with sufficient battery charge and signal, etc.

## Principles of managing birth at home

- Knowing how the midwife will be notified and whether there is a requirement to notify anyone else of the call out, e.g. labour ward or second midwife.
- Assessment on arrival: is labour progressing? Can the midwife leave and return later or rest in another room for a while? Is a second midwife needed for an imminent birth? This assessment should also include a history of the labour so far, with all assessments being recorded on a partogram or in the woman's records. Fetal and maternal wellbeing need to be established, abdominal examination is necessary; vaginal assessment may be according to the clinical indicators and the woman's wishes.
- Opportunity to establish a working area: space for equipment and resuscitation (portable, if possible), table for writing records, opportunity to inform second midwife of likely schedule (if not already contacted).
- Ongoing labour care: as for any labouring woman, including all assessments for labour progress, fetal and maternal wellbeing. It is likely that the woman will naturally be mobile and utilise the furniture and supporters around her for pain relief. She may also take regular baths or showers, eat and drink as she feels appropriate, pass urine as needed and use other techniques, e.g. the ironing, to help and distract. As labour progresses the midwife is more likely to observe the 'in on self' effect as the woman has less conversation and more of an intensity about her. The midwife will utilise the 'active inactivity' described above and is likely to begin intuitively to understand how the woman is progressing. If water labour or birth is planned the reader is encouraged to read Chapter 39.
- Second stage of labour: the woman is likely to push physiologically (see Ch. 34) using the furniture, etc. available to her; the midwife remains vigilant as to signs of second stage onset, fetal and maternal wellbeing and indicators of progress (see Ch. 34 for greater detail). The second midwife should ideally be called if not already present. The midwife should be mindful of her own care, e.g. back strain, when needing to adapt to the woman's position.
- Third stage of labour: many women may opt for expectant management at home; this requires that the midwife understands the physiology and is competent to undertake its management (see Ch. 35). The placenta remains the woman's property; however, often the midwife removes it from the home in a suitable container and disposes of it as for hospital births. If the

woman wishes to keep it she should be encouraged to bury it deeply in the garden or seek advice from Environmental Health. The midwife will need to improvise to examine the genital tract with sufficient light and visibility; equally if suturing is required chairs may be needed to act as lithotomy poles on which the woman places her legs and something firm may be needed beneath the woman's buttocks. All equipment is dealt with as for hospital births and returned to the hospital.

- Care of the newborn: there is little difference in the care of the newborn at home. If resuscitation is required the decision to call help is made swiftly and the midwife follows the usual guidelines (Ch. 60). Provision is made in the next 24–48 hours for a qualified person to undertake the neonatal examination.
- Transfer to hospital: the midwife must have referral systems and numbers in place; often referral is to the nearest consultant delivery suite or to a consultant obstetrician directly. Advice may also be sought from the supervisor of midwives and calls may be made directly to ambulance control on agreed numbers. Transfer to hospital is always made using an ambulance (often paramedic), and never by personal transport. GPs are often, by agreement, bypassed in such circumstances. A local protocol should clarify the procedure so it is rapid and direct. The woman may find referral very hard and it is appropriate to discuss the likely criteria with her in advance as well as at the time. Building a relationship, and therefore trust, with the woman antenatally is likely to make transfer a little easier for her. If an emergency transfer, it can be helpful to have a card written out (filling in the details at the last minute) that a member of the family can read from when speaking to ambulance control. Leaving the front door open and a light on can save valuable time. In some areas ambulance controls are notified in advance of the planned home births. If a paramedic attends, the midwife should be aware that the woman is still the midwife's 'case' and that full responsibility remains with the midwife, not the paramedic.
- Documentation: this is as thorough as for any hospital birth, including all discussions, referrals and actions. Partograms, birth notifications, etc. may all be left in the woman's home in advance.
- Other practitioners: occasionally women may bring in their own assistants such as aromatherapists. The midwife should ensure that, as the professional responsible, the woman and practitioner have sensible working limits and that if for any reason the midwife needs the therapy to stop, this is understood.
- Communicating when there are difficulties: occasionally women choose options that the midwife feels less comfortable about, for

example, poor lighting from candles only. Good preparation, continuity of care and opportunities to build a good trusting relationship with the woman in advance will smooth the management of such issues.

- Self-appraisal and audit: clinical governance ensures that the service is effective via audit, but this also aids midwives to appreciate the quality of their care and to review any areas that can be improved. Self-appraisal will help less experienced midwives to develop confidence in home birth management, along with the support of a supervisor of midwives.

## Role and responsibilities of the midwife

These can be summarised as:

- professional, thorough labour care undertaken in an unfamiliar environment but according to all rules and protocols that govern safe and effective practice
- recognising deviations from the norm and instigating referral.

## Summary

- Providing labour care at home for healthy women with a planned home birth can be a highly satisfying experience for the midwife and the family
- A range of new and existing skills are utilised; maintenance of skills such as resuscitation and emergency drills is essential
- Preparation, by all parties involved, contributes to the safety and delivery of care. This includes issues such as drugs, equipment, accessibility to other health care professionals and referral systems
- Many aspects of home care mirror hospital care but the midwife often needs to utilise her professional autonomy to the full. This is particularly the case when the unexpected occurs or the woman is outside of the low risk criteria.

## Self-assessment exercises

The answers to the following questions may be found in the text:

1. Summarise the current research relating to the safety of birth at home.
2. Compile a low risk criteria to identify women suitable for home birth.
3. Discuss the skills needed by the midwife to undertake safe home births.
4. List the items needed for a home birth.
5. Summarise the differences when caring for a labouring woman at home.
6. To whom will a midwife refer if a deviation from the norm occurs?

## REFERENCES

Cook M 2003 A 'beautiful' birth. MIDIRS Midwifery Digest 13(4):447–448

Floyd L 1995 Community midwives' views and experience of home birth. Midwifery 11:3–10

Hagelskamp C, Scammell A, Gray J et al 2003 Staying home for birth: do midwives and GPs give women a real choice? Midwives 6(7):300–303

Hodnett E D 1989 Personal control and the birth environment: comparisons between home and hospital settings. Journal of Environmental Psychology 9:207–216

Jones D 2003 Midwifery supervision and home births. Midwives 6(9):386–388

Kitzinger S 2001 Becoming a mother. MIDIRS Midwifery Digest 11(4):445–447

MCHRC (Maternal and Child Health Research Consortium) 1998 Confidential Enquiry into Stillbirths and Deaths in Infancy (CESDI), 5th Annual Report. Chapter 6. MCHRC, London

Olsen O 1997 Meta-analysis of the safety of home births. Birth 24:4–13

Olsen O, Jewell M D 2002 Home versus hospital births. Cochrane Database Systematic review 2003(1): CD000352

Reed B 2002 The Albany midwifery practice (2). MIDIRS Midwifery Digest 12(2):261–264

RCM (Royal College of Midwives) 2002:47 Home birth handbook, Vol. 1: Promoting home birth. RCM Trust, London

RCM (Royal College of Midwives) 2003 Home birth handbook, Vol. 2: Practising home birth. RCM Trust, London

# Chapter 39

# Principles of intrapartum skills — management of birth in water

The use of water as an analgesic in labour is anecdotally widely recognised. It can be used formally for the first, second and third stages of labour, either in a birthing pool in a hospital or birthing unit, or in a hired pool at home. Less formally, the standard bath or shower, at home or in hospital, is often used for pain relief, mainly in the first stage of labour. This chapter considers the significant issues in relation to birthing in water. A fuller understanding will be gained if it is read in conjunction with Chapters 30, 34, 35, 36 and 38.

## Learning outcomes

Having read this chapter the reader should be able to:

- highlight the current researched evidence
- discuss the advantages and disadvantages of water use in labour
- outline low risk criteria
- list the items of equipment necessary
- discuss the aspects of care pertinent to labouring in water
- discuss the midwife's role and responsibilities.

## Introduction

For various personal and managerial reasons, the incidence of water birth, while it may be increasing, is still small. Consequently, midwives may feel that they lack skill and experience in this aspect of care. MIDIRS (2003) advocate that evidence-based protocols should be available to all, including the women, and that midwives should have the opportunity to work alongside experienced colleagues until they feel able to practise themselves. Supervisors of Midwives play a crucial role in supporting midwives and in protecting the standards of care for women. Abbott (2004) is aware of situations where the NHS cannot provide midwives with sufficient skills and so independent midwives are contacted. Facilitating the woman's choice remains a significant issue.

## The evidence

While different aspects of water birth have been evaluated, the studies are often small and not randomised. Consequently, meta-analysis suggests that there is little difference in issues such as length of first stage, use of pain relief and incidence of perineal trauma, amongst others (Nikodem 2003). There are also outstanding questions (e.g. the overall rates of perinatal death) which make it more difficult to give women fully informed choices. MIDIRS (2003) suggest that there is still a need for large scale research. However, researchers such as Burns and Kitzinger (2001) and Garland and Jones (2000) believe that water birth is a safe and viable option, and can point to significant advantages.

### Advantages and disadvantages of water labour/birth

As with homebirth (Ch. 38) midwives have the opportunity to exercise their autonomy in a generally low intervention environment. The need to have confidence in the physiology of labour and the woman's ability to give birth naturally are significant features. The woman can utilise the buoyancy of the water to alleviate pain; she may also retain a greater sense of wellbeing and control, contributing to her good mental health postnatally. Anecdotally, there appears to be less perineal trauma from both episiotomy and tears.

### Who is suitable to use a birthing pool?

Historically, low risk criteria have been proposed; however Burns and Kitzinger (2001) suspect that under research conditions other issues such as hypertension or vaginal birth after caesarean could be included. At this time the following are proposed as safe criteria:

- established labour with spontaneous onset and no need for electronic fetal monitoring (EFM)
- uncomplicated pregnancy of >37 weeks' gestation (Burns & Kitzinger 2001).

Situations in which the use of water is contraindicated include:

- maternal dislike
- opiate use in labour
- induction of labour
- any known cause for concern for mother or fetus (Burns & Kitzinger 2001).

## Equipment

There should be space around the pool on each side and the means to fill, reheat and empty it. A sieve is useful to remove debris from the water and a mirror and torch may both be useful where lighting is dim. An aqua Doppler should be available. The midwife can also benefit from a kneeler or stool and the woman may appreciate a float to rest on. Midwives should protect themselves; for example, the woman can float to the surface for fetal auscultation, reducing the risk of damage to the midwife's back. The midwife must ensure, whether in hospital or at home, that the means to call for assistance and resuscitation equipment are all to hand. A mattress or other means of lying down comfortably should be available and a good supply of towels is essential. A bath thermometer may be integral to the design, otherwise one is required. A birthing stool may be helpful for land management of the third stage. Access to Entonox may be necessary. Pool use at home should include a trial run, ensuring that birthing partners are also comfortable with their role.

## Principles of care

### Assessments of maternal and fetal wellbeing
All labour observations and care are undertaken as for any other labour, including progress and wellbeing. The woman will need to leave the pool to pass urine and the midwife may decide in accordance with the other clinical signs as to the frequency and need for vaginal examinations. The aqua Doppler can be used throughout to assess fetal wellbeing. Contemporaneous records are maintained throughout and, in the event of a deviation from the norm, the woman is asked to leave the pool and a referral is made. The woman is encouraged to adopt positions that are comfortable. She may use Entonox, and other complementary therapies; it is important that she remains well hydrated.

### Water depth and temperature
The birthing pool needs to be able to accommodate water to the level of the woman's breasts when sitting. There is significant debate as to the water temperature; at this time Burns and Kitzinger (2001) recommend 35–37°C during the first stage of labour and 37–37.5°C in the second stage, providing that the mother is comfortable and neither too hot nor too cold. However, Anderson (2004) in her review of literature and physiology concludes that the woman's preference is the best guide to correct water temperature. It is often necessary to remove water when adding water for temperature adjustment purposes in order to retain a similar water level.

### The birth
A second midwife should be in attendance. The woman is likely to push physiologically and is more likely to have a 'hands poised' (McCandlish et al 1998) delivery (avoiding any stimulation to the

baby) with the midwife giving gentle verbal instruction, while utilising the mirror and possibly torch, to see advancement of the presenting part. It is not necessary to assess for the presence of the umbilical cord around the neck; interference can again cause premature stimulation. The baby should be born fully underwater, hence the need to retain the water level and to encourage the woman to keep her buttocks beneath the water. Once born the baby is brought to the surface without any unnecessary delay, where respiration can begin in air. As for any other birth, respiration difficulties necessitate clamping and cutting the cord, removing the baby to the resuscitation area and beginning the procedure (Ch. 60). It is noted (Anderson 2004) that often babies born in water appear to be blue for longer and take a few more moments to establish respiration (this may be linked to water temperature).

When bringing the baby to the surface, care should be taken in case of a short umbilical cord. Anderson (2000) cites a number of instances in which the cord has snapped on bringing the baby above the water level. Cord clamps should be readily available and the midwife should be alert to the need to act quickly. The baby should rest with its head above water, retaining its body heat, at approximately the level of the mother's uterus until management of the third stage begins.

### Third stage of labour

If clinically appropriate and desired by the woman, a physiological third stage can be completed in the pool. Blood loss may be harder to estimate and therefore the woman's clinical condition should be considered as part of the assessment. When convenient, the mother and baby are brought out of the pool and care continues as for any other birth (e.g. neonatal assessment, examination of the mother's genital tract, etc.). Garland and Jones (2000) suggest that higher rates of intact perineums have been observed when labouring in water. Abbott (personal correspondence, 2004) would agree, having experienced approximately 100 pool births with 100% intact perineums. If required, suturing would take place at a mutually convenient time to the mother and midwife.

### Infection control

As for any birth, measures are taken to maintain asepsis; however, there is often less intervention and so water cleanliness becomes one of the priorities. The sieve is used to remove any debris, but if the amount is significant, particularly following a vomit, it is advisable to ask the woman to leave the pool temporarily while decontamination takes place. Hired pools often have a disposable liner, but cleaning of the pool is also necessary. Plumbed pools should also be thoroughly cleansed after each use. Burns and Kitzinger (2001) recommend a chlorine-releasing agent of 10 000 parts per million; local protocols may approve other solutions, but they should all be effective against HIV and hepatitis B and C. Jacuzzi style pools should be avoided.

### Emergencies

The woman is asked to leave the pool quickly (and is usually very compliant!) and the management of the problem begins as for any other birth. In the event of shoulder dystocia, care should be taken not to knock the baby's head on the side of the pool.

## Role and responsibilities of the midwife

These can be summarised as:

- thorough, safe labour care as for any birth, but with added considerations for the comfort and safety of the woman, baby and midwife when using the medium of water for analgesia or birth
- contemporaneous record keeping.

## Summary

- Advocates believe that water increases mobility, soothes contraction pain and enhances the woman's feeling of control. Comprehensive researched evidence is still required
- Low risk protocols recommend which women can utilise water. Care is taken to ensure that the pool is appropriately filled; water temperature remains open to debate
- The baby is brought to the surface without delay; care is taken to avoid the cord snapping
- Infection control is a significant issue throughout and following the process.

## Self-assessment exercises

The answers to the following questions may be found in the text:

1. What is the current researched evidence with regard to the use of water for labour?
2. List the items of equipment necessary for birth in water.
3. Describe how the midwife would manage the second stage of labour in water.
4. List the considerations that a midwife should be mindful of when caring for a woman labouring in water.

## REFERENCES

Abbott L 2004 Personal correspondence. Online. Available: http://www.homebirths.net

Anderson T 2000 Umbilical cords and underwater birth. The Practising Midwife 3(2):12

Anderson T 2004 Time to throw the waterbirth thermometer away? MIDIRS Midwifery Digest 14(3):370–374

Burns E, Kitzinger S 2001 Midwifery guidelines for use of water in labour. OCHRAD, Oxford Brookes University, Oxford (eburns@brookes.ac.uk)

Garland D, Jones K 2000 Waterbirth: supporting practice with clinical audit. MIDIRS Midwifery Digest 10(3):333–336

McCandlish R, Bowler U, van Asten H et al 1998 A randomised control trial of care of the perineum during second stage of normal labour. British Journal of Obstetrics and Gynaecology 105(12): 1262–1272

MIDIRS 2003 The use of water during childbirth. Informed Choice leaflet (11) for professionals. MIDIRS, Bristol

Nikodem V C 2003 Immersion in water in pregnancy, labour and birth (Cochrane Review). Cochrane Library, Issue 1. Update Software, Oxford

Chapter **40**

# Assessment of the baby – assessment at birth

This chapter focuses on the principles of assessment of the baby, considering the different ways the condition of the baby is assessed at birth. The midwife is involved in assessing the baby as part of the care of the baby at birth. This provides an indication of how well the baby is making the adjustment to extrauterine life and whether any assistance is required.

**Learning outcomes**

Having read this chapter the reader should be able to:

- discuss the Apgar score and relate it to the need for the initiation of resuscitation
- describe the examination of the baby at birth, identifying how normal progress is recognised
- discuss the role and responsibilities of the midwife in relation to assessment of the baby at birth.

*Assessment at birth*

The assessment at birth is twofold: the first is an immediate assessment undertaken to assess the adjustment from intrauterine to extrauterine life, using the Apgar scoring system; the second is a complete physical examination to confirm normality and detect deviations from the norm.

# The Apgar score

Devised by Dr Virginia Apgar in the 1950s, this provides a means of assessing the condition of the baby at birth in relation to five variables – respiratory effort, heart rate, colour, muscle tone and reflex irritability. The score is initially assigned at 1 minute, to allow time for the changes to begin. Further scores are undertaken at 5 and 10 minutes. The score can be assessed more frequently if any of the scores are low and resuscitation is required, to provide an indication of the effectiveness of resuscitation measures undertaken (e.g. at 3 and 5 minutes). The 10-minute score provides an indication of future morbidity, with low scores associated with a poor neurological outcome.

Each variable is assigned a score of 0, 1 or 2, thus the baby is given a total score out of 10. A mnemonic, APGAR, can be used to remember the five variables (Table 40.1). A score of 7–10 at 1 minute suggests the baby is in a good condition. A score of 4–6 indicates moderate depression, requiring some degree of resuscitation. A baby who scores 0–3 is severely depressed and requires immediate resuscitation, possibly ventilation (Mead 1996).

It is difficult to anticipate which babies will have a low Apgar score at birth. Dijxhoorn et al (1986) suggest changes in the fetal heart rate do not compare well with Apgar scores at delivery. This may explain why some emergency caesarean sections undertaken because of serious concerns regarding the fetal heart rate deliver a baby with a total Apgar score of 9 or 10.

The Apgar score is a subjective scoring system and is therefore vulnerable to bias. Ideally it should not be assigned by the person undertaking the delivery. At the time of birth, the midwife delivering has to consider the condition of both the mother and the baby. This can result in retrospective scoring, influenced by subsequent events. Additionally, Letko (1996) suggests midwives could be less objective due to their involvement with the outcome.

Other factors can influence the score; for example, assessment of colour can be affected by lighting, skin pigmentation, haemoglobin levels and degree of peripheral perfusion (Letko 1996). Skin pigmentation generally develops from the fifth day of life in non-Caucasian babies (Silverton 1993); however, if the skin is darkly pigmented, the appearance can be assessed by observing the mucous membranes, the palms and the soles – these should be pink. The preterm baby is likely to have lower Apgar scores than the term baby due to neurological immaturity resulting in poor muscle tone, slower reflexes and a bluish-red colouring of the skin.

Table 40.1 The APGAR scoring system: the five classifications used and the criteria for scoring 0–2

| Sign | 0 | 1 | 2 |
| --- | --- | --- | --- |
| Appearance (colour) | Blue, pale | Body pink, limbs blue | All pink |
| Pulse (heart rate) | Absent | <100 | >100 |
| Grimace (response to stimuli) | None | Grimace | Cry |
| Activity (muscle tone) | Limp | Some flexion of limbs | Active movements, limbs well flexed |
| Respiratory effort | None | Slow, irregular | Good, strong cry |

### Assessing the score

- Observe the appearance, e.g. is the baby pink all over (2), is the body pink but the extremities blue (1), or is the baby pale or blue all over (0)?
- Estimate the heart rate by palpating the umbilicus or placing two fingers across the chest over the apex, count the rate for 6 seconds then multiply by 10. Determine whether the heart rate is above 100 (10 beats or more over the 6-second period) (2), under 100 (less than 10 beats in 6 seconds) (1) or absent (0). A baby who is pink, active and breathing is likely to have a heart rate above 100
- The response of the baby to stimuli should be noted. This could be in response to being dried or handled or, for a baby who is being resuscitated, it may be the response to facemasks or airways used. Determine whether the baby cries in response to stimuli (2), whether it is trying to cry but is only able to grimace (1) or whether there is no response (0)
- Observe the muscle tone of the baby by observing the amount of activity and degree of flexion of the limbs – are there active movements using well-flexed limbs (2), is there some flexion of the limbs (1) or is the baby limp (0)?
- Finally, observe the respiratory effort made by the baby – is it good and strong (often seen in conjunction with a crying baby) (2), is respiration slow and irregular (1) or is there no respiratory effort (0)?

| PROCEDURE | Apgar scoring |
| --- | --- |

- Ensure the lighting is sufficient to allow good visualisation of colour; have good access to the baby
- Note time of delivery, wait 1 minute then undertake first assessment, assess the five variables quickly and simultaneously, totalling the score
- Act promptly and appropriately accordingly to the score, e.g. a baby scoring 0–3 requires immediate resuscitation (it may already have commenced if the baby is obviously compromised at birth)
- Repeat at 5 minutes; the score should increase if previously 8 or below
- Repeat again at 10 minutes
- Document findings and act accordingly.

# Birth examination

The midwife is required to undertake a complete physical examination at birth to confirm normality and detect deviations from the norm (NMC 2004). This is usually undertaken within the first hour of birth. However, it is important not to allow the baby to become cold, and the examination may be delayed if the baby has a low temperature, or is unwell. While this examination should detect obvious abnormality, it can miss other abnormalities, particularly those that only become apparent in the first days of life. For this reason, a physical examination is also undertaken by the paediatrician or suitably trained midwife during the first 48 hours of life. The heart, lungs and hips are examined during this subsequent physical examination.

While it is not necessary to undertake the examination in exactly the same order as detailed below, it is important that the examination is thorough and complete; the midwife should develop a systematic approach to the examination.

## Principles of newborn examination

- Explain the procedure to the parents and gain their informed consent
- Wash and dry hands to minimise the risk of infection to the baby; gloves are worn if the baby has not yet been bathed
- Ensure adequate lighting to allow clear visualisation; have good access to the baby, preferably in the presence of one or both parents
- Check the baby is warm; to maintain the temperature only uncover the part of the baby being examined and re-cover quickly
- Examine the baby systematically and thoroughly.

### The head

Look for signs of moulding and caput succedaneum, as these may result in the head appearing asymmetrical and will influence the measurement of the head circumference. The head should be examined for visible signs of trauma (e.g. lacerations from a fetal scalp electrode, forceps marks) and for signs of bruising – this may increase the risk of physiological jaundice occurring.

Feel along the suture lines and fontanelles – are they of normal size and appearance? Widely spaced sutures may be indicative of a preterm baby, lack of moulding or hydrocephalus. Narrowly spaced sutures are usually a result of moulding. The posterior fontanelle often appears closed at birth due to the moulding. The anterior fontanelle should be palpated – a large fontanelle may be due to prematurity or hydro-cephalus, a small one is suggestive of microcephaly. If the fontanelle is raised, this may be due to raised intracranial pressure, while a depressed fontanelle is suggestive of dehydration – rarely seen at birth. Occasionally a third fontanelle can be felt between the anterior and posterior fontanelles that is suggestive of trisomy 21.

### Head circumference

The head circumference may be measured at birth, using the occipitofrontal circumference – the measurement around the occiput and forehead. However, due to the changes that occur at birth, this measurement is likely to change over the next 48 hours; for this reason, it is better to record the head circumference 2–4 days following birth (Johnston et al 2003).

### Shape of the face

The shape of the face should appear symmetrical; the size and position of the eyes, nose, mouth, chin and ears should be noted in relation to each other.

### Eyes

Examine the eyes to ensure two are present and assess their size, shape and any slanting. Cataracts may be noticeable by a cloudy appearance of the cornea. Any discharge should be noted; this is not normal and could be indicative of infection. The presence of conjunctival haemorrhage, usually acquired during the second stage of labour, should also be noted. The pupils should be examined and should appear round. Occasionally a keyhole shape is present (coloboma) which could be indicative of an underlying retinal defect.

### Nose

The shape of the nose and width of the bridge should be observed; this should be greater than 2.5 cm in the term baby. It is not unusual for the nose to be squashed at birth; if so, this should be noted, particularly if it is affecting the baby's ability to breathe. The nostrils should not flare; if they do, this is usually indicative of respiratory illness.

### Mouth

Observe the mouth; the lips should be formed and symmetrical. Asymmetry could be indicative of facial palsy. A small mouth may be due to micrognathia, often associated with underlying abnormality. The area between the lips and the nose should be examined for the presence of a cleft lip. The inside of the mouth should be visualised using a good light source; this is more easily achieved when the baby is crying or by pressing gently on the chin to encourage the baby to open his mouth. The palate should be observed for intactness, particularly at the junction of the hard and soft palate where a cleft palate may occur. Placing a finger inside the baby's mouth to feel around the palate is not recommended; while this may detect some cleft hard palates it is unlikely to detect a cleft soft palate. While looking in the mouth, the presence of white spots on the gums or palate (usually due to Epstein's pearls or teeth) should be noted, as should the length of the frenulum.

### Ears

Examine the ears to ensure two are present and they are fully formed, in the correct position. The ears of the term baby should contain enough cartilage to allow the ears to spring back into position when moved forward gently. The pinna should be well formed with defined curves in the upper part. Correct positioning of the ears is determined by tracing an imaginary line from the outer canthus of the eyes horizontally back to the ears; the top of the pinna should be above this line. Low set ears may be associated with an underlying chromosomal abnormality (e.g. trisomy 21). The external auditory meatus should be examined to ensure patency. The presence of accessory skin tags or auricles should be noted and may be associated with renal abnormalities (Rose 1994).

### Neck

Babies have short necks, which should be examined for symmetry. Move the fingers around the neck to detect the presence of any swelling (e.g. cystic hygroma, sternomastoid tumour). The baby should be able to move his head to both sides. Webbing is unusual and could be indicative of a chromosomal abnormality (e.g. Turner's syndrome); redundant skin folds at the back of the neck are suggestive of trisomy 21.

### Clavicles

Using the index finger, feel along the clavicles to ensure they are intact, particularly if there was a breech presentation or shoulder dystocia – both increase the risk of a fractured clavicle, resulting in little or no movement in the associated arm.

### Arms

Both arms should be the same length; this can be confirmed by straightening the arms down the side of the baby and comparing the two together. Both arms should be moving freely; spontaneous arm movements can be elicited by stroking the forearm or hand. Lack of movement may be associated with underlying trauma (e.g. fractures, nerve damage) or to poor motor control associated with neurological impairment. The number of digits should be counted and examined for the webbing between them. Polydactyly or syndactyly should be noted. The palm should be straightened and the number of palmar creases noted; a single crease might be associated with chromosomal abnormality (e.g. trisomy 21). Look at the nails for the presence of paronychia as these may become infected or get caught on bedding, causing them to tear and bleed.

### Chest

Examine the chest for symmetry of movement with respiration. The respiratory rate can be counted if needed and any signs of respiratory distress (e.g. sternal recession, intercostal recession) reported to the paediatrician immediately. The nipples and areolae should be well formed in the term baby and appear symmetrical on the chest wall but should not be widely spaced. Any accessory nipples should be noted. The breasts may appear enlarged; this is normal and of little significance unless there are signs of infection.

### Abdomen

Observe the abdomen, which should appear rounded and move in synchrony with the chest during respiration, inspecting the area to ensure it is intact and gently palpating to ensure there are no abnormal swellings. The umbilical cord should be securely clamped; this should be inspected to ensure there are no signs of haemorrhage.

### Genitalia

With boys, the length of the penis should be assessed; this is usually about 3 cm and the position of the urethral meatus confirmed. The foreskin should not be retracted as it is adherent to the glans penis and physically retracting it at this age can lead to phimosis. The scrotum should be gently palpated for the presence of two testes.

For girls, the vulva should be examined by parting the labia gently to ensure the presence of the clitoris, and the urethral and vaginal orifices. A mucoid discharge may be present which is normal.

### Legs

Examine the legs and feet to assess symmetry, size, shape and posture. Confirm that the legs are the same length by straightening them together and comparing the two. Both legs should be moving freely; lack of movement may be associated with underlying trauma (e.g. fractures, nerve damage) or to poor motor control associated with neurological impairment. The position of the feet in relation to the legs should be noted as both positional and anatomical deformities may cause the feet to be turned inwards or outwards, upwards or downwards. Some of these deformities will require corrective treatment. The shape of the feet should be noted, including oedema or a 'rocker bottom' appearance. The number of toes should be counted and examined for webbing between them by separating them; polydactyly or syndactyly should be noted.

### Spine

Examine the spine by turning the baby over, looking for any obvious abnormality such as spina bifida and also for any swelling, dimpling or hairy patches; these could indicate an abnormality of the spinal cord or vertebral column. Assess the curvature of the vertebral column by running the fingers lightly over the spine. This may be easier to do by straddling the baby over one hand, while using the other hand to feel the spine (ensure the head is supported). Gently part the cleft of the buttocks, look for any dimples or sinuses and confirm the presence of the anal sphincter.

### Skin

During the examination, the condition of the skin should be observed. The colour should be noted, as should the presence of any rashes or marks (e.g. birthmarks, bruising). Any obvious swelling or spots should be examined and recorded. A Mongolian blue spot may be evident in some babies, particularly those with an Asian or Black ancestry. This appears like bruising, usually over the sacral area. This should be observed over the next few days to enable the midwife to differentiate between the possibility of the discolouration being a bruise or a Mongolian blue spot.

### Elimination

The passage of urine or meconium should be recorded as it indicates patency of the renal and lower gastrointestinal tract respectively.

### Weight

The weight of the baby should be recorded in kilograms; this can be undertaken at the beginning or end of the examination provided the baby is warm.

### Length

The crown–heel length of the baby may be recorded; this is not routinely undertaken and is difficult to measure accurately. The length is measured in two stages using a non-stretchable tape measure: from the crown (top part of the head) to the base of the spine, and from the base of the spine to the heel. A second person may be required to straighten the legs. Alternatively, specialised calibrated equipment may be used providing a more accurate measurement. The head and feet must be in contact with the equipment, with the legs fully extended (Fig. 40.1).

**Figure 40.1** Measuring the length of the baby using specialised calibrated equipment (Adapted from Fraser & Cooper 2003)

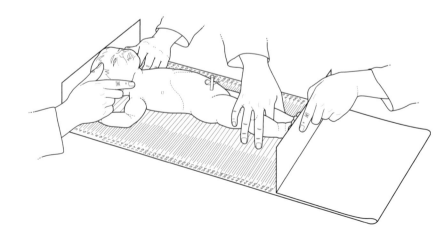

Once the examination is completed, the baby should be dressed and left comfortable either with the parents or securely in the cot. The findings should be recorded in the appropriate documentation, reporting any deviations to the midwife in charge or paediatrician. The parents should be informed of the findings.

## PROCEDURE    birth examination

- The procedure is explained to the parents and informed consent gained
- Wash and dry hands, put on gloves if required
- Ensure the lighting is good and the baby is warm
- Examine the baby methodically, beginning with the head, face and neck, then the clavicles, arms, hands, chest and abdomen; finally the genitalia, legs, feet and spine are examined
- The colour and activity of the baby are noted throughout the examination
- The passage of urine and meconium is recorded
- Other observations undertaken may include the head circumference, length and weight
- The baby is dressed following the procedure
- Discuss the findings with the parents
- Document findings and act accordingly.

## Role and responsibilities of the midwife

These can be summarised as:

- being able to competently assess the baby at birth, using the Apgar score, and understanding the significance of the score
- undertaking the birth examination thoroughly and competently, referring as necessary
- contemporaneous record keeping.

## Summary

- Assessment of the baby at birth is an important skill undertaken by the midwife
- Apgar scoring is quick and easy to undertake, but is subjective and influenced by factors such as lighting and skin pigmentation
- Birth examination is a thorough physical examination that detects obvious abnormalities; some abnormalities may not be apparent until the baby is older; subsequent examination should be undertaken as required.

**Self-assessment exercises**

The answers to the following questions may be found in the text:

1. How would a baby who scores 1 for each category of the Apgar score be recognised?
2. What factors influence the score awarded at birth?
3. Describe the top to toe examination of the baby undertaken by the midwife at birth.
4. What are the role and responsibilities of the midwife in relation to the assessment of the baby at birth?

## REFERENCES

Dijxhoorn M J, Visse G H A, Fidler V J et al 1986 Apgar score, meconium and acidaemia at birth in relation to neonatal neurological morbidity in term infants. British Journal of Obstetrics and Gynaecology 893:217–222

Fraser D M, Cooper M A 2003 Myles textbook for midwives, 14th edn. Churchill Livingstone, Edinburgh

Johnston P G B, Flood K, Spinks K 2003 The newborn child, 9th edn. Churchill Livingstone, Edinburgh

Letko M D 1996 Understanding the Apgar score. Journal of Obstetric, Gynaecological and Neonatal Nursing 25:299–303

Mead M 1996 The diagnosis of foetal distress: a challenge to midwives. Journal of Advanced Nursing 23:975–983

NMC (Nursing and Midwifery Council) 2004 Midwives rules and standards. NMC, London

Rose S J 1994 Physical examination of the full-term baby. British Journal of Midwifery 2(5):209–213

Silverton L 1993 The art and science of midwifery. Prentice Hall, New York

# Chapter 41

# Assessment of the baby — daily examination

This chapter considers the daily examination of the baby and the role and responsibilities of the midwife in relation to this. The midwife has a duty to ensure the optimum progress of the baby throughout the postnatal period. Providing the mother with the necessary advice regarding infant care (NMC 2004) facilitates this. To assist the midwife in offering the most appropriate advice, the day-to-day progress of the baby is sought by asking the mother about the baby's progress and by examining the baby as required. This examination is not a physical examination that mimics the birth examination; rather it assumes that obvious physical abnormalities have been detected. The daily examination seeks to confirm that normal progress is being made and that any deviations from the norm occurring since birth are detected early and treated.

## Learning outcomes

Having read this chapter the reader should be able to:

- describe the daily examination of the baby, identifying how normal progress is recognised
- discuss the role and responsibilities of the midwife in relation to daily examination of the baby.

## Principles of the daily examination

The examination should be undertaken methodically, ensuring the baby does not become cold, exposing only the part of the baby that is being examined. Access to the baby and good lighting are essential.

### Consent

As the baby cannot give consent for the examination, the midwife should explain the procedure to the parents and gain their consent. The examination should ideally be undertaken when one or both parents are present, as it enables discussion of the findings as the examination progresses and the parents can be asked pertinent questions that may influence the advice given to them regarding the care of their baby.

### Reduce infection risk

The baby is a 'compromised host' at birth, at risk from infection that can affect morbidity and mortality. It is important to wash hands prior to examining the baby to minimise the risk of infection to the baby. If contact with the baby's body fluids is likely, the midwife should apply gloves for self-protection.

### Behaviour

Discuss the activity of the baby with the parents, e.g. is the baby active, sleepy, contented, unsettled, does the baby cry a lot, what is the cry like, can the baby be pacified easily? The feeding pattern of the baby can be discussed and the number and type of wet and soiled nappies.

# Observation of the baby

Observe the baby, noting the colour of the skin, the respiratory pattern and movement of the limbs. The baby should appear pink all over, indicating good peripheral perfusion. When the baby has darkly pigmented skin, signs of peripheral perfusion can be assessed by observing the mucous membranes, the palms and the soles. Cyanosis with or without signs of respiratory distress should be reported to the paediatrician immediately. If the baby appears pale, this should be reported, as it could be indicative of underlying illness. It is not unusual for babies to develop physiological jaundice, seen as a yellow discolouration of the skin (and sometimes the sclera and mucous membranes). Physiological jaundice usually appears from the third day and may deepen over the next couple of days before beginning to subside by the seventh day. If the jaundice appears severe and widespread, especially if the baby is very sleepy or not feeding, the serum bilirubin level should be estimated. Clinical estimation of the degree of jaundice can be inaccurate and is influenced by the type of lighting, the reflective ability of objects around the baby and the peripheral blood flow (Johnston et al 2003). The respiratory pattern is noted, with a normal respiratory rate of 30–50 expected when the baby is at rest with no signs of respiratory distress. When the baby is active all four limbs should be moving.

### Head

Using the fingertips, feel along the suture lines and fontanelles. Moulding should have resolved within the first 24 hours of birth. The anterior fontanelle should be palpated, and should be level. If raised, this may be due to raised intracranial pressure; a depressed fontanelle is suggestive of dehydration. While feeling around the head, note any new swellings. A cephalhaematoma first appears between 12 and 36 hours and is likely to increase in size, taking up to 6 weeks to disappear. Any bruised or traumatised areas noted at or since birth should be examined to ascertain that healing is occurring and there are no signs of infection.

### Eyes

Inspect the eyes to ensure they are clear, with no signs of discharge. If a discharge is present, the eyes should be cleaned (Ch. 14) and a swab taken if indicated (Ch. 12). The parents should be shown how to clean the eye. Refer to the paediatrician if necessary.

### Mouth

The mouth should be looked at using a good light source and should be clean and moist; the presence of white plaques should be investigated as these could be indicative of a monilial infection. If the baby has fed recently, sucking blisters may appear on the lips. Although this gives the appearance that the skin is peeling from the lips, no treatment is needed.

### Skin

Skin colour should be assessed as discussed above. The skin should also be examined for any rashes, spots, bruising or signs of infection or trauma. Erythema toxicum appears as a blotchy red rash and is of little significance, as are milia. However, septic spots should be identified early and treatment instigated if required. Look also for areas of excoriation that may occur due to friction with bedding or clothes, or in cases of excoriation of the buttocks, may be due to an ammoniacal burn. The nails should be examined for paronychia.

### Umbilicus

The umbilical cord and umbilicus should be examined daily for signs of separation and to exclude infection (Ch. 14). The cord usually separates within 5–16 days; a small stump of cord may be left in the umbilicus, which should be examined daily. Early signs of infection may be detected by redness around the umbilicus; the cord may also smell offensive and become sticky.

### Weight

The baby often loses weight in the first few days that should be regained by the 10th day. The baby may be weighed on the third or fourth day to assess the amount of weight lost, but if the baby is thriving and feeding well, this is unnecessary. It is useful to weigh the baby at 10 days to ensure birthweight has been regained. While weighing the baby reassures the parents that the baby is thriving, it can also be a source of anxiety if the baby has lost weight or gains weight slowly.

### Following the examination

When the examination is complete, the baby should be redressed and the findings recorded in the appropriate documentation. The results should form the basis of advice given to the parents regarding the progress and subsequent care of the baby. Any deviations from the norm should be acted on accordingly and appropriate care instigated.

## PROCEDURE daily examination of the baby

- Begin by discussing the progress of the baby with the parents
- Explain procedure, gain informed consent
- Discuss the baby's behaviour and activity with the parents
- Wash hands, apply gloves if required
- Ensure there is good light and the baby is warm
- Observe the colour and general appearance of the baby
- Examine the head, eyes, mouth and umbilicus
- Weigh the baby if indicated
- Redress the baby
- Discuss the findings with the parents
- Document the findings and act accordingly.

### Role and responsibilities of the midwife

These can be summarised as:

- undertaking the daily examination thoroughly and competently, referring as necessary
- education and support of parents
- contemporaneous record keeping.

## Summary

- The midwife examines the baby daily as part of the care provided to the mother and baby during the postnatal period
- Although it is not as thorough as the birth examination, it provides an opportunity to discuss the progress of the baby and for advice and care to be offered as required.

### Self-assessment exercises

The answers to the following questions may be found in the text:

1. Describe the daily examination of the baby.
2. Which issues may be discussed with the parents to inform care?
3. When is a baby weighed and why?
4. What are the role and responsibilities of the midwife in relation to the daily examination of the baby?

REFERENCES

Johnston P G B, Flood K, Spinks K 2003 The newborn child, 9th edn. Churchill Livingstone, Edinburgh

NMC (Nursing and Midwifery Council) 2004 Midwives rules and standards. NMC, London

# Chapter 42

# Assessment of the baby – capillary sampling

This chapter considers capillary blood sampling from the baby. The most common method of obtaining blood samples from the neonate is via a heel prick (Barker et al 1994). The midwife undertakes this as part of routine screening, and also to detect or confirm deviations from the norm (e.g. serum bilirubin or serum glucose estimations).

## Learning outcomes

Having read this chapter the reader should be able to:

- describe the procedure for obtaining a capillary blood sample from the heel
- discuss the factors that may help or hinder the procedure
- discuss the role and responsibilities of the midwife in relation to capillary sampling.

## Underpinning anatomy

The blood is obtained from the capillaries contained within the skin. The arterial–venous network of the skin is located at the junction of the lower dermis and upper subcutaneous tissue. The skin should be punctured only to the depth of this junction to facilitate blood flow; a deeper puncture can have serious complications. If the calcaneus (heel bone) is punctured, there is a risk of osteochondritis or osteomyelitis resulting. The distance between the skin and bone can vary depending on where on the foot the measurement is taken (with the narrowest distance being at the posterior curve of the heel) and the weight and gestation of the baby.

Another consideration is the position of plantar arteries and nerves, which should be avoided. Puncturing the arteries can result in haemorrhage and increases the risk of introducing infection, which could result in septicaemia. Puncturing the nerves can result in permanent damage to the nerve.

Blumenfeld et al (1979) estimated the distance from the surface of the skin to the arterial–venous network to be 0.35–1.6 mm. Moxley (1989) reported on one study that demonstrated the distance from the skin to the bone to be 2.4 mm in the smallest baby (weight 560 g). Jain and Rutter (1999) suggested the distance between the skin and bone to be a minimum of 4 mm, with this reducing to 3 mm where the weight was <1560 g. There is some disagreement as to the maximum incision/ puncture depth. Usually this is up to 2 mm and never greater than 2.4 mm in the term baby. A shorter penetration may be indicated in the preterm or low birthweight baby.

### How to avoid puncturing the calcaneus, plantar arteries and nerves

- Use the lateral and medial portions of the heel as puncture sites
- Draw an imaginary line from midway between the fourth and fifth toes laterally and medially from the middle of the big toe as the calcaneus rarely extends beyond these (Fig. 42.1) (these points are also furthest away from the arteries and nerves)
- The correct depth of puncture can be achieved using a 'measured' lancet
- Select a new puncture site for each collection
- Use a good technique to avoid having to repeat the procedure.

# Neonatal blood screening tests

A number of screening tests are carried out, usually within the first week of life (commonly referred to as the Guthrie test). Other blood tests undertaken include bilirubin and glucose estimation. The following may be undertaken using the Guthrie form (the actual tests undertaken vary from centre to centre, with the exception of phenylketonuria):

**Figure 42.1** Heel sites for capillary sampling in the baby

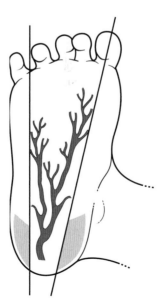

- phenylketonuria (PKU)
- maple syrup urine disease
- histidinaemia
- homocystinuria
- tyrosinaemia
- congenital hypothyroidism
- sickle cell disease
- cystic fibrosis.

### Guthrie test

The midwife is responsible for undertaking the test correctly and forwarding it to the appropriate test centre. The Guthrie test uses dried blood from sample spots on the Guthrie card 'blotting paper'. Usually four circles of blood (one drop of blood per circle) are required to undertake all the tests, with the number of circles varying with the different tests being undertaken (sometimes up to seven may be required).

One of the tests for phenylketonuria may involve the growth of the bacteria *Bacillus subtilis* on a culture medium. The growth of *B. subtilis* is inhibited if the baby is receiving antibiotics or if the foot is wiped with an alcohol-impregnated swab, possibly giving a false result.

Blood is taken from the fifth day of life, providing sufficient milk feeds have been ingested for the 48 hours preceding the test. A baby who is receiving antibiotics, or who is breastfeeding and whose mother is taking antibiotics, should still have the test. A note of this should be made on the form and the mother advised a repeat test might be needed. Alternatively, the test can be delayed for a couple of days if the antibiotic treatment is short term, but the test should not be undertaken until 48 hours after the treatment is completed.

If the test cannot be completed (e.g. insufficient blood on the card), it will have to be repeated. The test will also be repeated if the results are not within normal limits.

### Bilirubin estimation

A capillary sample may be taken to estimate the level of unconjugated bilirubin in the blood of a jaundiced baby. In some maternity units, the sample is then sent to the pathology laboratory, whereas other maternity units have the equipment (centrifugal machine) to undertake the test themselves. Usually two thin capillary tubes are filled with blood. Care should be taken to avoid getting air in the capillary tubes as this may result in the blood dispersing totally from the tubes during spinning, necessitating a further blood test.

### Blood glucose estimation

This is usually undertaken as a diagnostic test when hypoglycaemia is suspected or as a screening test in babies considered to be 'at risk' of developing hypoglycaemia. The midwife should be familiar with the equipment used to estimate the level of glucose in the blood. Increasingly blood glucose is being estimated via a venepuncture sample rather than a capillary sample as the results are more accurate.

## Equipment

The choice of equipment is usually between the automatic and the non-automatic lancet. The automatic devices may be reusable with disposable lancets or blades attached that puncture or incise the skin to a predetermined depth and are recommended for use. Automatic devices are considered to increase the volume of blood available and hence reduce the blood collection time and minimise haemolysis (Meehan 1998).

The devices are divided into two types: puncture and incision. Their action is slightly different in that the puncture devices deliver a small puncture wound to the skin whereas the incision devices make a clean straight incision into the skin. Some of the devices allow the midwife to choose the penetration depth; this is preferable when undertaking the procedure on a preterm or low birthweight baby.

## Factors to consider when undertaking capillary sampling

*Consent*

As the baby is unable to give consent, the procedure should always be discussed with the parents, whose consent is required prior to undertaking the procedure. The reasons for the test should be explained and also the significance of the results, particularly that they are not informed of a normal result with the neonatal screening tests. However, the need for a repeat test does not necessarily indicate an abnormality has been found; it is more likely that the first test was inadequate.

*Position and comfort of the baby*

The baby may be held either across the lap or against the shoulder by the mother, another person or the midwife undertaking the test. Alternatively, the baby can be laid on a flat surface (e.g. cot, changing mat on the floor). Upright positions are better as gravity can assist with the direction of blood flow and make it easier to collect the blood from the foot. Breastfeeding during the procedure places the baby in an ideal position. Whatever position is chosen, the baby should be held securely to prevent excessive movement of the foot, which may interfere with the collection of the sample, and to ensure that the person undertaking the test has hands free to hold the equipment, the foot and subsequently the card/testing equipment. It may be easier to wrap the baby in a blanket to prevent the baby's limbs moving too much, although some babies will object to this.

There are a number of behavioural responses to pain seen within the baby, which include facial expressions, body movements and crying characteristics. Facial expressions consisting of brow bulge, eye squeeze, nasolabial furrow and open lips can be seen in the majority of babies within 6 seconds of the heel prick. Facial expressions are considered more specific than body movements (which also occur in response to wiping the heel with a medicated swab) and crying (premature infants are less likely to cry) (Harrison & Johnston 2002). For many babies, however, this elicits a crying response with some becoming very distressed. This may inhibit blood flow as the leg muscles contract and impede circulation. Physiological responses including an increase in the heart and respiratory rate may also be seen, although it is not known if this is due to the pain of the procedure or the effects of being handled. The midwife should consider how the pain and discomfort can be reduced.

For the baby who is breastfeeding when the procedure is performed, very little pain symptomatology may be noticed, particularly when this is combined with skin-to-skin contact (Gray et al 2000). Not all studies confirm this although it is difficult to compare these studies; in Carbajal et al's (2003) study, breastfeeding was stopped 2 minutes before the procedure was undertaken.

Oral sucrose reduces the pain behaviour exhibited (Bilgen et al 2001, Overgaard & Knudsen 1999). While Stevens et al (2003) agree that sucrose is safe and effective, they suggest an optimal dose has not yet been identified and repeated use of sucrose in babies requiring several capillary samples should be investigated. Use of sucrose in the very low birthweight baby, where the condition is unstable or the baby is ventilated, also needs to be investigated further (Stevens et al 2003). Some parents may be opposed to the idea of administering sucrose to their baby; the midwife should be aware of alternative, more physiological methods of reducing the pain experience.

Overgaard and Knudsen (1999) found that making sure the baby was quiet and relaxed prior to the capillary sampling has a similar effect to sucrose administration.

The use of a local anaesthetic gel has been proposed for neonatal venepuncture (Moore 2001) and heel pricks (Bellini et al 2002) although Jain et al (2001) found it to be ineffective. If this is to be used it is important to ensure it is suitable for use in neonates and will not cause vasoconstriction as this will increase the difficulty in obtaining a sample and increase the pain felt by the baby.

### Use of alcohol–impregnated swabs

If an alcohol-impregnated swab is used, the area should be wiped for 30 seconds. It is important to ensure the area has dried before puncturing the skin. The swab should not be used when undertaking the Guthrie test. The mixture of blood and alcohol may cause a high glucose reading (Moxley 1989) and is therefore best avoided when testing blood glucose levels.

### Facilitating blood flow

Newborn babies have a sluggish circulation or vasoconstriction (acro-cyanosis) that may affect not only the amount of blood obtained but also the measurement of some blood tests. The baby should be kept warm, with only the foot exposed during the procedure. If the foot feels cool prior to the procedure, many midwives will warm the foot to facilitate blood flow. However, Barker et al (1996) found no advantage to warming the heel prior to sampling.

Holding the foot downwards encourages blood flow. If the blood is not flowing well, the heel may be gently squeezed and released. This should be undertaken carefully as excessive squeezing of the foot increases the risk of haemolysis and bruising due to haemodilution with interstitial fluid.

### Blood collection

The first drop of blood should be wiped away to avoid contamination from the skin. Petroleum jelly applied just below the puncture site will help the blood to collect in large globules, making collection easier.

- Guthrie test: using the card, ensure there is one large drop of blood per circle. Using more than one spot of blood may lead to an erroneous result. Blood should be applied from the top side of the card only
- Blood glucose: one large drop of blood is placed on to the reagent strip
- Bilirubin estimation: the end of the capillary tube is placed in the drop of blood and one finger is placed on the other end of the tube. The blood is drawn into the capillary tube and the finger removed to facilitate the passage of the blood down the tube, taking care not to allow the blood to spill out the other end. When full, the tubes are sealed, often with plasticine.

### Stopping the bleeding

When sufficient blood has been obtained, pressure should be applied to the site to cease blood flow and decrease the risk of haematoma for-mation and bruising. When the bleeding has stopped, a plaster may be applied, although this is not essential.

## Record keeping

This is particularly important if multiple tests are undertaken. The time and date of the test should be recorded as should the results when they become available. A record should be made of who has been informed of the results and any action to be taken. Complete all the information on the Guthrie card, particularly if the baby has been on antibiotics (or the mother if breastfeeding and taking antibiotics), or if the baby has had a blood transfusion during the past 48 hours. Most cards require the signature of the person who undertook the test so they can be informed if there are problems with the sample.

PROCEDURE   obtaining a capillary sample

- Gain informed consent from the parents; determine if they will be present and who will hold the baby
- Gather equipment:
  — suitable lancet
  — non-sterile gloves
  — alcohol-impregnated swab, if indicated
  — petroleum jelly, if indicated
  — collecting equipment
  — cotton wool ball or gauze swab
  — plaster to cover puncture site if required
  — portable sharps box
- Wash hands, apply gloves
- Position the baby appropriately, considering the comfort of the baby
- Inspect the foot to select the best site, avoiding underlying nerves and bone
- Encourage the baby to be calm and relaxed
- Wipe with alcohol-impregnated swab if indicated; leave to dry for at least 30 seconds
- Hold the ankle with the non-dominant hand with the foot flexed
- With the dominant hand pierce the skin with the lancet; put used lancet in sharps box
- Hold the foot downwards, wipe away the first drop of blood, apply petroleum jelly around the area the blood runs (but not over the puncture site)
- Allow the blood to form into large drops then collect the blood as required
- Using a cotton wool ball or gauze swab, apply pressure to the site; apply plaster if required
- Return the baby to the parents if they were not holding him during the procedure
- Dispose of equipment correctly and wash hands
- Discuss the results with the parents (when available)
- Document the results and act accordingly.

**Role and responsibilities of the midwife**

These can be summarised as:

- recognising the need for capillary blood sampling
- undertaking the procedure correctly and safely
- education and support of the parents
- contemporaneous record keeping.

## Summary

- Obtaining a capillary blood sample from the baby should be undertaken only when required, as there are risk factors associated with this procedure
- The midwife should be aware of the measures that can be taken to minimise the risks and ways in which blood flow can be promoted.

**Self-assessment exercises**

The answers to the following questions may be found in the text:

1. List the indications for undertaking capillary blood sampling.
2. When obtaining a capillary blood sample from the heel of the baby, how can the risk of damage to the underlying nerves and bone be minimised?
3. When obtaining a capillary blood sample from the heel of the baby, how can blood flow be encouraged?
4. Identify two factors that help and two factors that hinder the procedure of capillary sampling.
5. How can the amount of pain felt by the baby be reduced?
6. What are the role and responsibilities of the midwife in relation to capillary sampling?

## REFERENCES

Barker D P, Latty B W, Rutter N 1994 Heel blood sampling in preterm infants: which technique? Archives of Disease in Childhood (Fetal and Neonatal Edition) 71(3):206–208

Barker D P, Willetts B, Cappendijk V C et al 1996 Capillary blood sampling: should the heel be warmed? Archives of Disease in Childhood 74:F139–140

Bellini C V, Bagnoli F, Perrone S et al 2002 Effect of multisensory stimulation on analgesia in term neonates: a randomised controlled trial. Pediatric Research 41(4):460–463

Bilgen H, Ozek E, Cebeci D et al 2001 Comparison of sucrose, expressed breast milk and breast-feeding on the neonatal response to heel prick. Journal of Pain 2(5):301–305

Blumenfeld T A, Turi G K, Blanc W A 1979 Recommended site and depth of newborn heel skin punctures based on anatomical measurements and histopathology. Lancet 1:230–233

Carbajal R, Veerapen S, Couderc S et al 2003 Analgesic effect of breast feeding in term neonates: randomised controlled trial. British Medical Journal 326:13–15

Gray L, Watt L, Blass E M 2000 Skin-to-skin contact is analgesic in healthy newborns. Pediatrics 105(1):460–463

Harrison D, Johnston L 2002 Bedside assessment of heel lance pain in the hospitalized infant. Journal of Obstetric, Gynaecological and Neonatal Nursing 31(5):551–557

Jain A, Rutter N 1999 Ultrasound study of heel to calcaneum depth in neonates. Archives of Disease in Childhood 80:F243–245

Jain A, Rutter N, Ratnayaka M 2001 Topical amethocaine gel for pain relief of heel prick blood sampling: a randomised double blind controlled trial. Archives of Disease in Childhood (Fetal and Neonatal Edition) 84:F56–59

Meehan R M 1998 Heelsticks in neonates for capillary blood sampling. Neonatal Network 17(1):17–24

Moore J 2001 No more tears: a randomized controlled double-blind trial of amethocaine gel vs. placebo in the management of procedural pain in neonates. Journal of Advanced Nursing 34(4):475–482

Moxley S 1989 Neonatal heel puncture. The Canadian Nurse 85(1):25–27

Overgaard C, Knudsen A 1999 Pain-relieving effect of sucrose in newborns during heel prick. Biology of the Neonate 75:279–284

Stevens B, Yamada J, Ohlsson A 2003 Sucrose for analgesia in newborn infants undergoing painful procedures. Cochrane Library, Issue 3. Update Software, Oxford

Chapter **43**

# Assessment of the baby – developmental dysplasia of the hips

This chapter considers assessment for developmental dysplasia, including discussion of who should undertake the assessment, when and how.

**Learning outcomes**

Having read this chapter the reader should be able to:

- describe how the hips are examined to detect developmental dysplasia
- discuss the role and responsibilities of the midwife in relation to this screening test.

## Developmental dysplasia

Developmental dysplasia (congenital dislocation) of the hips occurs in 1–1.5 per 1000 births (Johnston et al 2003). The stability of the hips can be assessed at birth; some babies' hips will appear to be dislocatable while others are actually dislocated. It is important to detect this condition early to prevent long-term damage to the acetabulum that will result in shortening of the leg. While it may be difficult to detect dislocatable hips at birth due to the lax ligaments, all babies should be examined by a competent practitioner before they are discharged from the hospital. For babies born at home, this should be undertaken within the first 48 hours. While the paediatrician often performs this role, midwives are increasingly undertaking the examination, having undergone further training and assessment to be deemed competent (NMC 2004). If the hip is dislocatable, undertaking the test itself may be a cause of further damage. It is therefore very important that the test is done gently, but accurately, to avoid unnecessary repeat tests. Any baby who has a hip that is dislocatable should be referred to a paediatric orthopaedic surgeon.

Testing for developmental dysplasia of the hips involves looking at the appearance of the legs and the skin folds of the thighs, and then physically abducting the legs using either the Barlow or the Ortolani test, feeling for a palpable 'clunk' during the procedure. The range of abduction can also be assessed, as a limited range may be indicative of developmental dysplasia of the hip. However, ligamentous 'clicks' can be ignored as they are a normal finding at this time (Johnston et al 2003).

### Appearance of the legs and thigh skin folds

This is often part of the initial birth examination, but should be repeated prior to examination of the hips. The length of both legs should be the same; if one is shorter, this could be indicative of the head of the femur being located outside of the acetabulum. However, it can be difficult to measure the legs accurately. The legs should be held together and straightened as much as possible and the thigh creases should be symmetrical. Asymmetry is suggestive of developmental dysplasia, particularly if it is ascertained that this leg is shorter than the other. However, it should be remembered that bilateral developmental dysplasia can occur, in which case the thigh creases will appear to be symmetrical, as both femur heads will be displaced from the acetabulum. This assessment is not as reliable as the physical abduction tests, and therefore should not be used in isolation, but to provide further information to assist the diagnosis.

## Barlow's test

The rationale underpinning this test is to try to push the head of the femur out of the acetabulum in a backward direction. If achieved, this will be accompanied by a 'clunk' (Fig. 43.1). The normal hip is not dislocatable; no clunk will be felt.

### PROCEDURE    undertaking the Barlow's test

- Gain informed consent from the parents, undertaking the examination in the presence of one or both parents
- Wash hands; apply gloves if necessary
- Place the baby on a flat, firm surface, with good access to the baby
- Ensure the baby is warm, then undress the baby from the waist down, removing the nappy
- Position the legs in adduction
- Examining the hips one at a time, hold the knee and hip in a flexed position and place a thumb on the inner aspect of the thigh (over the inner trochanter) and the index and middle fingers over the outer part of the thigh (over the greater trochanter of the femur at the hip)
- Abduct the leg gently downwards to try to dislocate the hip by pushing down towards the supporting surface then gently pulling the leg upwards (if dislocatable, a 'clunk' is felt at this point as the

**Figure 43.1**    Barlow's test
(Adapted from Fraser & Cooper
2003)

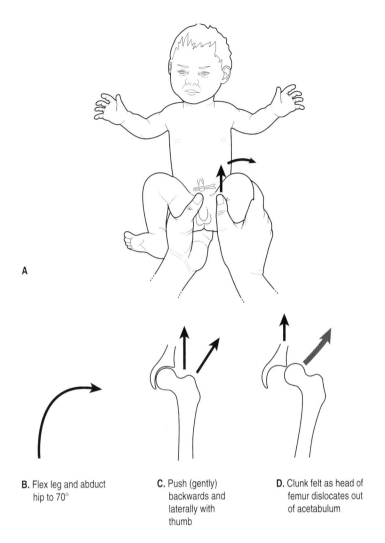

A

**B.** Flex leg and abduct
hip to 70°

**C.** Push (gently)
backwards and
laterally with
thumb

**D.** Clunk felt as head of
femur dislocates out
of acetabulum

head of the femur dislocates from the acetabulum and moves back towards it; this procedure is not possible if the hip is not dislocatable)

- Redress the baby
- Wash hands
- Discuss the findings with the parents
- Document the findings and act accordingly.

## Ortolani's test

The rationale for this test is that if the hip is unstable, the head of the femur will try to relocate in the acetabulum during the procedure as pressure is applied on the trochanter from behind, accompanied by a 'clunk' (Johnston et al 2003) (Fig. 43.2). The normal hip is not dislocatable; no clunk will be felt.

**Figure 43.2** Ortolani's test (Adapted from Fraser & Cooper 2003)

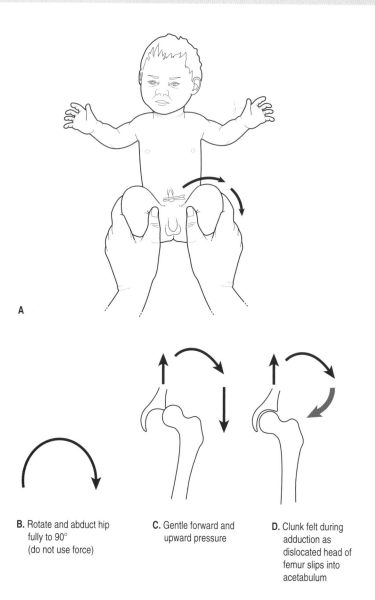

**A**

**B.** Rotate and abduct hip fully to 90° (do not use force)

**C.** Gentle forward and upward pressure

**D.** Clunk felt during adduction as dislocated head of femur slips into acetabulum

## PROCEDURE   undertaking the Ortolani's test

- Gain informed consent from the parents, undertaking the examination in the presence of one or both parents
- Wash hands; apply gloves if necessary
- Place the baby on a flat, firm surface, with good access to the baby
- Ensure the baby is warm, then undress the baby from the waist down, removing the nappy
- Examine the hips one at a time, taking hold of each leg, placing the thumb on the inner aspect of the thigh (over the inner trochanter) and the index and middle fingers over the outer aspect of the thigh (greater trochanter of the femur at the hip)

- Flex the knees and the hips 90° and abduct the leg gently (a 'clunk' is felt as the head of the femur dislocates from the acetabulum; if no clunk is felt, but the leg cannot be abducted fully, developmental dysplasia is also indicated)
- Redress the baby
- Wash hands
- Discuss the findings with the parents
- Document the findings and act accordingly.

### Role and responsibilities of the midwife

These can be summarised as:

- being able to undertake the procedure correctly and safely, if appropriately trained
- education and support of the parents
- referral as necessary
- contemporaneous record keeping.

## Summary

- The appropriately trained midwife or paediatrician should undertake assessment for developmental dysplasia prior to discharge from hospital, or within 48 hours of a home confinement
- There are two tests that can be used to assess the ability of the femur head to dislocate: Barlow and Ortolani.

### Self-assessment exercises

The answers to the following questions may be found in the text:

1. When would the midwife undertake the test for developmental dysplasia?
2. Describe the two methods of assessment.
3. What is the significance of the clunk?
4. What are the role and responsibilities of the midwife in relation to the assessment of developmental dysplasia?

### REFERENCES

Fraser D M, Cooper M A (eds) 2003 Myles textbook for midwives, 14th edn. Churchill Livingstone, Edinburgh

Johnston P G B, Flood F, Spinks K 2003 The newborn child, 9th edn. Churchill Livingstone, Edinburgh

NMC (Nursing and Midwifery Council) 2004 Midwives rules and standards. NMC, London

Chapter **44**

# Principles of infant nutrition – breastfeeding

More is learnt on an ongoing basis about the suitability of breast milk for human infants and the positive effects for the mother and child for short- and long-term health. However, MIDIRS (2003) cite evidence which suggests that only 20% of babies are exclusively breast fed at 3 months of age. This may be for many different reasons, but it is clear that midwives have a vital role in educating women as to the need for and method of breastfeeding. There is a wide range of detailed breastfeeding material published; this chapter focuses largely on the midwife gaining and developing the skills to facilitate correct breastfeeding. The physiology of lactation is reviewed, correct attachment at the breast is detailed and the role of the midwife is discussed.

| **Learning outcomes** | Having read this chapter the reader should be able to: |
|---|---|

- describe the anatomy of the breast and the physiology of lactation
- summarise the principles of correct breastfeeding
- discuss the recognition and significance of correct attachment at the breast
- describe the skills that the midwife needs to facilitate breastfeeding.

# Physiology of lactation

Understanding the anatomy of the breast and the physiology of lactation is one of the fundamental skills for facilitating successful breastfeeding:

- The glandular tissue is separated into lobes that are subdivided into lobules; within each lobule are alveoli, each of which is a cavity lined with acini cells surrounded by myoepithelial cells

- Each cluster of alveoli has lactiferous ducts that join with others to form lactiferous sinuses or ampullae. Milk collects in the ampullae that lie beneath the areola of the nipple. The lactiferous ducts open out onto the nipple. The nipples are lubricated by sebaceous glands
- Each breast functions independently; each has a rich blood and nerve supply.

Lactation is both the production and secretion of milk. The process begins at delivery when the placenta is expelled. The blood levels of oestrogen and progesterone fall, prolactin levels (from the anterior pituitary gland) rise, and milk production begins. Milk is manufactured by the acini cells. As the baby suckles, the stimulation causes the secretion of oxytocin from the posterior pituitary gland, which causes the myoepithelial cells to contract. Milk is forced along the ducts to the ampullae, and then forth into the baby's mouth as the baby actively feeds and removes the milk. This action of milk release is known as the let down reflex and is under neurohormonal control. Initially it may be an unconditioned reflex, but as time continues it may become conditioned (e.g. a response to the baby crying). It can be inhibited by anxiety; reassurance and encouragement are necessary to overcome this.

Prolactin influences milk production and oxytocin, milk secretion. Prolactin is released in higher amounts during night-time feeds. However, for lactation to be fully maintained, it is the effective removal of milk from the breast that sustains the milk supply. The supply is regulated according to the demand, i.e. the baby's appetite.

Due to the hormonal changes at delivery, lactogenesis occurs within 48–96 hours. For the woman who chooses not to breast feed the milk will gradually be reabsorbed. The breastfeeding mother will find that lactogenesis occurs more quickly as the suckling baby stimulates the supply. A successful first feed not only promotes lactation physiologically, but also indicates that breastfeeding is more likely to be successful in the longer term.

Colostrum is secreted from the breasts until lactogenesis occurs. Once lactation is established, the breast milk changes throughout the feed; the initial milk is the foremilk that is more watery and quenches the baby's thirst. The richer hindmilk follows as the baby continues to suckle, providing high calorie milk, essentially a meal in one breast (RCM 2002).

Consequently, successful breastfeeding relies upon two main principles, both of which are determined by the anatomy of the breast and the physiology of lactation:

1. Correct positioning and attachment of the baby at the breast to ensure that the milk is drained
2. Demand feeding, the baby taking as much or as little as he requires, when he requires, including night-time feeds, to maintain milk production.

# Factors that help

As a learned skill, breastfeeding can be difficult and stressful initially. Mothers need support; experienced friends and other groups such as the National Childbirth Trust can be as valuable as midwives. Maternity units that give consistent advice enable women to have confidence in their carers and the advice given. The 'Ten steps to successful breastfeeding' (UNICEF, cited RCM 2002) provide some of that consistency and suggest ways in which breastfeeding can be achieved and maintained:

1. There should be a written breastfeeding policy routinely communicated to all health care staff
2. All health care staff should be trained in the skills necessary to implement the policy
3. All pregnant women should be informed about the benefits and management of breastfeeding
4. Breastfeeding should be initiated within 30 minutes of giving birth (including birth by caesarean section where possible)
5. Mothers should be shown how to breast feed and maintain lactation even if separated from their baby
6. No food or drink other than breast milk must be given to a newborn unless medically indicated
7. Mothers and babies should be together for 24 hours a day (rooming in)
8. Encourage breastfeeding on demand
9. A breast-fed baby should not have a teat or pacifier
10. Encourage the establishment of breastfeeding support groups, available to mothers on discharge.

# Facilitating attachment

Women need to be able to understand the physiology of lactation and correct breastfeeding technique in order to cope for 24 hours a day at home. Consequently, the midwife should aim to assist the mother by giving instruction and verbal directions, rather than hands-on support (Inch et al 2003). Successful early feeds boost confidence as well as skills.

The woman should be comfortable and positioned so that her back is straight and her lap flat, so that the baby can be brought to the breast from below it (Inch & Fisher 1999). Pillows on her lap may be used to bring the baby to an appropriate height and a footstool may help to flatten her lap.

- The baby should approach the breast at the same angle as the breast and therefore should be turned towards the mother. The size of the breast will determine how far on his back he is. The hand opposite to the breast should support the baby with the palm behind the shoulders and index and middle fingers at the base of the skull. This allows the baby's head to extend slightly
- If it is necessary to support the breast a hand is placed against the ribs at the junction with the breast; this does not then interfere with the breast shape. A large or soft breast can be tilted up as the baby is put on, in order to correctly direct the nipple
- The baby's nose/top lip should be level with the nipple. The bottom lip will need to make contact as far away from the nipple as possible
- In order to accommodate the ampullae in the baby's mouth, it is important that the baby opens his mouth to a wide gape. The baby is brought towards the nipple so that the top lip touches the nipple and the mouth gapes (Fig. 44.1)
- The baby is then brought, with a swift but gentle movement (with no change in the angle or position) onto the breast so that the nipple is aimed at the upper third of the mouth, the bottom lip well away from the nipple. The baby will then have one-third nipple and two-thirds breast as his teat
- The baby begins sucking rhythmically almost immediately with quick short sucks that soon change to slow deep ones. The mother may experience a 'toe curling' session initially as the nipple is drawn out, but it should not be painful. Pain acts as the warning sign that the baby is not latched on correctly. Previously traumatised nipples may be uncomfortable initially, but should also improve after 10–20 seconds (Inch & Fisher 1999). If pain is evident the baby should be removed by placing the little finger in the baby's mouth to release the grip before drawing the baby away and beginning the process again.

For the baby that is latched on correctly, the mother/midwife may observe the following:

- As the baby sucks, his jaw moves; sometimes the ears can be seen to move with the jaw. Areola can be seen above the nipple, but little (depending on size) will be seen beneath the nipple
- Chin and breast are in close contact, the nose is free without the breast being held back
- Feeding is quiet (gulping indicates a poor fix) and reasonably lengthy. After the first week (Inch & Fisher 1999) it is rarely more than 40 minutes

Figure 44.1   The wide gape.
Note too, the slightly extended
head, proximity of top lip/nose
to nipple, position of bottom
lip and direction that nipple
enters the mouth

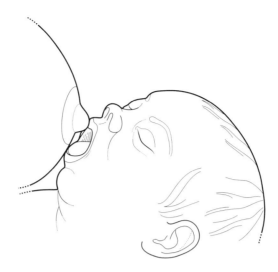

- The baby will suck and then pause, during which time he will remain on the breast. Sucking begins spontaneously within a few seconds, prompting is not required
- The baby will come off spontaneously when finished. A baby that continues to root may be assisted to latch on again, perhaps onto the other breast if the first one has been drained
- The baby will be satisfied, sleep peacefully between feeds, gain weight, and pass urine and normal stools
- The mother experiences the sensation of the breast being lighter and softer after feeding.

### Positioning

While needing to adapt the principles described above, the woman may choose to feed in any comfortable position. As the mother gains confidence she can experiment to find which positions suit both her and her baby. Night-time feeds, for example, may be managed lying laterally in bed. Midwives should be aware of the back strain that they can incur when assisting with breastfeeding and should practise within the safe moving and handling guidelines, working at the correct height without bending or twisting.

### Complications

Usually complications of breastfeeding are traced back to incorrect latching on. Insufficient milk supply, sore or cracked nipples and engorgement are all related to the feeding technique. If the baby is latched on correctly, the nipples will not be traumatised in any way, the milk will be drained properly so that engorgement does not occur and the supply of the milk will match the demand. Hence, these problems may be overcome with further support and education to ensure that the technique is appropriate. Inch and Fisher (1999) describe their breastfeeding clinic, noting that much information can be gained simply by observing the mother attaching the baby to the breast and advising on the technique.

### Expressing breast milk

Breast milk can be expressed, either by hand or by an electric or manual pump. The mother whose baby is nursed in intensive care, until the baby can breast feed for himself, often requires it. It is harder to maintain lactation when expressing and not breastfeeding due to reduced nerve stimulation of the nipple. The mother will require support and encouragement to express successfully. Manual expression needs to be learnt, otherwise equipment should be chosen that is easily sterilised. The milk may be kept for 24 hours in a fridge or frozen in a sterile container for up to 6 months.

### Role and responsibilities of the midwife

These can be summarised as:

- evidence-based practice with good communication to provide advice, support, encouragement and education to facilitate the woman's ability to breast feed (preferably with a 'hands off' approach from the midwife!).

## Summary

- Women can be empowered to breast feed successfully by midwives using their knowledge and supportive skills to give direction and guidance
- Correct attachment at the breast is vital, both to facilitate nutrition and to prevent breastfeeding problems
- The baby should demand feed and will draw the milk from the breast at his own pace.

### Self-assessment exercises

The answers to the following questions may be found in the text:

1. Describe the anatomy of the breast and how milk is formed.
2. Discuss how this information impacts on the success of breastfeeding.
3. Describe to a woman how to successfully attach her baby to the breast.
4. List the features that indicate a baby is correctly attached.
5. List the 'Ten steps to successful breastfeeding'.

## REFERENCES

Inch S, Fisher C 1999 Breastfeeding: getting the basics right. The Practising Midwife 2(4):35–38

Inch S, Law S, Wallace L 2003 Hands off! The Breastfeeding Best Start project (1). The Practising Midwife 6(10):17–19

MIDIRS 2003 Breastfeeding or bottle feeding? Informed choice leaflet (7) for professionals, 3rd edn. MIDIRS, Bristol

RCM (Royal College of Midwives) 2002 Successful breastfeeding, 3rd edn. Churchill Livingstone, Edinburgh

# Chapter 45

# Principles of infant nutrition — cup feeding

This chapter considers the correct technique for cup feeding. It is considered to be a viable alternative to using a teat for a breast-fed baby, but it is important that the technique is correct.

**Learning outcomes**

Having read this chapter the reader should be able to:

- discuss the indications for cup feeding
- describe the technique
- summarise the midwife's role and responsibilities in relation to cup feeding.

## Indications

Cup feeding allows the baby to take the milk from the cup at his own pace. It is always an interim measure, the aim being to successfully feed at some point, generally to breast feed. It is recognised to have three valuable uses:

1. As an interim measure for full-term babies for whom a feeding supplement may be required, or for whom breastfeeding is not yet established (the use of a teat may reduce the success of breast feeding; Lang 1994). Samuel (1998) describes the way in which babies mature their sucking action and cites examples of the ways in which cup feeding aided term babies that lacked that maturity and so were unable to feed initially
2. Constituents of milk may be retained along the walls of a nasogastric tube; tube use also bypasses the enzymes in the mouth that begin the process of digestion
3. For the preterm infant without sufficient suck/swallow coordination, who can easily tire if breast or bottle fed. Lang et al (1994) suggest it to be appropriate from 30 weeks' gestation. However, Freer (1999) demonstrated that preterm infants underwent greater physiological

instability when cup feeding than breastfeeding and so encourages caution.

It can be helpful in situations such as the special care baby unit, where expressed breast milk can be given in the mother's absence. Formula milk may also be given in this way if necessary. Samuel (1998) notes that less is taken from a cup than a bottle; the baby is therefore not overdistended and will not expect a large feed subsequently. The cups should be sterilised as for any other feeding equipment used for a baby (Ch. 46).

The baby should lap or sip, rather than having the milk poured into his mouth. The danger of aspiration into the lungs is possible if the baby is not permitted to control the flow. Thorley (1997) indicates a case study where poor technique reduced the infant's weight gain and caused aspiration. The procedure should not be hurried; the baby will feed at his own pace and should be permitted to demand feed.

Parents can be taught to cup feed easily and may gain greater confidence in relation to their subsequent feeding method, having had the opportunity to learn (Samuel 1998). It is highly likely that a term baby will dribble; parents should be prepared for this.

## PROCEDURE    cup feeding

- Ensure that the baby is alert and interested
- Gather equipment:
  - expressed breast milk
  - sterilised cup
  - bib/napkin
  - baby's records
- Wash hands
- Sit comfortably with the baby in an upright sitting position, well swaddled (to prevent hands knocking the cup) with the bib in place
- Direct the cup towards the baby's top gum with the level of milk touching his lips
- Retain the cup in this position; the baby will lap/suck, pause (as with any other feeding pattern) and commence lapping again when ready
- The baby will determine the pace and cease feeding when no longer hungry
- Wash and sterilise the cup, wash hands
- Complete documentation.

## Role and responsibilities of the midwife

These can be summarised as:

- recognising the need to use cup feeding as a valuable interim measure to support breastfeeding
- teaching a safe and correct technique
- support and encouragement of parents
- record keeping.

## Summary

- Cup feeding is a valuable interim measure; it is important that the baby and the cup are both positioned correctly and that the baby laps at his own pace.

## Self-assessment exercises

The answers to the following questions may be found in the text:

1. List the circumstances when cup feeding is indicated.
2. Describe how to cup feed a baby.
3. Summarise the role and responsibilities of the midwife when cup feeding.

## REFERENCES

Freer Y 1999 A comparison of breast and cup feeding preterm infants. Journal of Neonatal Nursing 5(1):16–20

Lang S 1994 Cup feeding – an alternative method. Midwives Chronicle 107(1276):171–176

Lang S, Lawrence C, Orme R 1994 Cup feeding: an alternative method of infant feeding. Archives of Disease in Childhood 71:365–369

Samuel P 1998 Cup feeding. The Practising Midwife 1(12):33–35

Thorley V 1997 Cup feeding: problems created by incorrect use. Journal of Human Lactation 13(1):54–55

Chapter **46**

# Principles of infant nutrition – sterilisation of feeding equipment

Babies should be protected against any potential sources of infection due to the immaturity of their immune system. Feeding equipment should be carefully sterilised; traces of milk can harbour and multiply bacteria quickly. The effects of gastroenteritis can be life threatening to a newborn baby and fungal infection can be difficult to treat. This chapter considers the correct use of the different sterilising techniques and the role of the midwife in relation to this.

## Learning outcomes

Having read this chapter the reader should be able to:

- describe all of the ways in which effective sterilisation can be undertaken
- discuss the role and responsibilities of the midwife.

## Sterilisation advice

Ackerley (2001) indicates that the advice given regarding sterilisation of feeding equipment needs to be given to all new mothers, regardless of feeding method at that time. Formula-feeding mothers need it immediately; breastfeeding mothers may or may not need it, but will have difficulty comprehending it fully if needing it when breastfeeding has failed (emotional distress) or tiredness is great. Equally, compliance with the advice is likely to be greater if the reasons for sterilisation are discussed as well as the methods. The midwife should teach the woman in a familiar environment using familiar equipment; care should be taken if the woman's first language is not English.

## Cleaning feeding equipment

All equipment needs to be thoroughly cleansed before being sterilised, regardless of sterilisation method. Retained milk will harbour bacteria and may survive the sterilisation process. This is the recommended cleaning technique (largely from Ackerley 2001):

- Dispose of a leftover feed within 90 minutes of starting
- Dismantle the bottle completely
- Wash all parts using hot soapy water and a bottle brush, or use a dishwasher
- Turn teats inside out and use the teat end of the bottle brush or a teat brush to clean all surfaces
- Squeeze water through teat holes
- Rinse items thoroughly under cold water tap to remove soap (Ellis & Kanneh 2000).

## Methods of sterilisation

Choices may be made according to convenience and costs, both of the initial outlay and of ongoing use. There are three different methods of sterilisation:

1. boiling
2. chemical
3. steam: microwave or electrical.

### Boiling

Boiling in the home can be a hazardous activity and therefore is often considered a short-term interim measure. Prolonged use of boiling may destroy the teats; boiling them alone for 5 minutes is acceptable. A large saucepan with a lid is required and a trivet in the base of the pan prevents the bottles from burning.

PROCEDURE    sterilisation by boiling

- Immerse the clean equipment fully in cold water in the saucepan, ensuring that there are no air pockets
- Put the lid on the pan and place on the heat; bring to the boil
- When clearly boiling, time for 20 minutes (Ackerley 2001); avoid adding anything else to the pan
- After 20 minutes, turn off the heat; leave undisturbed in the saucepan until required
- The equipment should be used within 12 hours (after 12 hours, or if any item is removed in the meantime, the process should be repeated)
- Care should be taken to avoid burns if the equipment is required before it has properly cooled.

### Chemical

Various preparations – tablets, liquids and crystals – are commercially available for chemical sterilisation, usually using cold tap water. However, it should be noted that sodium hypochlorite (often the chemical used) achieves a high level of disinfection rather than sterilisation

(Atkinson 2001). Metal parts of any description must not be placed in the fluid, but should be boiled. The manufacturer's instructions should be followed carefully, but they generally use similar principles.

PROCEDURE    **chemical sterilisation**

- A large enough container should be available with a well fitting lid
- Have thoroughly washed hands and a clean working surface
- Prepare the sterilising solution using the correct amounts of water and chemical to produce fluid of the correct concentration
- Fully immerse the clean utensils, ensuring there are no trapped air bubbles; put on the lid
- Leave the container undisturbed for 30 minutes (times may vary); if anything needs to be added to or removed from the solution during this time the 30 minutes begins again from the time of addition/removal
- Leave the container undisturbed until required
- When the equipment is required, wash hands, remove the items carefully, handling them by the aspects that will not come into contact with the baby or milk
- Either shake the excess off the equipment or, according to the directions, rinse them with recently boiled, cooled water (Ackerley 2001)
- Use them immediately
- Change the sterilising solution every 24 hours.

### Microwave
Non-metallic equipment can also be sterilised in a microwave using a specific microwave steriliser and suitable feeding equipment. Models vary, including some bottles that may be microwaved. The manufacturer's instructions should be followed carefully. It should be remembered that the timings often include standing time. The items should be resterilised if not used within 3 hours. Sterilising in a microwave without recommended equipment is inappropriate.

### Electric steam sterilisers
Feeding equipment can be sterilised by steam using an electric steriliser, for which the manufacturer's instructions should be followed carefully. The equipment does need to have complete contact with the steam and so should be loaded with open ends facing downwards. The cycle often lasts approximately 15 minutes; the items can be used immediately or left undisturbed until required.

## Recontamination

There are many ways in which feeding equipment can be recontaminated after sterilisation. Clean hands are essential, especially after changing nappies and toileting, food preparation and nose blowing

(Ackerley 2001). The work surface should be clean and uncluttered and as the feeds are prepared it is essential that no part that has contact with the milk or baby should be touched. Sterilised tongs are useful, especially to pull through the teats.

### Role and responsibilities of the midwife

These may be summarised as:

- careful education of the woman, with good documentation and ongoing review
- practising with research-based evidence.

## Summary

- There are four effective methods of sterilisation: boiling, chemical, microwave and electrical steam. Items must be thoroughly cleaned before sterilisation
- It is important that the technique is undertaken correctly whichever method is chosen; babies need to be protected from potential infection.

### Self-assessment exercises

The answers to the following questions may be found in the text:

1. Discuss why sterilisation of feeding equipment is necessary.
2. Describe how to sterilise feeding equipment when boiling.
3. Demonstrate how to sterilise feeding equipment using chemical sterilisation.
4. Discuss the different methods of steam sterilisation.
5. Summarise the role and responsibilities of the midwife in relation to effective equipment sterilisation.

### REFERENCES

Ackerley L 2001 Bottle feeding: how to give advice on hygiene. Professional Care of Mother and Child 11(6):152–155

Atkinson A 2001 Decontamination of breast milk collection kits: a change in practice. MIDIRS Midwifery Digest 11(3):383–385

Ellis M, Kanneh A 2000 Infant nutrition: part two. Paediatric Nursing 12(1):38–43

Chapter **47**

# Principles of infant nutrition – formula feeding

When a mother is advised not to breast feed or chooses not to, the midwife has an important role in facilitating successful infant nutrition using formula milk. This chapter considers the significance of correct feed reconstitution, potential dangers, feeding technique and the midwife's role and responsibilities. This chapter needs to be read in conjunction with Chapter 44 (breastfeeding) and Chapter 46 (sterilisation of feeding equipment).

---

**Learning outcomes**

Having read this chapter the reader should be able to:

- discuss the principles of correct formula milk preparation and the dangers of incorrect reconstitution
- describe how to feed a baby using formula milk
- summarise the role and responsibilities of the midwife.

---

## Formula feeding

This text does not have the scope to examine all of the evidence relating to feeding methods. However, it is clear that with only 20% of babies being exclusively breast fed at 3 months of age (MIDIRS 2003) a large proportion of the population are feeding with formula milk and therefore some of the longer term consequences are as yet unknown. Many short-term effects are known and these include dangers for the baby such as gastroenteritis, respiratory infections, ear infections, obesity, lesser developmental achievements and raised cholesterol in adult life. For the mother, there are higher risks of cancer of the breasts and ovaries and greater chances of hip fracture in later life (MIDIRS 2003). It is clear therefore that midwives have a significant responsibility in helping women to make the best feeding choice and to avoid some of the pitfalls with poor formula feeding techniques.

## Formula milks

Infant formula milks are generally either whey or casein dominant. Whey dominant is considered to be closer to human milk, while casein dominant may be more satisfying for the baby. Neither milk, however, can be compared with the suitability of breast milk for the newborn baby, despite advances to add prebiotics and the like to enhance immunity. Formula milk may be ready prepared, but is generally cheaper in powdered form for reconstitution. Other types of formula are available for particular circumstances (e.g. preterm babies, milk allergy, vegetarianism, organic preference); in many instances a paediatrician prescribes such a milk.

Each packet of formula milk powder is supplied with a plastic scoop that is suitable for use with that packet only. Reconstitution instructions should be followed correctly, the general rule being one level scoop of powder for each fluid ounce (28 mL) of water. The expiry date should be checked before the powder is used.

## Equipment required

The following equipment is suggested:

- six (to cover a 24-hour period) infant feeding bottles with tops, covers and teats. Wide necked bottles are often easier to clean. The scale on the side should be clearly visible. Standard flow teats are acceptable. The woman may make different choices later, according to her baby's needs
- sterilising equipment (Ch. 46)
- bottle and teat brushes (non-metallic)
- sterilisable tongs or tweezers
- plastic spatula or leveller if not integral in milk packet
- a kettle or means of boiling water.

## Feeding preparation

*Potential hazards*

Ackerley (2001) is clear that there are potential dangers of which midwives (and parents) should be aware. Gastroenteritis in babies is reported to cost the NHS £35 million per year (MIDIRS 2003), hence the need to focus on correct preparation of formula feeds. Dangers include:

- unclean equipment that has been not been properly sterilised and is then recontaminated (see Ch. 46 for additional guidance)
- a reconstituted feed is a breeding ground for bacteria and so needs to be:
  1. cooled rapidly. The water alone may cool at room temperature, but if containing the milk powder then additional measures are needed. The bottle can be placed in a mug or jug of cold water

with ice cubes, or under cold running water. Commercial can or bottle coolers can also be used

2. stored below 5°C. A fridge thermometer is useful; feeds should not be kept in the door but in the body of the fridge

3. reheated rapidly. The bottle is placed in a mug or jug of boiling water, shaken gently and tested after 2 minutes. The boiling water may need replacing and care should be taken with other young children around

- While microwaving is not recommended for reheating formula feeds, Ackerley (2001) recognises that it is frequently used. Therefore the recommendation is to heat the feed for 10-second bursts only, shaking and testing after each one, repeating as necessary. The lid should be loosened before microwaving

- Incorrect reconstitution of feeds can lead to obesity, electrolyte imbalance and constipation (excess powder) or malnutrition (insufficient powder)

- Unfinished feeds need to be disposed of within 90 minutes of starting and the equipment needs washing immediately.

### Preparation of formula milk

There are several important principles:

- Equipment must be freshly sterilised and ready to use, hands should be washed, surfaces should be clean and uncluttered and, if possible, undivided attention should be given to the task. Avoid recontaminating the equipment by sneezing, etc.

- The water should be boiled once. The bottle is filled to the appropriate level *before* the powder is added; this is best judged at eye level

- Either: (A) cool the water in the fridge (maximum 24 hours), making up the feed moments before needing it (warm the water or the feed; some powders will reconstitute in cold water), or (B) cool the water at room temperature, make up all the feeds and store in the fridge for up to 24 hours. Option A is considered to be the safer option (Ackerley 2001)

- The scoop of powder should be level, not tightly or loosely packed, but filled and levelled. The powder is added to the water, the top or teat and cover are applied (sterilised tweezers are helpful) and the milk is shaken gently to ensure appropriate mixing of the contents

- The instructions must be followed completely, but in general, that for 3 fluid ounces of milk there would be 3 fluid ounces of water and 3 level scoops of powder

- Prior to use, the feed should be at room temperature or above (up to 33°C; see above). The temperature should be checked before it

is given to the baby by testing a few drops on the inside of the woman's wrist. The milk should be warm, but not hot
- Discard unfinished feeds immediately (see above).

# Feeding technique

The principles of demand feeding should be upheld: the baby will feed when hungry, taking as much or as little as desired. Babies fed with formula milk often have a regular feeding pattern, approximately 4 hourly, but this may vary. Feed times should be enjoyable and relaxed, when either parent can feed. The baby should be held securely, close to his parent, in a similar position to breastfeeding, so that eye contact can be maintained.

The teat needs to be over the baby's tongue and the bottle tipped up far enough for air to be excluded from the teat. The teat should administer regular drops, rather than a stream of milk (Ellis & Kanneh 2000). The baby will suck and pause, retaining the teat in his mouth. A bib may catch any of the dribbles. The baby may be winded once or twice during the feed, often by just sitting the baby upright. Rubbing or patting of the back may assist winding. Occasionally a small amount of milk is regurgitated with wind; this is a normal process. A baby should never be left to 'prop' feed alone; the danger of choking is enormous.

The baby will cease feeding when he has had sufficient milk. The midwife should record the amount of feed taken, the total amount over a 24-hour period acting as an indicator of sufficient nutrition. The baby should be settled between feeds, gain weight and pass urine and stools normally. The stool may be firmer and slightly more offensive than that of a breast-fed baby.

Increasing the amount of feed is necessary when the baby is draining the full amount in the bottle. An additional ounce is reconstituted.

**Role and responsibilities of the midwife**

These can be summarised as:
- practising evidence-based practice with regard to knowledge of formula milks, their reconstitution and storage
- education and support of parents to ensure safe and successful infant nutrition and feeding technique
- recognition of a healthy formula-fed infant, correct record keeping.

## Summary

- It is important that formula milk is reconstituted, stored and warmed correctly and that sterilised equipment is used
- The midwife has an important role in assisting parents to develop a safe and satisfying feeding technique, and in recognising a healthy formula-fed baby.

| Self-assessment exercises | The answers to the following questions may be found in the text: |
|---|---|

1. Describe how to assist parents to successfully feed a baby using formula milk.
2. Describe how a feed is correctly reconstituted.
3. Discuss the possible dangers of incorrect reconstitution, cooling, storage and warming.
4. Summarise the midwife's role and responsibilities when caring for a woman and baby when the baby is being fed with formula milk.

## REFERENCES

Ackerley L 2001 Bottle feeding: how to give advice on hygiene. Professional Care of Mother and Child 11(6):152–155

Ellis M, Kanneh A 2000 Infant nutrition: part two. Paediatric Nursing 12(1):38–43

MIDIRS 2003 Breast or bottle feeding. Informed choice leaflet (7) for professionals, 3rd edn. MIDIRS, Bristol

# Chapter 48

# Principles of infant nutrition — nasogastric feeding

Nasogastric tubes (NGTs) may be used in both adults and babies. They are, as the name suggests, a tube which passes through the nose, into the oesophagus and through into the stomach. They have two main uses:

1. placing food or medication into the stomach
2. removing substances from the stomach (e.g. if 'mucousy').

This chapter considers, for a baby, nasogastric tube insertion, feeding or lavage and removal.

## Learning outcomes

Having read this chapter the reader should be able to:

- discuss when a nasogastric tube is indicated for a baby
- describe how one is inserted and removed safely
- describe how a baby is fed using a nasogastric tube
- describe how to undertake gastric lavage
- summarise the role and responsibilities of the midwife.

## Considerations

The inexperienced midwife must be trained and supervised before undertaking the procedure. Nasogastric feeds may be undertaken for babies in ward areas, special care baby units or occasionally at home. It is the most unnatural way of feeding, with an obvious, unsightly tube attached to the face, with greater dangers of gastric reflux and vomiting. Therefore, while it has a significant place for the baby that is unable to gain nutrition any other way, it should be used only when really necessary. The midwife has a responsibility to teach and support parents as they care for their baby and carry out this aspect of care.

For short procedures such as gastric lavage (p. 366) the tube may be inserted and removed; if it is required over a longer period it must be securely attached across the baby's cheek.

| PROCEDURE | **inserting a nasogastric tube** |

- Gain informed consent from the parents and gather equipment:
  — sterile nasogastric or Ryles tube, size FG 6 (for a baby weighing >1.7 kg)
  — sterile 5 mL syringe
  — tape
  — pH indicator blue litmus paper
  — non-sterile gloves
  — stethoscope
- Position the baby in a good light and a safe place, e.g. in the cot or held by an assistant; swaddle tightly so that hands are kept from the face
- Wash hands and apply gloves
- Measure the distance from the ear to the nose and then from the nose to the xiphisternum (Fig. 48.1), noting the distance markers on the tube
- Pass the tube through the smaller nostril, gently but smoothly; if resistance is felt, stop and try the other nostril, observing the condition of the baby throughout. Stop and remove the tube if there is any gasping or cyanosis
- Once the tube has been passed through the appropriate length, hold the tube in place, attach the syringe and withdraw approximately 0.5 mL of gastric aspirate
- Test the aspirate with the pH indicator litmus paper; blue will turn to pink in the presence of gastric acid. If the aspirate is hard to withdraw, the tube may have been occluded by mucus on insertion; 1–2 mL air may be injected first and then the aspirate withdrawn
- Once the position is confirmed, tape the tube in place across the baby's cheek
- If there is insufficient gastric secretion to use the litmus paper test, then 2.5 mL of air may be gently syringed down the tube, while listening over the baby's stomach with a stethoscope. The air entering the stomach should be clearly audible. This procedure should only ever be completed with air, *never water*, in case the tube is in the lungs. If there is ever any doubt as to where the tube is, it should be either removed and the procedure repeated or checked with an x-ray
- Dispose of equipment correctly
- Wash hands
- Document and act accordingly.

**Figure 48.1** Measuring the length of the nasogastric tube prior to insertion: measure from ear to nose, then from nose to xiphisternum, noting the distance markers on the tubing

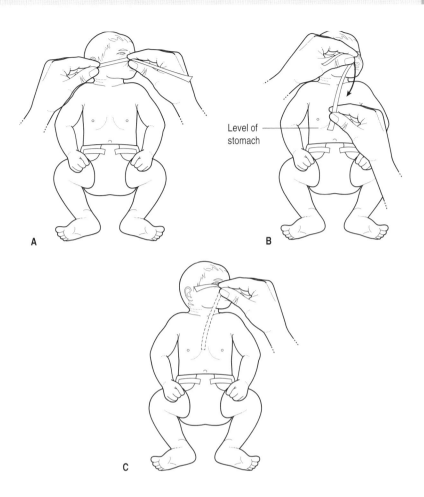

A

B

Level of stomach

C

# Administering a tube feed

This type of feeding technique will only be used if there is a specific indication. Breast or formula milk may be used. The amount may be specifically prescribed or calculated based on the baby's daily requirements according to weight, gestation and age. The feed is usually intermittent (bolus); the tube is flushed after each administration and the milk stored and prepared in a sterile way. Continuous infusion is sometimes indicated.

| PROCEDURE | administering a tube feed |

- Gain informed consent from the parents and gather equipment:
  — sterile syringes, 2 mL, 5 mL and 20 mL
  — pH indicator/blue litmus paper
  — milk, at room temperature
  — non-sterile gloves
  — sterile water for oral use

- Position the baby in a good light and a safe place; the baby may be cuddled by one of his parents and interaction should take place as for any other kind of feed
- Wash hands and apply gloves
- Using the 2 mL syringe, establish that the tube is correctly in the stomach by extracting and testing the gastric aspirate using the pH indicator or blue litmus paper (according to local protocol)
- Remove the plunger from the 20 mL syringe, attach the syringe to the tube, but occlude the tube by compressing it gently
- Pour the required amount of milk into the syringe, holding it in an upright position
- Release the occlusion on the tube so that the milk begins to flow into the stomach
- Regulate the flow by occluding and pausing if it is too fast. The feed should be leisurely and enjoyable, as for any other feed
- Observe the baby's condition throughout and stop the procedure if necessary, e.g. coughing, vomiting, hypoxic or bradycardic episodes
- Follow the feed with 3 mL of sterile water drawn up using the 5 mL syringe to cleanse the tube once the feed is completed (Naysmith & Nicholson 1998)
- Close off the tube, dispose of the equipment and wash hands
- Complete the records.

## Gastric lavage

Gastric aspirate may be sent for microscopy, culture and sensitivity if the baby requires an infection screen. A nasogastric tube is inserted, a small amount of aspirate withdrawn and the tube removed. This contrasts with gastric lavage, which may be undertaken when the baby is 'mucousy', having swallowed much mucus at birth, and is therefore unable to feed. The mucus is removed from the stomach using a sterile water 'washout' (some babies will vomit it themselves).

### PROCEDURE  gastric lavage (baby)

- Gain informed consent from the parents and gather equipment:
  — sterile nasogastric tube
  — non-sterile gloves
  — pH indicator/blue litmus paper
  — disposable receiver
  — sterile water for oral use (at room temperature or up to 33°C)
  — sterile syringes, 5 mL and 20 mL
- Wash hands and apply gloves
- Insert the tube. Confirm correct position in the stomach using 5 mL syringe and pH indicator (p. 364)

- Draw up 10 mL sterile water into the 20 mL syringe. Attach to the tube and plunge it steadily down into the stomach. Draw back the 10 mL immediately; mucus is also seen
- Dispose of it into the receiver
- Observe the baby's condition throughout and stop the procedure if necessary
- Plunge down and withdraw the next 10 mL of water in the same way
- Continue the process until no further mucus is seen (2–3 times)
- Remove the tube (see below) and dispose of equipment correctly
- Wash hands
- Document findings
- Continue to observe the baby and his feeding pattern.

# Removal of a nasogastric tube

Local protocols will indicate the length of time a nasogastric tube may be retained. Mears (2001) highlights the physiological distress to preterm babies when having a tube changed. She notes that a tube may be left in situ for 5–7 days rather than 2 days. Equally, to avoid the trauma of unnecessary reinsertion, ensure that removal is definitely indicated before removing it. Unfortunately, babies frequently remove their own nassogastric tubes unless the tube is well secured!

## PROCEDURE    removal of a nasogastric tube

- Obtain informed consent; position the baby in a good light and a safe place
- Wash hands and apply gloves
- Remove the tape from the face
- Pull out the tube smoothly and quickly, place into a bag for disposal (the baby may sneeze)
- Check the tube is complete, dispose of equipment correctly and wash hands
- Complete documentation and act accordingly. Ensure that the baby feeds normally following the procedure.

## Role and responsibilities of the midwife

These can be summarised as:

- completing the techniques competently, seeking informed consent from parents, educating and supporting them
- observation of the baby during and following the procedure; referral if necessary
- contemporaneous record keeping.

## Summary

- Nasogastric tubes may be used to feed babies in special circumstances or to withdraw aspirate from the stomach
- The tube must be confirmed to be in the stomach before any fluid is run through it
- The condition of the baby must be observed throughout.

---

**Self-assessment exercises**

The answers to the following questions may be found in the text:

1. Discuss when a nasogastric tube may be required for a baby.
2. Describe how to safely insert a nasogastric tube and complete a milk feed.
3. Describe how to remove a nasogastric tube.
4. Describe how to complete a gastric lavage.
5. Summarise the role and responsibilities of the midwife in relation to each of these aspects of care.

---

### REFERENCES

Mears M 2001 Changing nasogastric tubes in the sick and preterm infant: a help or hindrance? Journal of Neonatal Nursing 7(6):202–206

Naysmith M R, Nicholson J 1998 Nasogastric drug administration. Professional Nurse 13(7):424–427

Chapter **49**

# Principles of phlebotomy and intravenous therapy – maternal venepuncture

Venepuncture is the puncturing of a vein with a needle, usually to obtain specimens of blood for laboratory analysis, but may also include the administration of drugs intravenously in an emergency. The ability of a midwife to undertake venepuncture facilitates individualised and holistic care for the woman from the same practitioner. This chapter considers the indications for venepuncture, the rationale for correct preparation and the procedure. The role and responsibilities of the midwife are summarised.

## Learning outcomes

Having read this chapter the reader should be able to:

- discuss the indications for venepuncture
- describe how venepuncture is undertaken safely
- discuss the rationale for the choice of vein and equipment used
- summarise the role and responsibilities of the midwife.

## Indications

- Antenatal 'booking' bloods
- Assessment of full blood count and presence of rhesus antibodies during pregnancy. Further repeats if rhesus negative blood group, with Kleihauer test after delivery
- Other tests may be taken if there is an existing disease, e.g. thyroid function tests, blood glucose monitoring, anti-epileptic drug levels, or if other conditions are suspected, e.g. sickle cell anaemia, thalassaemia, hepatitis B
- Antenatal screening tests for fetal normality, e.g. alphafetoprotein
- Cross-matching prior to blood transfusion, or sometimes prior to operative delivery.

This is not an exhaustive list, but it does indicate that women are often asked to give blood specimens. Fear of needles or of fainting can be real fears; midwives should be sensitive to both the physical and psychological aspects of the skill. Simulated practice may be valuable to the novice, as may the opportunity to observe others, work under their supervision and maintain the skill once learnt.

## Suitable sites

Blood is always taken from a vein, never an artery. Arterial blood is only ever sought by medical staff in specific circumstances (e.g. for blood gas analysis). The physiological additional blood volume during pregnancy and the general body warmth of the pregnant woman both create vasodilatation, making venepuncture easier than with many other groups of people. Being healthy, their veins are also often in a good condition.

The midwife should appreciate the anatomy of the arm below the elbow. The basilic, median cubital and cephalic veins are all appropriately placed in the antecubital fossa and are suitable sites for effective venepuncture (Fig. 49.1). Understanding the anatomy is also important to ensure that arteries and nerves are avoided. The skin should be free from inflammation and bruising.

### Choosing a vein

While veins are often visible nearer to the skin surface, such obvious ones are not always suitable for venepuncture. It is better to palpate a vein, aided by the use of a tourniquet that obstructs the venous return. The woman can be asked to clench and unclench her fist a couple of times to increase the prominence of the vein, but this isn't always necessary and can affect the results. Veins are generally bouncy and full. Often women will know from past experience which are their 'good' veins. Palpating the vein also allows the midwife to avoid two other structures:

- valves, which are seen as 'nodules' within the vein and make specimen collection both very difficult and painful if venepuncture is attempted *below* the valve
- arteries, which have a palpable pulse.

### Skin preparation

As an aseptic procedure, the skin should be cleansed with either a 70% chlorhexidine preparation or an alcohol-impregnated wipe. Dougherty and Lister (2004) suggest proper cleansing of the area is required (>30 seconds), rather than swift wiping which only serves to disturb the skin bacteria. The skin should be given at least 30 seconds to air dry and the vein should not be repalpated. The need to prevent infection entering the veins is very important.

**Figure 49.1** Suitable veins for venepuncture (Adapted with kind permission from Williams 1995)

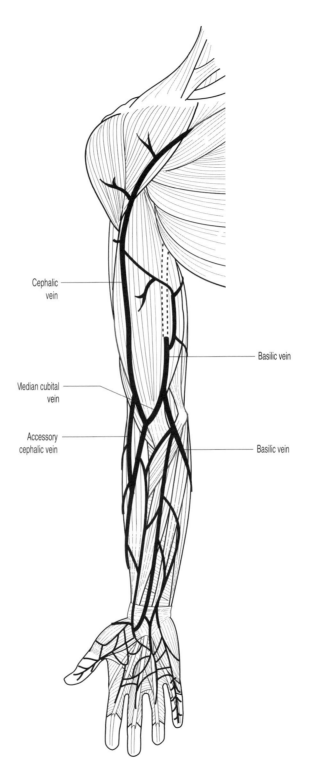

Cephalic vein

Basilic vein

Median cubital vein

Accessory cephalic vein

Basilic vein

## Equipment

Equipment should be:

- sterile and used in such a way as to maintain asepsis
- ideally a closed vacuum system that also protects the midwife from contact with body fluids.

Closed systems (e.g. Vacutainer) use a vacuum so that as the vein is punctured and the 'syringe'/bottle is applied to the system, there is no leakage of blood. The procedure is adapted according to the equipment used. Syringes and needles increase the risk of contamination and needlestick injuries. Midwives should be familiar with the system used in their practice area, along with the bottles, forms and transport means.

It is advisable to wear gloves, particularly if inexperienced in venepuncture. Sharps boxes should be used correctly and a used needle should *never* be resheathed (see Ch. 9 for discussion re: new protection devices).

---

**PROCEDURE** **maternal venepuncture**

- Gather equipment:
  - receiver and sharps box
  - Vacutainer needle (green 21 g) and sheath or alternative
  - appropriate specimen bottles
  - 70% alcohol-impregnated wipe or 70% alcohol and dressing pack
  - sterile gloves
  - antiseptic hand rub
  - sterile cotton wool ball
  - tourniquet
  - adhesive plaster
  - specimen request form
- Gain informed consent; ensure the woman is comfortable, with her arm supported in an accessible position; good light is required
- Wash hands
- Apply the tourniquet approximately 5 cm above the antecubital fossa; encourage the woman to clench and unclench her fist a couple of times if necessary
- Identify the chosen vein by palpation, retaining the site of entry in the 'mind's eye'
- Apply hand rub and sterile gloves
- Cleanse the skin thoroughly (>30 seconds); wait for it to dry (>30 seconds)
- Assemble the Vacutainer system, gently unsheathing the needle when ready

- Using the non-dominant hand, apply slight tension to the skin below the point of entry (this will anchor the vein)
- Insert the needle into the vein at a 30° angle; be decisive but not too firm
- Insert the vacuumed bottle and watch it fill; remove when flow stops (fill subsequent bottles if necessary)
- If blood does not appear the needle may be 'nudged' a little further in, or withdrawn a small amount (if no blood is seen, or the woman is in acute pain, remove the needle, collect new equipment and try another site)
- Release the tourniquet, withdraw the needle and then apply pressure using the cotton wool ball to the puncture site for the next minute (the woman should be encouraged to do this, if able). Keep arm horizontal
- Apply plaster if required
- Dispose of sharps and equipment correctly
- Wash hands
- Label the specimen bottles and request form; send the specimen to the laboratory. Ensure that the results are acted upon on return
- Document and act accordingly.

### Bruising

Bruising can occur if the needle is removed before the tourniquet is released. It may also be worsened if the woman is asked to bend her arm when applying pressure to the puncture site.

### Role and responsibilities of the midwife

These can be summarised as:

- undertaking the procedure competently and safely
- education and support of the woman
- referral if necessary
- contemporaneous record keeping.

## Summary

- Venepuncture is a skill that all midwives should be able to complete competently
- It is an aseptic procedure that ideally uses a closed vacuum system so that there is no contact with body fluids
- Specimens should be in the correct bottles, labelled and dispatched, and the results acted upon accordingly.

**Self-assessment exercises**

The answers to the following questions may be found in the text:

1. List the occasions when a woman may be asked to supply a blood specimen.
2. Describe how to locate a suitable vein for venepuncture.
3. Which anatomical structures should be avoided?
4. What equipment is required to complete the technique safely?
5. Demonstrate how to undertake venepuncture correctly.
6. Summarise the role and responsibilities of the midwife when undertaking venepuncture.

## REFERENCES

Dougherty L, Lister S 2004 The Royal Marsden Hospital Manual of Clinical Nursing Procedures, 6th edn. Blackwell Publishing, Oxford

Williams P L (ed) 1995 Gray's Anatomy, 38th edn. Churchill Livingstone, Edinburgh

# Chapter 50

# Principles of phlebotomy and intravenous therapy – intravenous cannulation

As one of the vascular access devices, peripheral intravenous cannulae are commonly sited and cared for by midwives. A peripheral cannula is sited into a vein for the purposes of infusing fluids or administering medicines via the intravenous route. Performing the skill requires training, supervised practice and ongoing maintenance. This chapter considers the skills of siting and removing an intravenous cannula, and the role and responsibilities of the midwife are discussed.

## Learning outcomes

Having read this chapter the reader should be able to:

- discuss the indications for cannulation
- describe how the site is selected and the equipment chosen
- describe a safe cannulation technique
- describe the correct removal of an intravenous cannula
- summarise the role and responsibilities of the midwife.

## Considerations for the childbearing woman

The additional blood volume in pregnancy and higher body temperature usually mean that the veins are prominent and are therefore easier to gain access to.

## Indications

- Fluid replacement or drug administration in an emergency
- Administration of whole blood or blood products
- For drugs that need careful control, e.g. Syntocinon infusion
- In preparation for a potential complication or operative delivery, e.g. trial of scar, multiple or breech birth
- Fluid administration with epidural analgesia.

# Choice of site

Correct choice of site considers:

- Structures to avoid:
  - the dominant arm
  - areas that are painful, bruised, tortuous, thrombosed or inflamed
  - areas with compromised circulation, oedema or fracture
  - joints, valves in the vein (seen as bulges), bone, ligaments, muscle, nerves or tendons
  - arteries, particularly those that run in unexpected directions.
- Try to choose:
  - a vein (identified by its lack of pulse and the ability to empty and fill by occluding and releasing it digitally)
  - a vein in good condition that can be palpated in the lower half of the arm, e.g. dorsal venous network (back of the hand) and cephalic and basilic veins of the forearm (Fig. 50.1).

## Asepsis and use of standard precautions

Infection (systemic or localised) is one of the highest risks of cannulation. It is of considerable significance that it is an aseptic procedure. The cannula should be sterile and for single use. All sharps should be disposed of correctly in a sharps box. If required for long-term use the cannula should be changed every 72–96 hours.

Skin cleansing is recommended with at least a 70% alcohol swab (Dougherty & Lister 2004), ensuring that the skin is cleaned for at least 30 seconds; a rapid 'one wipe' of the skin may cause more harm than good as the skin flora are merely disturbed. Ideally, chlorhexidine 2% in 70% alcohol should be used as this has a lasting effect (RCN 2003). The skin should be cleansed working from the inside outwards. It should air dry for about a minute before the cannulation is commenced. The vein should not be repalpated after the skin has been cleansed.

## Use of local anaesthetic

As an uncomfortable procedure, the use of topical or injected local anaesthetic should be considered. Often topical analgesia needs up to an hour to be effective, making it difficult to use if the cannula needs to be inserted quickly (Coates 1998). A small amount of local anaesthetic such as lidocaine (lignocaine) may be injected intradermally (Ch. 23) at the proposed puncture site, with cannulation taking place once it is effective (3–5 minutes). The prescription will be under patient group direction, but extreme care should be taken so that the lidocaine (lignocaine) does not enter the bloodstream when cannulating. Intravenous lidocaine (lignocaine) can be dangerous.

Figure 50.1  (A) Veins of the forearm; (B) veins of the hand (Adapted with kind permission from Williams 1995)

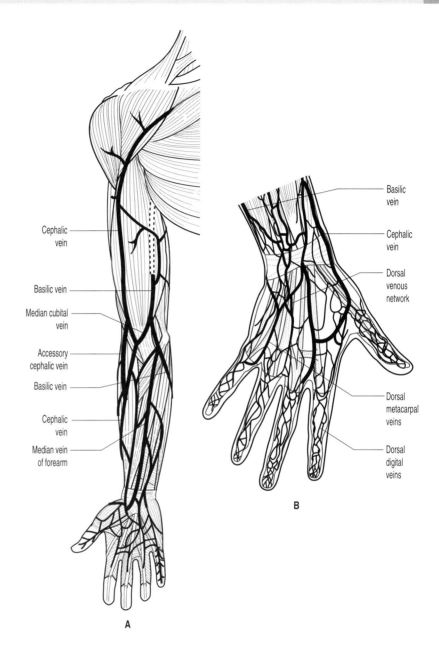

# Choice of equipment

A cannula should be a suitable size for both the vein and the fluid that is to be infused. A large bore cannula should be used for the childbearing woman – sizes 14 or 16 g.

Cannulae may vary slightly according to the manufacturer, but generally consist of a polyurethane piece of tubing with a hub, into which there is a bevelled needle (stylet), also with a hub. Wings may be attached for ease of securing the cannula and there may or may not be a needleless injection port (Fig. 50.2). The cannula should be flushed with 0.9% sodium chloride twice a day, if it is only to be used intermittently, and secured with a semi-permeable occlusive dressing (Snelling & Duffy 2002). A poorly dressed cannula increases the risks of leaking, tissuing (extravasation), infection, air embolism and trauma.

| PROCEDURE | intravenous cannulation |
|---|---|

If topical analgesia is to be used the vein would be selected, the cream applied and the vein covered; the procedure would commence 45–60 minutes later.

- Gain informed consent, ensure privacy and gather equipment:
  — appropriately sized sterile cannula
  — semi-permeable occlusive dressing
  — 70% alcohol swab or dressing pack and chlorhexidine 2% in 70% alcohol
  — sharps box
  — tourniquet
  — sterile gloves and hand rub
  — local anaesthetic with sterile needle and syringe, if used
  — intravenous infusion or 0.9% sodium chloride (with sterile needle and syringe) for flushing
  — disposable sheet
- Wash hands
- Position the arm so that it is supported, in a good light, with the disposable sheet beneath it
- Apply the tourniquet approximately 5 cm above the antecubital fossa so that the veins can fill, but arterial flow is not obstructed; ask the woman to clench her fist a few times to encourage the veins to fill
- Select the most likely vein by palpation; inject intradermal local anaesthetic into the skin if required, in the region of anticipated cannula entry
- Use hand rub and apply gloves

**Figure 50.2** Intravenous cannulation (Adapted with kind permission from Nicol et al 2000)

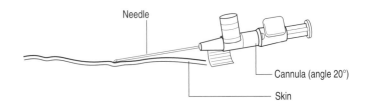

Needle

Cannula (angle 20°)

Skin

- Cleanse the skin thoroughly for at least 30 seconds; allow it to air dry for at least a minute
- Immobilise the vein by supporting the skin below the insertion point, with slight tension, using the non-dominant hand
- Insert the cannula at an angle of approximately 20°; as the vein is entered a flashback of blood is seen in the hub
- Reduce the angle of insertion almost to skin level, advance the cannula slowly a few millimetres further, pause and withdraw the needle halfway; a second flashback will be seen along the cannula
- Gradually advance the cannula into the vein, up to the hub, while simultaneously withdrawing the needle until almost withdrawn, remembering to remain at the same depth, following the direction of the vein. Release skin traction
- Release the tourniquet, gently occlude the vein above the cannula and withdraw the needle completely. Dispose of needle into sharps box
- Aseptically either attach the administration set, take blood specimens or flush and cap off the cannula
- Secure carefully with the dressing
- Ensure the woman is aware of ongoing care of the cannula, asking her to report any adverse effects
- Dispose of the equipment correctly and wash hands
- Complete records and ensure ongoing care of the cannula and/or infusion (see Ch. 51).

Failure to succeed sometimes means that the cannula has been pushed through the vein wall. If unsuccessful for a second time an experienced colleague should be sought. Repeated failed attempts are distressing to the woman and reduce the number of suitable veins.

# Removing a peripheral cannula

Cannula removal is much more pleasant for the woman than insertion. The midwife should ensure that it is to be removed before doing so!

## PROCEDURE   removal of a cannula

- Gain informed consent and gather equipment:
  — sterile gloves
  — sterile gauze and tape
  — disposable sheet
  — sharps box
- Wash hands

- Position the arm so that it is supported, with the disposable sheet beneath it
- Loosen the tape around the cannula
- Open the gauze, apply gloves
- Begin to withdraw the cannula from the vein; prepare to place the gauze immediately over the puncture site as the cannula is withdrawn
- Apply continuous pressure to the puncture site for at least 1 minute
- Place the cannula into the sharps box
- Secure the gauze with tape once satisfied that bleeding has stopped
- Ensure the woman is comfortable
- Wash hands
- Observe the site later for signs of bleeding or infection
- Complete records.

### Role and responsibilities of the midwife

These can be summarised as:

- correct selection of site, use of equipment, insertion and removal of peripheral cannula
- appropriate training and maintenance of the skill
- education and support of the woman
- ongoing care and observation of the site
- correct documentation.

## Summary

- Peripheral intravenous cannulation is an uncomfortable, invasive technique
- The midwife should be appropriately trained and able to maintain the skill
- It is an aseptic procedure, using the correct sized cannula for the vein and nature of the fluid
- The site is chosen with care, avoiding arteries and joints but choosing the basilic or cephalic veins of the hand and forearm.

### Self-assessment exercises

The answers to the following questions may be found in the text:

1. Discuss the indications for cannula insertion.
2. Describe how to choose a correct site for peripheral intravenous cannulation.
3. Discuss the type of equipment selected.
4. Describe and demonstrate how a cannula is inserted correctly.
5. Describe how to remove a cannula correctly.
6. Summarise the role and responsibilities of the midwife when inserting and removing a peripheral intravenous cannula.

## REFERENCES

Coates T 1998 Venepuncture and intravenous cannulation. The Practising Midwife 1(10):28–31

Dougherty L, Lister S 2004 The Royal Marsden Hospital Manual of Clinical Nursing Procedures, 6th edn. Blackwell Publishing, Oxford

Nicol M, Bavin C, Bedford-Turner S et al 2000 Essential nursing skills, 2nd edn. Mosby, Edinburgh

RCN (Royal College of Nursing) 2003 Standards for infusion therapy. RCN, London

Snelling P, Duffy E 2002 Developing self directed training for intravenous cannulation. Professional Nurse 18(3):137–142

Williams P L (ed) 1995 Gray's Anatomy, 38th edn. Churchill Livingstone, Edinburgh

Chapter **51**

# Principles of phlebotomy and intravenous therapy – intravenous infusion

This chapter focuses on the skills involved with the setting up, monitoring and discontinuation of an intravenous infusion, including reference to the types of solution commonly used and the monitoring of fluid balance. These are skills primarily used in the hospital setting for the childbearing woman and the baby. For the woman, having an intravenous infusion in progress can be debilitating, affecting her mobility and independence. She may require assistance in caring for herself and for her baby. It can also alter her body image.

**Learning outcomes**

Having read this chapter the reader should be able to:

- discuss the indications for an intravenous infusion
- describe the different types of fluid solution commonly used for an intravenous infusion
- describe the formula for calculating the flow of an intravenous infusion
- discuss the midwife's role and responsibilities in relation to intravenous infusion therapy
- discuss how fluid balance is monitored and the significance of this.

## Definition

An intravenous infusion is the introduction of sterile fluid into the blood circulation. When intravenous therapy is expected to be short term, access to the circulation is usually via the veins of the back of the hand, wrist or lower arm. If intravenous therapy is expected to be long term, lasting several days or weeks, the subclavian vein or internal jugular vein is the usual site of cannulation. The latter is rarely used in midwifery. Prior to commencing an intravenous infusion, cannulation is required (Ch. 50). Due to the risk of infection it is important to use a no-touch technique throughout.

## Indications

- Maintenance of fluid, electrolyte and nutrient balance when oral fluids or food are withheld or not tolerated, e.g. pre- and post-operatively
- Hypovolaemia, e.g. haemorrhage, shock, dehydration
- Administration of drugs, e.g. Syntocinon.

## Equipment

### Intravenous administration set

These are sterile prepacked sets consisting of a long piece of tubing with a drip chamber and trocar at the top end and a nozzle at the bottom end that connects to a cannula. Around the tubing is an adjustable roller clamp that alters the flow of fluid (Fig. 51.1). There are two main types used in midwifery – one for the administration of clear fluids and one for blood transfusion, the latter having a double chamber and a filter.

Burette sets or volume control devices are used when an infusion pump is unavailable, to obtain greater control over the flow rate. The drip chamber is calibrated, with a clamp above and below the chamber, and is filled with the amount of fluid to be infused during 1 hour. The flow rate is calculated according to the drop factor (varies according to manufacturer's instructions) and the amount prescribed. It will require refilling each hour. As it limits the amount of fluid transfused, it reduces the risk of the woman receiving too much fluid too quickly.

The use of a closed system of infusion will reduce the risk of infection; with each connection that is added to the infusion line, the

**Figure 51.1** An intravenous administration set (Adapted with kind permission from Jamieson et al 2002)

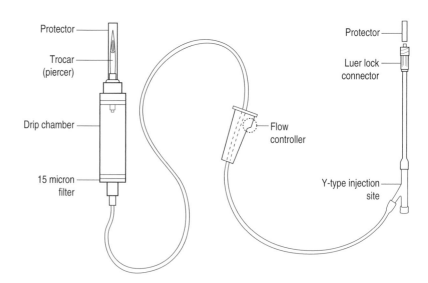

Protector

Trocar (piercer)

Drip chamber

15 micron filter

Flow controller

Protector

Luer lock connector

Y-type injection site

infection risk increases. For example, three-way taps used between the cannula and infusion line are difficult to keep clean and can act as a reservoir for microorganisms which multiply in the warm, moist environment, increasing the risk of infection (Dougherty & Lister 2004).

### Infusion pumps

A variety of infusion pumps are available that adjust the infusion flow electronically, administering a prescribed amount of fluid over a set time. The midwife should know how the infusion pump works and ensure it is properly maintained.

### Syringe pumps

Syringe pumps may also be used for the administration of drugs, e.g. insulin (Ch. 26).

## Intravenous fluid

Intravenous fluid can be one of a variety of solutions (Table 51.1) with different types of containers used, e.g. soft plastic bag, glass bottle, semi-rigid plastic (polyfusor). Glass containers have a rubber bung covered by a sterile seal that is removed and wiped with an alcohol-impregnated swab just prior to insertion of the trocar from the top end of the infusion set. To facilitate flow of the fluid, a sterile air inlet needle is inserted through the rubber bung to equalise the pressure within the bottle. Sterile scissors should be used with the semi-rigid container to

Table 51.1  Intravenous infusion solutions commonly used in midwifery

| Solution | Example | Indication for use |
| --- | --- | --- |
| Crystalloid – isotonic solutions (same tonicity as blood) | 0.9% Sodium chloride 5% Dextrose | To compensate for fluid loss from diarrhoea and vomiting by expanding the circulating volume |
| Crystalloid – hypotonic solutions (lower particle concentration than plasma) | 0.45% Sodium chloride | To compensate for fluid loss by moving fluid into intracellular spaces Used if sodium intake restricted |
| Crystalloid – hypertonic solutions (higher tonicity than plasma) | 20% Dextrose | To compensate for fluid loss by moving fluid from intracellular to extracellular spaces Used to correct hypoglycaemia |
| Colloids – undissolved particles (protein, starch, sugar) too large to pass through capillary walls | 5% or 25% Albumin | Draws fluid from interstitial and intracellular spaces Used when crystalloid solutions are ineffective |
| Plasma expanders Colloid fluids | Dextran, Gelofusine | To expand plasma volume by drawing fluid from interstitial spaces |
| Blood and blood products | Whole blood, packed cells | To maintain circulatory volume, increase particular blood components |

cut off the end of the entry conduit. The trocar is inserted into this tube and twisted to ensure a good fit.

### Checking the infusion solution prior to administration

A doctor must prescribe the solution, which is checked by two people, one of whom should be a qualified midwife, nurse or doctor to ensure the correct infusion is given to the correct woman. The midwife should check:

- the woman's name and unit number
- the prescription – type of infusion fluid and amount to be infused, which should be accurately written up and signed
- the fluid should be examined for signs of discolouration, cloudiness or sediment and the container examined for signs of contamination
- the batch number should be recorded on the drug chart.

# Calculating the flow rate of the intravenous fluid

The midwife should refer to the administration set being used for details of the number of drops per mL, referred to as the drop factor. Commonly the drop factor is 20 for clear fluids and 15 for blood. It is important to ensure the fluid is infused over the correct period of time to prevent over- or under-infusion, both of which can have serious consequences. The following formula is used to calculate the number or drops per minute:

$$\frac{\text{Volume of solution (mL)} \times \text{number of drops/mL (drop factor)}}{\text{Required infusion time (minutes)}}$$

For example, if 500 mL Hartmann's solution is prescribed over a 4-hour period, using an administration set with a drop factor of 20, the flow rate will be:

$$\frac{500 \times 20}{240} = 41.67 = 42 \text{ drops per minute, approximately.}$$

### Use of an infusion pump

This should be used according to the manufacturer's instructions. Generally the following formula can be used to calculate the rate (mL/hour):

$$\text{Rate (mL/hour)} = \frac{\text{Volume (mL)}}{\text{Time (hour)}}$$

For example, if an infusion pump is to be used to administer 500 mL Hartmann's solution over 4 hours, the rate should be set at:

$$\frac{500}{4} = 125 \text{ mL/hour}$$

| PROCEDURE | commencing an intravenous infusion using a fluid bag |

- Gain informed consent and gather equipment:
  — administration set
  — infusion solution
  — sterile or clean receiver
  — hand rub plus sterile or non-sterile gloves
  — infusion stand
  — infusion pump if required
  — dressing, if required; preferably a clear dressing to allow good visualisation of the cannulation site
- Wash hands
- Open the administration set and close the roller clamp below the drip chamber
- Remove cover from the top end of the tubing and from the infusion bag, without touching either opening
- Insert the trocar into the fluid bag
- Suspend the fluid bag from an infusion stand
- Gently compress the drip chamber to partially fill it
- Remove the cover from the other end of the tubing and place over the receiver, taking care not to touch it
- Slowly release the flow control clamp to fill the tubing with fluid
- Remove any air bubbles by running the fluid into the receiver without touching the sides of the receiver
- Close the roller clamp
- Replace the cover on the end of the tubing until ready to connect to the cannula
- When required, apply hand rub and gloves, occlude the vein, remove the cover and connect the tubing to the cannula
- Adjust the flow rate accordingly using the roller clamp
- Apply dressing if required
- Dispose of equipment correctly and wash hands
- Commence a fluid balance record
- Document and act accordingly.

### Changing the administration set

The administration set can be changed every 48–72 hours as this is not associated with an increased risk of phlebitis or infection (Fuller 1998, RCN 2003). The exceptions to this are if a blood transfusion has been administered (change the tubing every 12 hours or following every second unit of blood; McClelland 2001) or the administration set has had a number of manipulations. Also, the tubing should be changed immediately if it becomes occluded or damaged and each time the cannula is replaced. The procedure is the same as above.

### Changing the intravenous solution

Prior to the fluid bag emptying completely, the next solution should be checked ready for use. Speakman (1999) suggests this should be when there is less than 50 mL of fluid left to infuse. The fluid should be checked as discussed above. Before changing the solution, close the roller clamp, ensuring the drip chamber is half full. After handwashing, the midwife should remove the tubing trocar from the fluid bag and insert it into the new solution. The roller clamp should be opened and the flow rate adjusted. Record keeping is completed as appropriate.

### Ongoing care of the intravenous infusion

- The rate of flow should be closely observed to ensure the correct amount of fluid is being infused. The rate of flow can be influenced by the position of the arm or hand, particularly when the joint is flexed. The height of the infusion bag will also affect the rate; raising it increases the rate
- The infusion site should be monitored at least once a day to ensure there are no complications, e.g. infection, phlebitis (RCN 2003), and the cannula is still in situ and patent
- The cannula should be flushed regularly (every 24–48 hours) or following administration of intravenous medication (Fuller 1998) with 0.9% sodium chloride to reduce the risks of thrombus formation and colonisation from microorganisms. If the last 0.5 mL of the flushing solution is administered as the syringe is being withdrawn from the cannula port, a positive backflow of blood into the cannula is created; this is thought to prevent clotting at the site (Fuller 1998)
- The equipment should be monitored to ensure it is working properly
- The woman should be assessed regularly to ensure there are no complications arising, including phlebitis, thrombophlebitis, infection, pain, haematoma, air embolism (Campbell & Lunn 1997).

# Monitoring fluid balance

To ensure the woman is tolerating the amount of fluid being infused a fluid balance chart should be commenced at the beginning of the infusion and maintained throughout. This is a method of measuring the amount of fluid taken into the body through the intravenous and oral routes, and comparing it with the amount of fluid lost from the body in urine. Normally intake and output balance; however, if the amount of fluid taken in exceeds the amount excreted, water intoxication can result. Failure to excrete the excessive fluid load will result in rapid expansion of the body fluid compartments. Cardiac failure can ensue, characterised initially by increasing dyspnoea and peripheral oedema, unless fluid intake is restricted. A reduction in plasma osmolarity and oedematous cells can also result in convulsions and coma if the brain cells swell. If output exceeds intake, dehydration with shrinkage of cells and tissues can occur. An output of 500 mL daily is required to excrete the solutes that require elimination.

A fluid balance chart is divided into two sections – intake and output. These are further divided into oral and intravenous fluids for intake. Output includes urine, vomit, diarrhoea, nasogastric drainage and loss from drains. Blood loss should also be recorded. The midwife should carefully measure the amount of fluid actually drunk by the woman and the amount of solution infused, keeping a cumulative total of the intake. All forms of fluid output should also be carefully measured and recorded, again with a cumulative total. This allows for a very quick assessment of the fluid balance status of the woman. It should be remembered that these charts do not take into account fluid obtained from food or insensible fluid loss. The midwife should total the intake and output at the end of a 24-hour period, document this in the appropriate records and act on the results accordingly.

## Role and responsibilities of the midwife

These can be summarised as:

- being responsible for commencing the intravenous infusion, using a no-touch technique to minimise the risk of infection
- ongoing care of the woman with an intravenous infusion, ensuring it is running correctly, replacing the infusion fluid according to the prescribed regimen, monitoring the condition of the woman for any adverse effects and assisting her with day-to-day activities
- recognising the significance of fluid balance
- contemporaneous record keeping.

## Summary

- An intravenous infusion is a means of giving fluid or drugs directly into the circulation
- It is not without risk and careful assessment of the woman is required during the procedure
- It is debilitating for the woman who will require assistance in caring for herself and her baby.

## Self-assessment exercises

The answers to the following questions may be found in the text:

1. What are the indications for an intravenous infusion?
2. Describe the main categories of infusion solutions used in midwifery.
3. How is an intravenous solution commenced, once cannulation has occurred?
4. What is the formula for calculating the flow rate of an intravenous infusion?
5. What are the responsibilities of the midwife during an intravenous infusion?
6. How is fluid balance recorded and why is this important?

## REFERENCES

Campbell T, Lunn D 1997 Intravenous therapy: current practice and nursing concerns. British Journal of Nursing 6(21):1218, 1220, 1222, 1224–1228

Dougherty L, Lister S (eds) 2004 The Royal Marsden Hospital manual of clinical nursing procedures, 6th edn. Blackwell Publishing, Oxford

Fuller A 1998 The management of peripheral IV lines. Professional Nurse 13(10):673, 677–678

Jamieson E M, McCall J M, Whyte L A 2002 Clinical nursing practices, 4th edn. Churchill Livingstone, Edinburgh

McClelland B 2001 Handbook of transfusion medicine, 2nd edn. The Stationery Office, London

RCN (Royal College of Nursing) 2003 Standards for infusion therapy. RCN, London

Speakman E 1999 Fluid, electrolyte and acid–base balances. In: Potter P A, Perry A G (eds) Fundamentals of nursing concepts, process and practice, 4th edn. Mosby, St Louis, p 835–889

Chapter **52**

# Principles of phlebotomy and intravenous infusion – blood transfusion

This chapter examines safe blood transfusion of women (not babies) and the midwife's role and responsibilities. Blood grouping, the dangers of transfusion and suitable equipment are all discussed in detail.

**Learning outcomes**

Having read this chapter the reader should be able to:

- define blood transfusion, listing its likely uses in the maternity care setting
- discuss why O rhesus negative blood is the universal donor and AB positive the universal recipient
- discuss in detail the role of the midwife when caring for a women receiving a blood transfusion, citing the PACK mnemonic (Bradbury & Cruickshank 2000).

### Definition

Whole blood or components of blood are introduced into the venous circulation, usually for the purposes of treating a clinical abnormality. Shortage of red blood cells results in hypoxia and the circulatory system needs to have sufficient blood within the vessels to sustain blood pressure, heart rate and all other circulatory functions. The DoH (1994) recommends using whole blood quickly for the management of massive obstetric haemorrhage. Maternity units have two units of O rhesus negative blood available for immediate transfusion to any woman while awaiting cross-matched blood, such is the significance of blood transfusion in saving lives.

Blood transfusion can be a controversial treatment: it is the transfer of live tissue from one person to another. Some religious groups will refuse transfusion. Despite careful screening there is the possibility of disease or antibody transmission and blood is an expensive treatment that may vary in its availability. However, the responsibility for safe and effective transfusion rests with all health professionals, especially those directly administering it, e.g. the midwife (Shamash 2002).

## Indications

Indications for transfusion include:

- hypovolaemia, e.g. after a significant haemorrhage
- low haemoglobin
- clotting disorders
- exchange transfusion for the fetus or baby
- certain blood diseases.

Blood can be administered in different forms: whole blood, packed red cells (plasma removed), platelet concentration, fresh frozen plasma, white blood cells and cryoprecipitate (clotting factors). Other less common preparations are also available.

## Blood groups

Blood groups are defined as A, B, AB or O rhesus negative or positive. The group is determined by the presence of an antigen on the red cell surface and an antibody in the serum. Individuals with group A, for example, have A antigens on their surface and B antibodies in the serum (Table 52.1).

An incompatible blood donation initiates the antigen–antibody reaction, causing red blood cells to agglutinate (clump together); this is a serious transfusion reaction, potentially leading to kidney failure and death. Blood group O is known as the universal donor (having no antigens for antibodies to fight), while group AB is known as the universal recipient (having no antibodies to fight foreign antigens). 85% of the population have an additional antigen on their red cells, the rhesus factor. If rhesus positive blood is introduced into a rhesus negative person, antibodies then form, with a haemolysing effect on the next introduction of rhesus positive blood. Therefore the true universal donor is O rhesus negative (Rh−) and the true universal recipient is AB rhesus positive (Rh+). It should be noted that the presence of maternal antibodies (e.g. anti-D, anti-Kell, etc.) can have life-threatening consequences to the fetus and as such care must be taken to screen maternal blood before 12 weeks' gestation to identify any potential problems (Anderson 2004).

Table 52.1 Antibodies/antigens of the blood groups

| Group | Antigen | Antibody |
|-------|---------|----------|
| A | A | B |
| B | B | A |
| AB | AB | None |
| O | None | AB |

## Safe protocols

There are considerable dangers associated with blood transfusion (see below). Williamson et al (1999) indicate that a large proportion of the problems are associated with incorrect checking procedures. The British Committee for Standards in Haematology (BCSH 1999) task force has recommended national guidelines that cover all aspects of transfusion care. Bradbury and Cruickshank (2000) summarise these as PACK:

- **P**atient and pre-transfusion checks
- **A**sepsis and apparatus
- **C**hecking and clerical procedures
- **K**eeping vigilant with accurate records.

### Patient and pre-transfusion checks

- A full history must be taken of any previous transfusions, transplants, pregnancies and current medication to identify any possible risk factors for this transfusion. Full information should be given, allowing the woman to make an informed decision for consent (where appropriate) prior to the blood being cross-matched
- The initial blood sample should be taken from the woman after she has been verbally identified, as well as identified with her notes and, ideally, identity bracelet. The bottles should be labelled in her presence with her full name, date of birth (DoB), gender, hospital number (I.D.) and signature of staff taking the sample. The request form is equally thorough and the sample dispatched correctly
- When ready, the blood is collected from the blood fridge within 30 minutes of commencement of transfusion (blood that has been out of the fridge for longer should be reported to the haematologist for their decision as to whether to proceed). The blood collection slip should be checked against the blood, including the woman's name, DoB and I.D. number. Its removal should be signed for in the blood register with the time and staff signature. Blood should be handled and transported carefully; some areas have a specific collection box. All staff that collect blood should be trained and fully aware of their responsibilities.

### Asepsis and apparatus

- Strict asepsis is adhered to throughout the transfusion. The midwife screens the blood visually before the transfusion is commenced to exclude colour changes, bubbles, leakage or clotting – these may indicate bacterial contamination
- The cannula in the vein should be 19 gauge or larger as blood cells are damaged by compression
- While similar to intravenous giving sets, blood transfusion sets have a double chamber that acts as a filter to debris (Fig. 52.1). The recommended filter is a 170 micron filter, but larger transfusions may

**Figure 52.1** Blood transfusion giving set; note the filter and double chambers (Adapted with kind permission from Jamieson et al 2002)

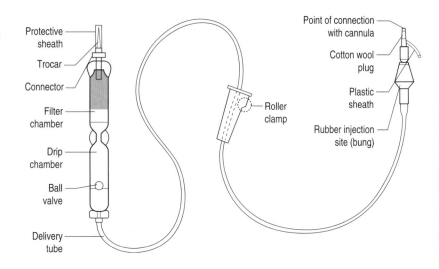

have an additional filter placed between the blood and the giving set. The giving set should be changed after 12 hours and on completion. It is not necessary to prime the giving set with normal saline (Atterbury & Wilkinson 2000) and glucose should not be administered before or after a transfusion through the same cannula

- The fragile nature of blood cells means that using infusion pumps is inappropriate. This may change, but currently infusions run according to how they are set manually. A blood administration set generally administers blood at 15 drops per mL (whereas standard intravenous administration sets are 20 drops per mL), but this should be confirmed on the packet (Anon. 1999). A unit of blood should be completed in 5 hours. The infusion rate (drops per minute) is calculated accordingly:

$$\frac{\text{Amount to be transfused (mL)} \times 15 \text{ (i.e. drops in each mL)}}{\text{Hours for transfusion in minutes}}$$

e.g. if one unit of 500 mL is to transfuse over 4 hours, what is the infusion rate?

$$\frac{500 \times 15}{240}$$

Answer: 31 drops per minute approximately.

- For transfusions of 4–6 units running slowly, warming is not necessary. For more or faster than 50 mL/kg/hour, or through a central line, a blood warmer is used. Blood is never placed into hot water, microwaved or put on radiators. Pressure bags or specific pumps may sometimes be used for rapid transfusions, but the fragility of blood should be remembered.

## Checking and clerical procedures

- Local protocols will dictate whether it is one midwife plus one other, or a midwife alone who checks the details and therefore administers the transfusion. This should be in accordance with NMC (2004) Guidelines for the Administration of Medicines. Any incident, e.g. incompatible transfusion given, should be reported confidentially to SHOT (see references).
- Checking must be meticulous, with the details of the woman, blood group and unit numbers all agreeing on the blood unit, patient records, prescription chart and blood issue/compatibility form, along with the woman's identity. She should be asked to give her name, address and DoB, rather than being asked: 'Are you Mrs Smith?' Any discrepancies whatsoever should be referred to the haematologist before the transfusion is commenced. The checking should be at the bedside.

## Keeping vigilant with accurate records

- The dangers of blood transfusion are discussed below; the midwife must be vigilant in looking for signs and symptoms throughout
- There is little evidence as to the frequency of observations while a blood transfusion is running. However, given that serious reactions can occur within the first 10–15 minutes, it is prudent to:
  — undertake a full set of baseline observations before the transfusion commences including temperature, pulse, respiration and blood pressure
  — repeat these after 15 minutes, with the transfusion running slowly for that time
  — observe the woman carefully and to repeat the observations at any time that she may complain of any changes in how she is looking or feeling
  — repeat them frequently if any changes in vital signs are noted
  — complete a full set of observations on completion of the unit
  — treat each new unit in this way
- An unconscious woman will not be able to report changes in how she is feeling and therefore observations and visual checking are needed frequently
- Records must be thorough; time commenced and fluid balance must be included along with the ongoing observations. The compatibility form should be available throughout and kept in the woman's records
- The blood bag may be retained on completion according to local protocols, often for 48 hours, in case of adverse reaction
- In accordance with standard precautions, the giving set is disposed of into a sharps box
- Haematological screening is completed the following day, e.g. full blood count and urea and electrolytes.

# Dangers of blood transfusion

- Transfusion incompatibility: signs of haemolytic reactions include fever, flushing, shivering, rigors, loin pain, headache, chest pain, tachycardia, tachypnoea, hypotension, haematuria, haemorrhage, oliguria, anxiety and possible death. Usually a rapid reaction, within a few mL of transfusion. *Action*: stop transfusion, maintain venous access with normal saline, call medical aid urgently, resuscitate the woman
- Circulatory overload: women have an increased blood volume in pregnancy (1.5 L extra) making it easier to overload their circulatory system if they are not hypovolaemic; fluid gathers in the lungs (pulmonary oedema) resulting in dyspnoea, hypertension, tachycardia, cough and raised central venous pressure. May be seen during or after transfusion. *Action*: stop transfusion, call medical aid, administer oxygen and diuretic
- Febrile reaction: as much as possible, white cells are removed from donated blood, but after a large transfusion women can have a significant febrile reaction. This includes hyperpyrexia, rigors, sweating and tachycardia. Onset is often within 30–90 minutes and it can mimic a haemolytic reaction. *Action*: stop transfusion, call medical aid, exclude haemolytic reaction. If transfusion is to continue, antihistamines and steroids may be needed
- Allergic reaction: the severest type of reaction is anaphylaxis (Ch. 21); it can occur within 30 minutes, exhibiting rash, wheezing, shortness of breath and hypotension. *Action*: stop transfusion, call medical aid (urgently if anaphylaxis), resuscitate using adrenaline (epinephrine) and steroids
- Thrombophlebitis, air embolism, iron overload, hypothermia, excess potassium and reduced calcium are other dangers that can occur, either with or following the transfusion. For any untoward sign medical aid is called.

### Slow-running transfusion

The infusion may stop if the vein goes into spasm from the cold blood. A warm compress may dilate the vein and encourage blood flow. Occlusion of the cannula may be overcome with gentle flushing using 0.9% sodium chloride. However, if time has elapsed the blood may have clotted in the tubing and a new administration set will be required. The woman should be supplied with the call bell and be encouraged to ring if she has any difficulties or thinks that the transfusion has stopped.

---

PROCEDURE    administering a blood transfusion

This procedure applies for transfusions of 4–6 unit size. Massive transfusions of larger numbers incur some different issues such as warming, rapid transfusion and central venous pressure (CVP) monitoring.

- Gain informed consent, collect blood from the blood fridge. A flushed cannula should already be in place. Wash hands
- Approach the woman with her records, the blood and all equipment needed. Confirm identity and undertake the thorough checking procedure (discussed above)
- Complete and record baseline vital sign observations (see above)
- Prime a blood administration set: close the clamp, pull back the tabs to expose the entry portal and insert the giving set. Turn the bag upside down, open the clamp, squeeze the blood through the first chamber and a third of the way through the second chamber. Close the clamp. Re-invert the bag, hang up, open the clamp and run through so that blood comes to the end of the line (Atterbury & Wilkinson 2000). Aseptically attach to the cannula
- Establish that the woman is comfortable and the call bell is within reach
- Transfuse the first 50 mL over the next 10–15 minutes, observing the woman closely
- Complete records
- After 15 minutes complete a full set of observations and adjust the flow rate
- Observe the woman throughout and call the obstetrician if anything untoward occurs; complete observations as necessary (see above)
- Complete a full set of vital sign observations on completion of the unit
- Commence the second unit (if prescribed) by removing the first bag and replacing it with the new one. Undertake all observations and adjustments to flow rate as for the first unit
- When the transfusion is complete, apply gloves, remove the administration set, dispose of correctly and, according to local protocol, either send the blood bag back to the blood bank or retain it for 48 hours in case of adverse reaction (see above)
- Complete records
- Repeat blood tests are taken the following day.

## Other considerations

As an expensive, potentially hazardous treatment, practitioners are asked to consider if blood can be used minimally and other techniques such as iron therapy employed (Shamash 2002). Equally, infection transfer can be reduced by autologous transfusion – one's own blood donated 3–4 weeks in advance (Godfrey 2000). While both of these practices may be of limited use in maternity care, nevertheless the midwife needs to appreciate the need to help women maintain good haemoglobin levels pre- and post-delivery, to manage ante- and postpartum haemorrhages quickly and efficiently and therefore to consider reducing the overall need for blood transfusion.

## Summary

- Blood transfusion is valuable in saving lives; blood should be correctly cross-matched and checked to avoid incompatible transfusions and should be stored and transfused correctly
- There are dangers associated with blood transfusion; the midwife should maintain careful observation of the woman throughout.

**Self-assessment exercises**

The answers to the following questions may be found in the text:

1. What is a blood transfusion?
2. When may a blood transfusion be necessary?
3. Describe the components of other blood products that can be transfused.
4. Which blood group and rhesus factor is the universal donor? Why is this?
5. Which blood group and rhesus factor is the universal recipient? Why is this?
6. Describe the process that protects the woman from receiving an incompatible transfusion.
7. Describe how the midwife would recognise that haemolysis was occurring.
8. If a unit of blood containing 420 mL were to be transfused over 3 hours how many drops per minute would it flow at?
9. When does the midwife assess vital sign observations during a transfusion?

## REFERENCES

Anderson T 2004 Blood transfusion: the hidden dangers. The Practising Midwife 7(3):12–16

Anonymous 1999 Calculating drug dosage. Nursing Standard 13(28): insert, 2 pages (unnumbered)

Atterbury C, Wilkinson J 2000 Blood transfusion. Nursing Standard 14(34):47–52

BCSH (British Committee for Standards in Haematology, Blood Transfusion Task Force) 1999 The administration of blood and blood components and the management of transfused patients. Transfusion Medicine 9:227–238

Bradbury M, Cruickshank J P 2000 Blood transfusion: crucial steps in maintaining safe practice. British Journal of Nursing 9(3):134–138

DoH (Department of Health) 1994 Report on confidential enquiries into maternal deaths in the United Kingdom 1988–1990. HMSO, London

Godfrey K 2000 In the bag. Nursing Times 96(14): 26–29

Jamieson E M, McCall J M, Whyte L A 2002 Clinical nursing practices, 4th edn. Churchill Livingstone, Edinburgh

NMC (Nursing and Midwifery Council) 2004 Guidelines for the administration of medicines. NMC, London

Shamash J 2002 Blood counts. Nursing Times 98(45):23–26

SHOT (Serious Hazards of Transfusion initiative) Online. Available: http://www.shotuk.org

Williamson L M, Lowe S, Cohen H et al 1999 Serious hazards of transfusion (SHOT) initiative: analysis of the first two annual reports. British Medical Journal 319:16–19

Chapter **53**

# Principles of moving and handling

Manual handling accidents have far-reaching implications, not only for the midwife who is unable to work in both the short and sometimes the long term and who may suffer pain and disability, but also for employers, in terms of time lost from work and large financial compensation packages paid out to employees (Cowell 1998, Stevens 2004, White 1998). In 1998 a nursery nurse was awarded £78 000 in compensation following a lifting injury which resulted in severe damage to her back and an inability to work for 4 years (Tolley 2000).

Injuries can occur through the use of incorrect lifting techniques, inappropriate lifting and moving as well as adopting poor posture for procedures such as delivery and assisting with breastfeeding. This chapter focuses on the principles of moving and handling, considering how the risk of injury can be minimised, and employers' and employees' responsibility in relation to this. Relevant anatomy of the spine is discussed and related to both lifting and posture, and how injury can occur. There is a vast amount of literature and legislation relating to manual handling which is added to regularly, hence it is not possible to cover this in detail. This chapter provides an overview of manual handling and the reader is advised to read other texts and visit the Health and Safety Executive website (www.hse.gov.uk) for further information.

| **Learning outcomes** | Having read this chapter the reader should be able to: |
|---|---|

- discuss the responsibilities of both the employer and employee in reducing the risk of injury occurring when moving or handling
- describe the anatomy of the spine and related structures, relating this to the mechanics of moving and handling
- identify situations that place the midwife at increased risk from a moving and handling injury
- discuss how lifting should occur, should it be required
- describe how a good posture can be achieved.

Back injuries appear to be more common in newly qualified and very senior staff. Blue (1996) suggests this may be due to acute trauma in newly qualified staff, but could be a result of the cumulative effect of smaller traumatic episodes, combined with reduced physical fitness, for older, more senior staff. Both employers and employees have a responsibility to make every effort to reduce the risk of injury occurring. For employees this could include maintaining their own fitness levels; back injuries occur less frequently in people who are physically fit and undertake high energy activities on a regular basis (e.g. swimming and running) (Blue 1996).

# Anatomy of the spine

The spine, or vertebral column, is responsible for maintaining the upright posture of the body, provides flexibility of movement and protects the spinal cord. The spine consists of 33 separate bones or vertebrae – 24 moveable and 9 fused vertebrae (Fig. 53.1):

- seven cervical vertebrae: C1–C7 (the neck)
- twelve thoracic vertebrae: T1–T12 (the upper trunk)
- five lumbar vertebrae: L1–L5 (the lower trunk)
- five fused sacral vertebrae: S1–S5 (the sacrum)
- four fused coccygeal vertebrae (the coccyx).

The vertebrae articulate with their immediate neighbours, with muscles attached, and the thoracic vertebrae meet with the ribs. The coccyx articulates with the sacrum at the sacrococcygeal joint. Each vertebra has a main body, situated anteriorly, that acts as a shock absorber as the posture changes. The size of the body varies throughout the vertebral column, beginning small with the cervical vertebrae, increasing in size to the lumbar vertebrae. Behind the body is the vertebral foramen, a large central cavity that contains the spinal cord, with nerves and blood vessels passing from here, out through spaces between the vertebrae.

A flexible intervertebral disc connects the vertebral bodies to each other. These discs, which have a fibrocartilage outer layer surrounding an inner semi-solid centre, assist with absorbing shock from movement and affect the flexibility of the spine. The vertebrae and discs are supported by ligaments that help to maintain the vertebrae in position and limit the amount of stress transmitted to the spine by restricting excessive movement. The ligaments do not produce as much support for the lumbar vertebrae, creating an inherent weakness in this area. The lumbar vertebrae experience higher levels of stress when the back is bent and the knees kept straight while lifting than when keeping the back straight and the knees bent (Kroemer & Grandjean 1997). This stress increases significantly if the back is twisted, as can occur when leaning over a bed.

**Figure 53.1** Vertebral column-bones and curves (Adapted with kind permission from Wilson & Waugh 1996)

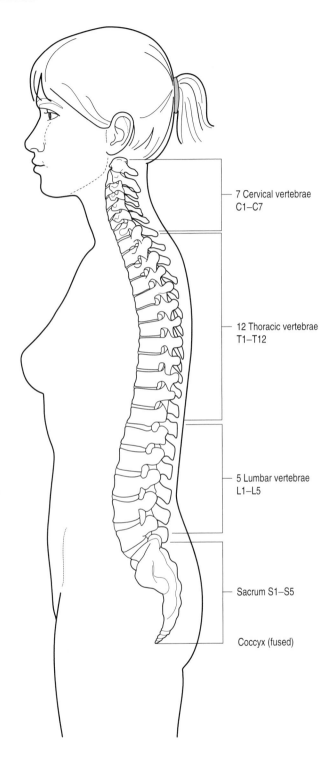

7 Cervical vertebrae
C1–C7

12 Thoracic vertebrae
T1–T12

5 Lumbar vertebrae
L1–L5

Sacrum S1–S5

Coccyx (fused)

The vertebral column is not straight, but has four curves (see Fig. 53.1):

- cervical curve (convex curve anteriorly)
- thoracic curve (concave curve anteriorly)
- lumbar curve (convex curve anteriorly)
- sacral curve (concave curve anteriorly).

The first three curves are important in relation to posture; when they meet in a midline centre of balance, weight distribution is balanced and a healthy posture ensues, protecting the supporting structures from injury (Blue 1996).

# Considerations for moving and lifting

There are four important categories that should be considered in relation to moving and lifting, as these can affect the likelihood of an injury occurring (HSE 1992):

1. the task
2. the load
3. the working environment
4. the individual.

## The task

Does the task involve:

- holding an object or load away from the trunk?
- twisting or stooping?
- reaching upwards?
- using large vertical movements?
- carrying an object for a long distance?
- strenuous pushing or pulling?
- repetitive handling?
- insufficient rest or recovery?
- unpredictable movement of an object, e.g. carrying fluids?

## The load

Is the load or object:

- heavy?
- bulky?
- difficult to hold?
- unstable, e.g. fluid?
- intrinsically harmful, e.g. sharp?

### The working environment

Within the environment, are there:

- constraints on posture?
- poor or slippery floors?
- variations in levels?
- poor lighting conditions?

### The individual

Does the job:

- require an unusual capability, e.g. in relation to weight of load?
- cause a hazard to anyone with a health problem?
- cause a hazard to anyone who is pregnant, or who has had a baby within the past 2 years?
- require special information or training?

A positive answer to any of these questions indicates that a risk assessment should be undertaken prior to any moving or lifting activities, with the aim of reducing the risk of injury as far as possible.

## Principles of lifting

It is inevitable that some lifting will occur, mainly relating to equipment; lifting people is not usually part of the midwife's role. There are variations in the maximum weight an individual can lift. Women generally have lower lifting strength than men and an individual's physical capability is affected by age and health (HSE 1998). Lifting strength increases until the early 20s with a gradual decline seen thereafter. The HSE (1998) suggests this becomes more significant from the mid-40s onwards with the risk of manual handling injury being highest 'for employees in their teens and 50s and 60s'. The maximum weight one should lift is also affected by whether the individual is standing or sitting, with the latter lifting a significantly lower weight than the former. It is also influenced by whether the elbows are bent or straight and the position of the object to be lifted – higher weights are more permissible if at waist height than if at head or feet height. Pregnancy will also affect the maximum weight a woman should attempt to lift (Tolley 2000). It is therefore important to take these factors into account when undertaking a risk assessment.

Stevens (2004) points out, however, that no-lift policies imposed by employers are, in several circumstances, illegal. For example, the midwife has a duty of care to manually lift an immobile woman away from danger such as fire if this is the only method of removal available, or to move the woman if she is unable to relieve pressure on her body and is at increased risk of pressure ulcer formation (Ch. 57). To reduce the risk of injury, the midwife needs to understand the principles involved.

The normal adult has an imaginary 'centre of gravity' that is close to the base of the spine when standing in an upright symmetrical position. The feet form the base, and a vertical line drawn through the centre of gravity will reach the floor halfway between the feet, between the balls and heels (the baseline). This determines the person's balance and how far the position can be altered by leaning or reaching before balance is lost (Pheasant 1991). A body that experiences prolonged periods of imbalance may suffer stress and strain to the muscles of the trunk and abdomen, and – if not relieved – injury and pain (Jamieson et al 2002). Imbalance can be reduced by keeping the centre of gravity within the baseline, achieved by widening the foot stance.

The vertebral column supports the weight of the head, neck, arms, hands and upper trunk. As the weight of the upper body increases so does the force placed on the spine. If an object is being carried, the spine is compressed further. The acts of walking, bending and twisting the trunk also increase the force placed on the spinal column, particularly the intervertebral discs. So, when moving an object that also requires the midwife to walk, bend or twist, considerable force is placed on the intervertebral discs.

To minimise the risk of injury when lifting a load, the spine should be straightened, in alignment with the head (which should be raised), the knees relaxed and the base widened. The load should be held as near to the body as possible (Fig. 53.2). When lifting with a rounded back, curvature of the lumbar spine results, applying asymmetrical pressure on the

**Figure 53.2** Position of spine when lifting a load

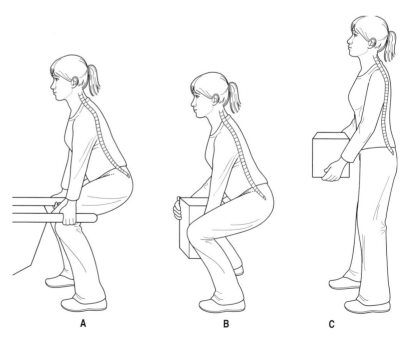

A          B          C

intervertebral discs. If continued, the pressure can result in the disc erod-ing, resulting in a 'slipped' disc. This is where the outer layer ruptures and the centre of the disc herniates through the gap to press on the spinal nerves or their roots. Damage to the surrounding tissues can also occur. In severe cases, the prolapsed discs can compress the spinal column.

It is also important to ensure that the object being lifted is kept as close to the body as possible. The compression forces increase with both the weight of the object and the further away from the body it is held, and directly affects the amount of stress placed on the lumbar spine (Kroemer & Grandjean 1997).

Blue (1996) recommends using the entire hand when lifting as this encourages a better grip on the object and reduces the need for unnec-essary movements to readjust the grip. The use of handles can also encourage a better grip on an object.

Within the maternity setting most women are mobile, with a very small minority requiring assistance with mobility, although Mander (1999) suggests immobility and impaired mobility will increase due to changes in obstetric practice (e.g. epidural analgesia). Mobility should be encouraged as far as possible, as this not only reduces the incidence of injury to the midwife, but also promotes physical wellbeing in the mother. When this is not possible, the use of appropriate moving and handling equipment is important. For women who need assistance to move up the bed, devices such as monkey poles are useful. The woman should be reminded to bend her knees and flex her head towards her chest to reduce the shearing effect. The midwife can press against the woman's feet to prevent them slipping while she is moving up the bed. It is useful to discuss this with the woman prior to surgery whenever possible and to watch her practise moving herself up the bed following these principles. When women need to be moved from one bed to another (e.g. following caesarean section), sliding devices should be used. These are slid underneath the woman and allow her to slide between the two surfaces with minimal effort from the midwives (Fig. 53.3). The woman can also be advised to turn on her side and push herself upright with her hand, using the elbow nearest the bed as a prop. Once sitting upright, it will be easier for the woman to get up from the bed unaided, particularly if the bed is lowered so that her feet are placed on the floor.

Therefore, when lifting or moving is unavoidable, the midwife should ensure that:

- mechanical aids are used whenever possible
- the feet are widened to maintain balance
- the back is straight to prevent unnecessary pressure on the interver-tebral discs
- the knees are bent to reduce the pressure on the vertebral column

**Figure 53.3**    Slide placed underneath woman

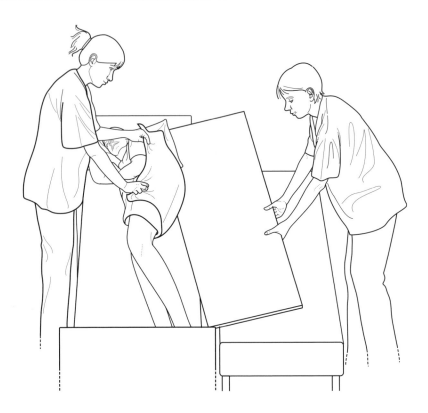

- the object being lifted is kept close to the body, grasping the object between the knees if being lifted from the floor
- the body is not twisted or rotated when lifting or lowering the object
- sufficient numbers of people are involved to ensure the maximum load per person is not exceeded. These people must understand the correct technique and be able to work as a team, with one member acting as the coordinator and directing the proceedings.

# Correct posture

The midwife may also sustain injury through bad posture, particularly if prolonged, when strain is placed on the muscles of the back. Situations where this can occur include:

- sitting for long periods (including driving)
- supporting a labouring woman
- delivery
- perineal suturing
- assisting with breastfeeding.

### Sitting
When sitting with the back straight, the pelvis is tilted forward and the posture is maintained by the muscles, which can tire quickly. The

pressure on the intervertebral discs is increased compared with a standing position. To reduce the need for muscle effort, slouching can occur. This allows the pelvis to rotate backwards and the posture and weight of the trunk are maintained more by the ligaments than the muscles. While this is effective in reducing the workload on the muscles, it doubles the force placed on the intervertebral discs, compared with the upright position (Pheasant 1991). The pressure can be reduced by using a chair with a good back rest; the pelvis rotates backwards, as for the slouched position, but the spine flexes again when it comes into contact with the back of the chair. This results in less pressure being placed on the intervertebral discs, which can be reduced further by the use of a pad in the lumbar region, possibly to a pressure that is 30–40% lower than when in a standing position (Pheasant 1991).

### Stooped posture

The midwife may have a stooped posture, where the trunk is inclined forward in situations such as delivery and assisting with breastfeeding. In this situation the weight of the upper body is supported by post-vertebral muscles. Contraction of these muscles can result in the intervertebral discs becoming compressed.

### Asymmetric posture

The midwife may adopt an asymmetric posture involving side bending when delivering a woman in an alternative position, particularly if she is upright or on all fours and the midwife is on the floor. This again increases the pressure on the spine and predisposes to injury. Whenever the midwife is required to adopt an unusual position, careful consideration should be given to maintaining a symmetric posture and not to maintain the position for long periods to avoid undue pressure on the muscles and ligaments.

## Employers' responsibilities

The Manual Handling Operations Regulations 1992 (HSE 1992) require employers, as far as is reasonably practicable, to remove the need for employees to undertake manual handling where there is a risk of injury. Employers are required to undertake a risk assessment for any situation in which manual handling may be required. This should take place before the situation arises to give the employer sufficient time to take measures to reduce the risk of injury to employees (e.g. use of appropriate equipment). Each employer should have a safer patient handling policy, manual lifting should be avoided and manual handling should only occur if it does not involve lifting most or all of a person's weight (RCN 1996).

## Employees' responsibility

In relation to risks at work, employees have a duty to cooperate with their employers in relation to safe manual handling. They should inform their managers of any situations that could be considered to put them at risk of injury. They also have a responsibility to ensure they make full use of equipment provided for manual handling. Employees must know how to use the equipment properly, attending appropriate training sessions to update and maintain their knowledge and skills.

### Role and responsibilities of the midwife

These can be summarised as:

- informing the employer of any situations in which a risk assessment should be undertaken
- using moving and handling equipment correctly
- knowing how to lift a load correctly
- being able to achieve a good posture in whichever position is undertaken
- recognising the situations in which the midwife is at risk of injury from poor posture and taking steps to reduce the risk of injury.

## Summary

- Incorrect moving and handling techniques can cause serious damage to the physical health of the midwife
- The midwife should not be involved in lifting another person, but should use appropriate equipment for this purpose
- The midwife is at risk of physical injury when adopting a poor posture.

### Self-assessment exercises

The answers to the following questions may be found in the text:

1. What are the responsibilities of the midwife and the employer in relation to moving and handling?
2. Describe the anatomy of the spine and associated structures that are involved in the mechanics of moving and handling.
3. Identify five situations from clinical practice that place the midwife at increased risk from a manual handling injury.
4. When lifting a load, how can the risk of injury be reduced?
5. How can the midwife achieve a good posture and what is the significance of a poor posture?

## REFERENCES

Blue C L 1996 Preventing back injury among nurses. Orthopaedic Nursing 15(6):9–19

Cowell R 1998 Equipment for moving and handling patients. Professional Nurse 14(2):123–127, 129–130

HSE (Health and Safety Executive) 1992 Manual handling guidance on regulations; manual handling operations regulations. HMSO, London

HSE (Health and Safety Executive) 1998 Manual handling. Manual handling operations regulations 1992; guidance on regulations. HMSO, Norwich

Jamieson E M, McCall J M, Whyte L A 2002 Clinical nursing practices, 4th edn. Churchill Livingstone, Edinburgh

Kroemer K H E, Grandjean E 1997 Fitting the task to the human: a textbook of occupational ergonomics, 5th edn. Taylor and Francis, London

Mander R 1999 Manual handling and the immobile mother. British Journal of Midwifery 7(8):485–487

Pheasant S 1991 Ergonomics, work and health. Macmillan, Basingstoke

RCN (Royal College of Nursing) 1996 Introducing a safer handling policy. RCN, London

Stevens D R 2004 Manual handling and the lawfulness of no-lift policies. Nursing Standard 18(21):39–43

Tolley 2000 Health and safety at work handbook 2000, 13th edn. Tolley, Croydon

White C 1998 How to prevent injury caused by moving and handling. Nursing Times 94(34):57–60

Wilson K J W, Waugh A 1996 Ross and Wilson anatomy and physiology in health and illness, 8th edn. Churchill Livingstone, Edinburgh

# Chapter 54

# Principles of perioperative skills

Unfortunately surgery may result in fatality. Women may undergo caesarean section (CS), but can also attend theatre for procedures such as
manual removal of placenta, perineal repair, abscess drainage and cervical suture removal. NICE (2004) lists the estimates of risks and benefits
of CS, for which there are few benefits listed! The midwife has a significant role in caring safely for the woman before, during and after surgery.

This chapter considers care prior to elective and emergency surgery,
intraoperative care and postoperative recovery care. It focuses largely
upon caesarean section, but the principles may be applied to other
types of surgery.

Care in theatre is specialised care, requiring cooperative teamwork
between all the professional groups involved. The midwife may take
on a number of different roles (e.g. pre- or postoperative care, theatre
scrub nurse or runner, recovery care).

## Learning outcomes

Having read this chapter the reader should be able to:

- discuss thorough preoperative care prior to elective and emergency CS
- summarise the general principles of intraoperative care
- discuss recovery and post CS care
- summarise the midwife's responsibilities in each role.

## Reducing CS rates

Reducing the risks of surgery is a significant aspect of care. If, however,
the need for surgery itself can be reduced, this is highly advantageous.
NICE (2004) recommend an increase in homebirth, external cephalic
version for a singleton breech, continuous labour support, partogram
use, availability of fetal blood sampling for suspected fetal distress,
induction of labour post maturity and consultation with a consultant
prior to surgery.

# Preparation for surgery

Delivery by caesarean section is very different from vaginal delivery, but is still nevertheless the precious birth of someone's child. Some women may anticipate operative delivery to be useful in helping them to avoid the pain of labour and so psychologically prepare for surgery and the recovery afterwards. Other women may feel cheated of a labour experience and feel deeply distressed at being delivered by caesarean section, particularly if it is an emergency. Emergency surgery can also be a frightening experience in which the woman may fear for her life or that of her baby. Psychological care before, during and afterwards are all vital components of care.

# Physical preparation for elective surgery

Many of the physical complications that occur during or after surgery can be reduced or eradicated by careful preoperative preparation. It can be helpful if there is a routine checklist so that none of the aspects are missed.

### Consultation with obstetrician and anaesthetist

Elective CS should be undertaken after 39 weeks' gestation to reduce the baby's risks of respiratory disorder. Each woman should be seen by an obstetrician (see above) and anaesthetist prior to surgery. Other members of the multidisciplinary team may also be included (e.g. a physiotherapist). The woman's health, reason for surgery and suitability for chosen anaesthetic are all assessed. NICE (2004) recommend offering all women regional anaesthesia (spinal or epidural), the risks being less than with a general anaesthetic. Equally, all women should give both verbal and written consent; clearly this can only be after thorough discussions of the risks and benefits of the CS. Women who seek CS for social and not clinical reasons may be denied their request or referred for a second opinion.

A full blood count will confirm the haemoglobin level. Other haematology screening is not routinely required (NICE 2004) for healthy women with uncomplicated pregnancies. Obviously, this is reviewed for each individual woman; some women will require blood to be grouped and saved or cross-matched prior to surgery. High risk CS (e.g. placenta praevia) must take place where there are blood transfusion services readily available. Other investigations may be ordered (e.g. chest x-ray). The midwife will undertake an antenatal assessment and baseline vital sign observations. Allergies (e.g. to latex, antibiotics, etc.) should be carefully documented. Postoperative care and analgesia are discussed. Some of these aspects of care may be completed at a prior clinic appointment so that the woman arrives on the day with all of the preparations completed.

### Care of the gastrointestinal tract

Fasting prior to surgery is indicated so that the risk of aspiration is reduced. It takes approximately 6 hours for the stomach to be empty from food, and 2–3 hours for fluids (Scott et al 1999). However, pregnancy, labour, some drugs (e.g. pethidine) and anxiety can all delay gastric emptying; nevertheless starvation for periods of longer than 6 hours is unnecessary and distressing for the woman. Antacid therapy or $H_2$ antagonists are given so that the gastric acid will be less acidic and reduced in volume, respectively. This is prescribed preoperatively; an antiemetic may also be included to reduce nausea. An intravenous (I.V.) infusion will be sited prior to the surgery, particularly if preloading is required for regional anaesthesia. Good hydration also reduces the risks of thromboembolism.

### Premedication

Premedication are drugs administered prior to surgery in preparation for, or as part of, the anaesthetic. They may be prescribed in any form according to need – relaxant, antiemetic, analgesic, etc. The most likely premedication in the maternity setting are the antacid/$H_2$ antagonists described above. Other drugs would be administered with caution, anticipating their transfer across the placenta. It becomes important therefore that a premedication is given at the prescribed time, and that the anaesthetist is informed if for some reason the surgery does not then happen at the expected time.

### Skin preparation

In an attempt to reduce postoperative wound infections, preoperative skin preparation is indicated. This is discussed in Chapter 56 (postoperative wound management), but remains a largely inconclusive science. The woman, as a minimal requirement, should take a shower. She will wear a gown, without any underwear, particularly noting that bras may reduce chest expansion and have metal components that may interact with other theatre equipment. She is asked not to use deodorant or talcum powder, both of which may be flammable. All make-up is removed, so that the actual colour of her nail beds and mucous membranes may be seen in order to recognise any cyanosis. Hair removal from the wound site remains controversial; shaving is technically contraindicated due to the abrasions of the skin and the likely increase of wound infection. Hair may be clipped or a depilatory cream used, but often a small number of pubic hairs are shaved immediately below the site for incision, as close to the surgery time as possible.

### Care of bladder and bowels

Constipation may be a problem postoperatively after fasting and being immobilised; it is therefore better for the bowel to be emptied preoperatively. Glycerin suppositories may be administered the evening before surgery if necessary (Ch. 25). A residual or indwelling catheter may be used to prevent any trauma or overdistension to the bladder during surgery and is sometimes inserted prior to transfer to theatre, or at the time of surgery (Ch. 16).

### Thromboembolic prophylaxis

Death from pulmonary embolism (following deep vein thrombosis – DVT) is a serious risk for childbearing women who have experienced surgery or any period of immobility. This is discussed in detail in Chapter 58, but correctly sized compression stockings should be applied prior to surgery, particularly for women with higher risk factors (e.g. obesity or varicose veins). Early mobilisation and a subcutaneous heparin regimen will be commenced postoperatively.

### Identity and removal of prosthesis

All prostheses are removed prior to surgery (e.g. contact lenses, false limbs, dentures, etc.). Hearing aids may be retained depending upon the surgeon/anaesthetist. Capped teeth are noted if general anaesthesia is to be administered due to the risk of being dislodged and inhaled. Metallic jewellery is removed, but wedding rings are usually taped securely in place. Identity bands are worn, especially if the woman is likely to be unconscious, and identity bands are often prepared in advance for the baby.

### Record keeping

The midwife will ensure that all of the physical and psychological preparation is recorded contemporaneously.

## Emergency surgery

Preparation for emergency surgery should include all of the above, but is often carried out much more quickly. Fasting, for example, is not possible. Antacids and antiemetics are administered, and if necessary, i.e. before general anaesthetic, the stomach contents may be removed using a wide bore nasogastric tube. The reader will appreciate that the speed required means that the preparation may be seen to be less thorough than for elective surgery, and therefore there are higher intraoperative and postoperative risks from emergency surgery.

## Intraoperative care

The midwife's role will vary in this setting depending upon which of the roles is undertaken. Theatre care is very detailed; general principles are summarised below, but the reader is encouraged to consider other literary sources. The following general principles should be upheld in theatre:

- The most important person present is the woman. Her dignity and safety should be maintained whether awake or anaesthetised
- Her safety is paramount, whether that is her internal safety:
  - maintenance of her airway and respirations: with a general anaesthetic this includes using preoxygenation, a cuffed endotracheal (ET) tube, cricoid pressure (Fig. 59.1, p. 455), rapid sequence induction and mechanical ventilation. A protocol will exist should intubation fail; the anaesthetist and operating departmental practitioner (ODP) will instigate this
  - pulse oximetry monitoring is used throughout to detect any hypoxia regardless of type of anaesthesia (Ch. 7)
  - the theatre table should have a tilt of 15° to avoid aortocaval occlusion
  - blood pressure is monitored throughout and maintained by adjusting the fluid volume; fluid balance is essential
  - asepsis is maintained throughout to reduce the risk of infection; I.V. antibiotics are offered routinely (cephalosporin or ampicillin) to reduce postoperative infection (NICE 2004)
  - known allergies should be accommodated; a latex-free trolley is often available in theatre for affected women
- or her external safety:
  - care of the immobile or unconscious woman: safety upon the operating table, care of numb limbs and pressure areas (Ch. 57), attention to temperature maintenance, prevention of burns from diathermy equipment, care of infusion lines, monitors, etc.
- Theatre work is teamwork, for which all members of the team should be able to recognise their limitations and call in more senior or expert help if needed. The DoH (1998) indicates that often consultant level expertise is either not called or called too late, and that sometimes the severity of the situation is not recognised by junior staff. Anaesthetists should be supported by skilled help, e.g. ODP. Communication should be good between all team members, especially if laboratory or haematology support is required (DoH 1998)
- Theatre is a sterile environment in which strict surgical asepsis is maintained. Scrubbed persons wear sterile gowns and gloves, all of which are applied after scrupulous hand hygiene. The rear of the gown is handled at the edges by the person fastening it, but the front remains totally sterile. Drapes (often disposable) are used to establish a sterile field; these are only touched by a scrubbed person. All of the items within the sterile field should be sterile and are opened and transferred in such a way as to retain their sterility. Everyone in the theatre environment moves around in such as way as to maintain the integrity of the sterile field. The air is scavenged and – as a restricted area – only people wearing theatre clothing and footwear

are permitted. External sources of potential infection, e.g. shoes, are prohibited.

- Theatre should also be appropriately stocked with all of the necessary equipment: drugs and anaesthetic gases, anaesthetic machine, monitors, resuscitation equipment, I.V. fluids and infant resuscitaire, amongst other things

- Staff should also protect themselves, working under the protection of the health and safety legislation, use of extensive standard precautions – e.g. masks with visors, aprons, wellingtons, etc. – and moving and handling requirements. Those with close patient contact may choose to double glove (especially if HIV is an issue)

- Swabs, needles and instruments are all counted initially. The circulating midwife also counts the swabs and needles; these are recorded on the board where the scrub midwife can see them. Any additional items that are opened during the surgery are added to the information on the board. As the wound is closed swabs, needles and instruments are checked and counted; the scrub midwife uses the circulating midwife again to establish that the final count equates with the original one. This ensures that nothing has been retained inside the wound. Contemporaneous records should be completed; these may include a theatre register or anaesthetic record

- CS under regional anaesthesia means that the woman will be fully able to appreciate all that's happening. She and her partner's wishes can be respected, e.g. she may be able to lift the baby from her abdomen herself, silence may be requested so that the mother's voice is the first one heard by the baby, immediate skin-to-skin contact may be possible and early breastfeeding should not be ruled out (Coggins 2003). Equally, being awake can be a time of heightened anxiety. Care should include preparing her for the environment and the sensations (pushing and pulling, but not pain) that she may experience

- For the woman having a general anaesthetic, there is a heightened sensitivity to sound as the anaesthetic is administered. She will also require repeated and ongoing reassurance as she recovers, drifting in and out of sleep

- Specific guidance is given within the NICE guidelines (NICE 2004) as to the surgical techniques that reduce pain and infection. These include issues such as transverse abdominal incision, blunt incision of the uterus, avoiding forceps, use of I.V. oxytocin and controlled cord traction for placental delivery, uterine suturing in two layers within the abdomen, non-suturing of the visceral or parietal peritoneums or subcutaneous tissue (unless >2 cm) and avoidance of superficial wound drains

- Care of the baby: resuscitation equipment and personnel should be on hand if there has been a general anaesthetic or fetal compromise.

Care should be taken to label the infant and to maintain body temperature.

# Postoperative care

This should be completed in a recovery area where there is immediate access to oxygen, suction, resuscitation equipment, monitors, emergency call bells and appropriately skilled one-to-one staff.

After a general anaesthetic an airway is usually inserted following extubation by the anaesthetist. The woman should remove this spontaneously as she regains consciousness.

Postoperative care, particularly that given during the recovery period, encompasses all of the following, whichever type of anaesthetic has been administered:

- maintenance of the airway, with or without oxygen therapy
- assessment of respirations, heart rate, blood pressure and temperature
- use of pulse oximetry for oxygen saturation with assessment of colour
- correct positioning, care of numb limbs and pressure areas
- assessment of consciousness
- assessment of levels of pain, care of patient-controlled analgesia (PCA) (Ch. 26)
- care of I.V. infusion/blood transfusion and fluid balance
- care of wound (and drain if appropriate)
- observation of loss per vaginam
- care of urinary catheter/urinary output
- return of sensation following regional anaesthesia
- time with the baby and opportunities to feed.

## Observations

All vital sign observations will be completed at 5-minute intervals initially. As time passes and all other observations remain within normal limits the frequency of observations may be reduced to every 15 minutes, 30 minutes, etc. They should be half hourly for at least 2 hours and hourly thereafter until satisfactory (NICE 2004). After approximately 1 hour the woman should be conscious, comfortable, semi-recumbent if appropriate and able to tolerate sips of water. She will remain in the recovery area until the anaesthetist and midwife are satisfied that she may be transferred to the ward area. All of the care listed above is ongoing throughout recovery care. Record keeping is particularly important, and the midwife should have access to calling the anaesthetist and obstetrician at any time if any deviations from the norm are noted.

### The baby

The baby is cared for accordingly, noting that babies born in theatre:

- are often cooler
- need to be fed as soon as possible
- should be labelled before leaving theatre
- are more likely to experience respiratory distress.

### Other issues

Consideration is given to the partner and their needs. The midwife also ensures that the placenta and membranes are assessed as for any other delivery. Cord blood is taken if the woman is rhesus negative and an umbilical artery pH is performed if there was fetal compromise. Birth registers, etc. are completed as for any other birth.

### Ongoing care

Psychologically, there is relief and enjoyment of the new baby, but it may be tinged by pain, immobility, distress (if rapid emergency or major complications were present) and frustration that progress appears slow. In the days following the surgery the woman will appreciate sensitive and individualised midwifery care and should have the opportunity to review her care and future pregnancies with her obstetric team.

Postoperative care, while individualised, will probably include attention to hygiene and oral care, thromboembolic prophylaxis (see above), vital sign observations, pressure area care, urinary output and analgesia.

For analgesia, NICE (2004) recommend diamorphine as the initial analgesic of choice, noting that PCA offers the woman good pain relief. Non-steroidal anti-inflammatory drugs can also be given concurrently and continued after the opioids have stopped. Where diamorphine or morphine has been given intrathecally, the midwife will need to assess respirations hourly for 24 and 12 hours respectively (NICE 2004). Opioids given epidurally or via PCA require hourly respiration rate observations throughout the treatment and for 2 hours after discontinuation. Good pain relief is essential to the woman's recovery.

Sips of water are given are given within the first hour of surgery. Thereafter the woman may eat or drink as she wishes (NICE 2004). Intravenous infusion is discontinued when appropriate, often the following day. The urinary catheter is removed when appropriate and voiding encouraged (see Ch. 16); this should be at least 12 hours after the last regional analgesia. Early mobilisation is encouraged and naturally the woman will require support and care with her baby, particularly to establish breastfeeding. While this is often a motivating factor for the woman after CS, the midwife should ensure that the woman is having sufficient rest and is not over-tired.

The wound may be uncovered after showering and will be cared for as discussed in Chapter 56. Haemoglobin estimation may be completed on the third postoperative day after postnatal diuresis has occurred. The midwife should be sensitive to the woman's emotional state, noting that she has undergone two significant life experiences – having a baby and major surgery. Standard postnatal assessment is a part of each day's care in conjunction with specific postoperative needs.

Discharge from hospital will depend upon the woman's progress and social support; it may be from 24 hours to 3–4 days. Post-surgery advice includes the avoidance of lifting and driving until free of discomfort, effective contraception for at least 1 year and attendance for assessment (usually with the obstetrician) at the end of the puerperium.

Audit of CS care is recommended in order that units can both provide quality care and reduce the CS rate.

### Role and responsibilities of the midwife

These can be summarised as:

- evidence-based practice throughout
- preoperative care to reduce intra- and postoperative complications
- skilled care within theatre and recovery
- comprehensive postoperative care
- effective multidisciplinary teamwork and recognition of limitations where appropriate
- referral when indicated
- contemporaneous record keeping.

## Summary

- Theatre care is detailed and specialised; childbearing women have increased risk factors including aspiration, aortocaval occlusion and thromboembolism
- Preoperative preparation should include consent, identity, care of the gastrointestinal and urinary tracts, skin preparation, removal of prostheses, thromboprophylaxis and psychological support; good preoperative care can reduce the intra- and postoperative risks
- Intraoperative care considers the woman to be the highest priority for maintaining her internal and external safety. This comprises many aspects of care
- Postoperative care focuses on vital sign observations, airway and consciousness, pain relief, assessment of wound and haemorrhage, care of infusions, bladder care, adaptation to parenthood and feeding and psychological support.

| Self-assessment exercises | The answers to the following questions may be found in the text: |
|---|---|

1. Discuss the requirements and rationale for preoperative preparation prior to emergency caesarean section. Compare and contrast this with preparation for elective surgery.
2. Summarise the general principles of conduct and care in the theatre environment.
3. Discuss the midwife's role and responsibilities to the woman before, during and following caesarean section.
4. Describe the care that the midwife gives to a woman in the immediate and ongoing recovery period after a caesarean section under regional anaesthesia.
5. List other occasions when it may be necessary for childbearing women to undergo surgery.

## REFERENCES

Coggins J 2003 Caesarean birth: a birth none-the-less! MIDIRS Midwifery Digest 13(1):76–79

DoH (Department of Health) 1998 Why mothers die. Report on Confidential enquiries into Maternal Deaths in the United Kingdom 1994–1996. The Stationery Office, London

NICE (National Institute for Clinical Excellence) 2004 Caesarean section: Clinical Guideline 13. NICE, London

Scott E, Earl C, Leaper D et al 1999 Understanding perioperative nursing. Nursing Standard 13(49):49–54

Chapter **55**

# Principles of wound management — principles of wound healing

This chapter focuses on the principles of wound healing, by describing briefly the process of wound healing and will consider factors that influence the process. The midwife should understand the principles of wound healing that underpin the care provided in relation to wound management. Recognition of the normal healing process is essential and a knowledge of the factors that influence wound healing is fundamental to the care of a woman with a wound.

Surgical wounds occur as a result of operative delivery, when the abdominal skin, fat, muscles, peritoneum and uterus are incised, or during an episiotomy, when the perineal skin, muscles and vaginal wall are incised. Non-surgical perineal wounds may occur when the perineal tissues tear during delivery or as a result of nipple trauma due to inappropriate latching of the baby. A wound may also result when the skin is punctured, e.g. during venepuncture, capillary sampling, application of a fetal scalp electrode, administration of an intramuscular or subcutaneous drug, cannulation.

## Learning outcomes

Having read this chapter the reader should be able to:

- describe the process of wound healing, identifying how the different phases can be recognised
- discuss the factors that enhance or hinder wound healing
- discuss the complications associated with wound healing.

## Physiology of wound healing

Healing of wounds begins following any injury to the body; an intact skin provides an efficient first line of defence against invading organisms. Wounds whose edges are in apposition (e.g. surgical wounds) heal quickly by first or primary intention. Deeper, gaping wounds take longer to heal by secondary intention.

There are four phases of wound healing:

1. haemostasis
2. inflammation
3. proliferation
4. maturation.

The length of time to progress through these phases varies for each wound and can be influenced by factors such as wound size, suturing, the clinical condition of the person and infection.

### Haemostasis

This vascular phase begins immediately there is tissue damage. Vasoconstriction occurs to minimise bleeding and assist with initiating the coagulation process. A fibrin clot forms, temporarily closing the wound. While the clot is forming, blood or serous fluid may exude from the wound as the body tries to cleanse the wound naturally.

### Inflammation

The blood vessels around the wound dilate, causing localised erythema, oedema, heat, discomfort, throbbing and sometimes functional disturbance. Macrophages clear the wound of debris in preparation for new tissue growth. A small necrotic area forms around the wound margin where the blood supply was interrupted. Epithelial cells from the wound margin move under the base of the clot, the surrounding epithelium thickens and a thin layer of epithelial tissue forms over the wound. As the clinical signs of the inflammation phase are similar to those of infection it is important the midwife can distinguish between a wound that is healing normally and one that is infected. Provided the wound is clean, this phase lasts about 36 hours, but is prolonged in the presence of infection or necrosis (Flanagan 1996).

### Proliferation

This phase involves the growth of new tissue through three processes:

- granulation
- wound contraction
- epithelialisation.

During granulation, capillaries from the surrounding vessels grow into the wound bed. At the same time, fibroblasts produce collagen fibres, providing the framework for new connective tissue formation. Collagen increases the tensile strength and structural integrity of the wound. Healthy granulation tissue has a bright red, moist, shiny appearance, a 'pebbled' looking base and does not bleed easily.

Once the wound is filled with connective tissue, fibroblasts collect around the edges of the wound and contract, pulling the edges together. A firmer, fibrous epithelial scar forms as the fibroblasts and collagen fibres begin to shrink, resulting in contraction of the area and obliteration of some of the capillaries. This only occurs with healthy tissue that has not been sutured.

During epithelialisation new epithelial cells grow over the wound surface to form a new outer layer, recognised by the whitish-pink, translucent appearance of the wound. The process is enhanced in a moist, clean environment.

### Maturation

Once epithelialisation is complete, the new tissue undergoes a time of maturation when it is 're-modelled' to increase the tensile strength of the scar tissue. In Caucasian skin, the scar initially appears red and raised, and then with time changes to a paler, smoother, flatter appearance. Scar tissue in darkly pigmented skin has a lighter appearance initially when compared with Caucasian skin. Mature scar tissue is avascular and contains no sweat or sebaceous glands or hairs. This phase can take up to 2 years to complete and may be the reason why some wounds that appear to have healed suddenly break down (Keast & Orsted 1998).

This healing process also occurs around sutures. When the sutures are removed, the epithelial cells can be dislodged and may be visible on the sutures as debris.

Wound healing by secondary intention occurs with deeper, wider wounds, whose edges cannot be brought into apposition. Inflammation may be chronic, with more granulation tissue forming at the expense of collagen during proliferation. Granulation tissue gradually fills the wound with re-epithelialisation beginning at the edges. Healing by secondary intention takes longer, resulting in more scar tissue forming.

## Factors that influence wound healing

- Nutritional status: an adequate intake of protein, vitamins A and C, copper, zinc and iron is required. Proteins supply amino acids, essential for tissue repair and regeneration. Vitamin A and zinc are required for epithelialisation, and vitamin C and zinc are necessary for collagen synthesis and capillary integrity. Iron is required for the synthesis of haemoglobin which combines reversibly with oxygen to transport oxygen around the body
- Smoking: smoking interferes with the uptake and release of oxygen to the tissues, resulting in poor tissue perfusion
- Increasing age: this affects all phases of wound healing due to impaired circulation and coagulation, slower inflammatory response and decreased fibroblast activity
- Obesity: fatty tissue can have an inadequate blood supply, resulting in slower healing and decreased resistance to infection
- Diabetes mellitus: impaired circulation and tissue perfusion can occur in diabetes mellitus. Additionally, hyperglycaemia can inhibit phagocytosis and predispose to fungal and yeast infection

- Corticosteroids: raised levels of plasma corticosteroids may result from stress, steroid therapy or disease. It delays both the inflammatory and immune responses, resulting in delayed wound healing and a predisposition to infection
- Drugs: anti-inflammatory drugs suppress protein synthesis, inflammation, wound contraction and epithelialisation
- Impaired oxygenation: a low arterial oxygen tension may alter collagen synthesis and inhibit epithelialisation. Poor tissue perfusion may occur in the presence of hypovolaemia or anaemia. Oxygen is necessary for fibroblast activity
- Infection: infection causes increased inflammation and necrosis, which delays wound healing. If there is a deep wound infection, the wound may need to be kept open to avoid re-epithelialisation occurring over the infecting organisms as this is likely to result in abscess formation
- Wound stress: prolonged or violent vomiting, abdominal distension or laboured respirations may cause sudden tension on the wound, inhibiting the formation of collagen networks and connective tissue.

## Complications of wound healing

### Haemorrhage

Haemostasis usually occurs within several minutes of an acute wound occurring. However, bleeding may occur if a bleeding point is not tied off, as a result of the clot or suture dislodging or infection, and may occur internally and externally. Internal bleeding can lead to haematoma formation.

### Infection

Infection usually appears within 2–3 days following a traumatic injury or 4–5 days following a surgical wound. The wound site will appear red, swollen and painful. There may also be weeping from the wound, usually a yellow, green or brown discharge depending on the infecting organism which may also be malodorous.

### Dehiscence

If an acute wound does not heal properly the layers of skin and tissue can separate, usually during the proliferation phase. Separation can be partial or complete. It occurs more commonly where there is greater strain on the wound and decreased vasoconstriction (e.g. obesity), and particularly with abdominal wounds, if a sudden strain is placed on the wound (e.g. coughing, sitting up).

### Evisceration

This is a rare medical emergency that occurs when the visceral organs begin to protrude through the separated wound layers.

*Fistula*

This may occur as a result of poor wound healing, possibly resulting from infection.

### Role and responsibilities of the midwife

These can be summarised as:

- understanding the physiology of wound healing and application of this to practice, particularly when observing wounds
- appreciating the factors that influence wound healing
- referral if indicated
- contemporaneous record keeping.

## Summary

- Wound healing occurs by primary or secondary intention
- There are four phases of wound healing that can be affected by various factors
- Mature scar tissue can take up to 2 years to form; during this time the wound can break down.

### Self-assessment exercises

The answers to the following questions may be found in the text:

1. Describe the four phases of wound healing.
2. How would the midwife distinguish between a wound that is healing normally and one that is infected?
3. Describe the three processes involved with proliferation.
4. How would the midwife recognise healthy granulation tissue?
5. Discuss the factors that enhance or impair wound healing.
6. What complications are associated with wound healing?

### REFERENCES

Flanagan M 1996 A practical framework for wound assessment 1: physiology. British Journal of Nursing 5(22):1391–1397

Keast D H, Orsted H 1998 The basic principles of wound care. Ostomy/Wound Management 44(8):24–31

# Chapter 56

# Principles of wound management — postoperative wound management

Wound management aims to promote healing of the tissue, and also to prevent infection. Infection is costly, not only in terms of resources, but also for the debilitation suffered by the woman. Wounds are classified according to their nature (Briggs 1997); the midwife is generally likely to see clean contaminated wounds, i.e. surgically closed wounds that have involved the genitourinary tract (e.g. lower segment caesarean section – LSCS).

Effective wound management includes consideration of other factors such as the environment and the woman's preoperative health and preparation. This chapter focuses on LSCS wound management – the role of preoperative preparation, method of closure, wound dressings and cleaning, removal of sutures, clips, staples and drains. The reader is advised to consider other chapters – for example, Chapter 11 (asepsis), Chapter 37 (perineal repair), Chapter 54 (perioperative skills) – in order to appreciate holistic management.

## Learning outcomes

Having read this chapter the reader should be able to:

- discuss the factors that reduce wound infection
- discuss the evidence for wound management
- summarise care of the wound following caesarean section
- describe how to dress a wound, remove sutures, clips and staples
- describe how to empty, dress and remove a wound drain.

## Preoperative considerations

Childbearing women who are healthy and enter hospital only a short time before their planned surgery have a lesser risk of wound infection than those who are unwell and have longer hospital admission times. Being anaemic or having an existing infection reduces wound healing.

Preoperative showering is considered to be more helpful than bathing, and should be considered the night before, using chlorhexidine 4% (Byrne et al 1991). However, both the solution used and the timing/number of the showers is open to further investigation before being conclusive (Simmons 1998). Emergency surgery reduces the option for this; it may also mean that the membranes have been ruptured for some time with or without labour, a factor that may, anecdotally, also increase the postoperative risk of infection.

Hair can harbour bacteria and may make dressing removal very uncomfortable. Hair removal also remains an unresolved issue. Simmons (1998) suggests that hair should be retained unless in the way, but also recognises that if removal is required, shaving is the most harmful way of doing it. Clippers or depilatory creams are less likely to cause skin abrasion. Skin abrasions allow microorganisms to enter the skin and increase the likelihood of wound infection. If shaving is necessary, it should be done carefully and as near to the time of surgery as possible.

# Intraoperative care

The surgery itself is performed under controlled environmental conditions and strict surgical asepsis is maintained. The operating time for a caesarean section is often less than 1 hour and the surgery is relatively straightforward. Enkin et al (2000) indicate the value of a single dose of systemic broad spectrum antibiotic therapy during caesarean section to reduce infection risks. NICE (2004) make other recommendations (e.g. use of one surgical knife rather than two, nonclosure of the subcutaneous tissue space, etc.), all of which are aimed at reducing unnecessary activity and the incidence of wound infection.

## Skin preparation

The skin of the operative site is cleansed; it is inconclusive as to the nature of the lotion that should be used. Cruse and Foord (1980) found little difference in the infection rate with the use of soap and alcohol-based products compared to povidone-iodine or chlorhexidine.

## Wound closure

Wound closure may be undertaken using suture material, staples or clips. Suturing may be continuous or interrupted, and wound drains may be used. The purpose of wound closure is to bring the skin edges together in apposition so that the natural healing process can begin. There appears to be little research into the most effective type of wound closure; it is noted that it may vary according to the type of tissue or wound. Bucknall (1981) indicated that silk produced a greater tissue reaction than nylon for abdominal wounds. As a foreign substance in the tissue, only the minimal amount of suture material with a minimal inflammatory response should be used to promote wound healing. LSCS wounds are often closed with one continuous nylon (prolene) suture or with clips or staples. NICE (2004) indicate that superficial wound drains should be avoided for caesarean section wounds.

### Wound dressings

The wound dressing protects the wound from external infection (until natural healing has begun) and from catching on clothing. It is able to absorb any excess exudate from the wound, but should create an environment in which wound healing can be promoted. It is likely that for a caesarean section wound the dressing chosen will be a low adherent dressing, one that has an absorbent pad, but one that maintains humidity and a protective cover (Dale 1997).

## Postoperative wound care

### Cleaning and dressing wounds

A wound that has skin edges in good apposition will begin to heal quickly, reducing the risk of wound infection (Briggs 1997). Assessment of a wound should consider the clinical condition of the woman, the timing and nature of the surgery and the appearance of the wound. The decision to redress a wound must also include whether wound cleaning is indicated. Cleaning a wound may perform two functions:

1. remove wound debris
2. remove sloughy or necrotic tissue (Fletcher 1997).

Morison (1992) suggests that cleaning a wound when neither of these criteria applies can damage the new delicate tissue and can remove the naturally present mild exudate.

Noe and Keller (1988) indicated that it was safe from the first postoperative day for wounds sutured with nylon to be washed with soap and water. Meers et al (1992) agree, suggesting a clean dressing technique using water and non-sterile gloves, as opposed to an aseptic technique, for sutured wounds that need redressing.

If the wound requires further cleaning, Flanagan (1997) suggests the use of isotonic saline (0.9%) at body temperature. Tap water may also be considered. The question of when a wound dressing should be changed remains unanswered. It would appear sensible to make a daily *assessment*, but not to disturb the wound by cleaning or redressing it unless necessary.

### Dressing techniques

Briggs et al (1996) indicate that wound dressing is largely a ritualistic practice. Dougherty and Lister (2004) argue that gloved hands cause less trauma than forceps and that foam is kinder on the tissues than cotton wool or gauze. Increasingly, irrigation of wounds is recommended rather than swabbing (Cunliffe & Fawcett 2002) but it can be difficult to appreciate the pressure necessary for effective irrigation. Krasner (1992) recommends using an 18–19 gauge needle and 35 mL syringe at full pressure to achieve 8 pounds per square inch, using normal saline (Dealey 1999). Cunliffe and Fawcett (2002) cite studies which suggest as much as 250–500 mL of fluid may be needed to correctly irrigate. Pre-prepared canisters, etc. may be available; however, using a shower head may be an alternative but the literature is not conclusive. The evidence related to other aspects – tape, scissors, 'clean' and 'dirty' hands, trolleys, flowers, curtains, etc. – appears to be inconclusive. What is clear is that hand hygiene needs to be scrupulous and that the hygiene of the whole environment has an effect on infection rates (Briggs et al 1996).

For a woman with a LSCS wound, the following principles are suggested, but the reader is encouraged to be aware of the increasing evidence:

- The theatre dressing can be removed after 24 hours
- The woman should shower daily, the wound being dried gently and loose cotton clothing being worn
- The wound should be assessed then, and on every postoperative day after that, until care is discharged or transferred. It should be noted that obesity increases the risks of infection (Enkin et al 2000)
- Suture/clip/staple removal is planned (described below)
- If the wound is exuding excess fluid or can catch on the clothing, a dressing should be applied, otherwise the wound may be left uncovered
- If a wound requires redressing it should be with a suitable non-adherent dressing that retains moisture
- If a wound requires cleansing and redressing it should be with a clean technique, using body temperature (warmed slightly) normal saline or tap water, using either irrigation or foam swabs, and a suitable dressing
- If a wound appears infected a wound swab may be taken and a referral made. An aseptic dressing technique should be used. Assessment may be made in conjunction with the obstetrician or infection control adviser.

PROCEDURE  **aseptic dressing technique**

(Adaptations may be made for a clean technique)

- Gain informed consent and establish that redressing is indicated
- Collect the equipment on a clean dressings trolley/clean surface at home:

— hand rub, sterile gloves

— apron

— sachet of 0.9% sodium chloride at room temperature or tap water (depending on local protocol)

— sterile dressing pack with disposable bag and suitable dressing

— 18–19 gauge needle with 35 mL syringe and sharps bin

- Position the woman appropriately, maintaining privacy and dignity
- Apply apron and wash hands while the assistant opens the outer layer of the pack
- Open the inner wrapper of the pack touching only the edges of the paper; the assistant slides the sterile gloves onto the sterile field (Ch. 11)
- Loosen the existing dressing, place the disposable bag over the hand and remove the dressing (see Nicol et al 2000)
- Invert the bag, with the dressing inside and attach it to the side of the trolley as a refuse bag
- Use hand rub and apply gloves
- Assess the wound; if cleaning is indicated, the assistant pours the cleansing solution into the tray
- Cleanse the skin around the wound with foam
- Then either (depending on local protocol):
  a. clean the wound with foam and gloved hands, passing the swab from the 'clean hand' to the 'dirty hand' (see p. 101); wipe with the 'dirty hand', using each swab to wipe once only, wiping from areas of discharge outwards. Discard the swab, repeat as necessary; *or*
  b. hold a piece of gauze at the dirtier end of the wound and irrigate with the syringe and needle or canister, from clean to dirty, catching the fluid in the gauze
- Dry the surrounding skin
- Apply and secure the dressing
- Dispose of equipment correctly
- Ensure the woman is comfortable; discuss findings and ongoing care with her
- Return the trolley to the clean area, washing it down if required
- Wash hands
- Document findings and act accordingly.

## Removal of sutures, clips or staples

The decision to remove sutures, clips or staples is taken according to the assessment of healing of the wound. Sutures are removed when the wound has healed, i.e. skin edges in close apposition without signs of infection; this is often 5–10 days after surgery. Sutures that are retained for too long can delay wound healing. Suture removal is an aseptic procedure: a clean dressings trolley should be used in the hospital setting; a clean surface is utilised in the home. A receptacle is required to place clips or staples in so that they can be disposed of correctly in the sharps bin. If the wound gapes after any of the sutures have been removed the midwife will refer the woman before removing them all, and may apply an adhesive suture in the meantime. Obviously, only non-absorbable sutures need to be removed.

### Removing sutures

The aim of correct suture removal is to ensure that no part of the external suture is taken through internally:

- Lift and hold the external part of the suture with forceps using the non-dominant hand
- Cut beneath the knot as near to the skin as possible using scissors or stitch cutter in the dominant hand (Fig. 56.1A)
- Remove the suture by pulling it gently through the skin

This principle applies whether the sutures are interrupted, continuous or subcuticular. A continuous suture requires the midwife to lift, cut and pull through repeatedly, until the end of the suture is removed. Subcuticular suturing that is held in place with a bead should have the bead removed at the distal end of the wound so that on removal the suture is pulled from the end nearest to the midwife. The removal should be smooth; the woman may experience the pulling sensation rather than discomfort.

### Removing staples

- Hold the staple remover as if a pair of scissors
- Insert the lower blade directly under the staple
- Squeeze the handles together; the staple will be lifted from the skin as it concertinas (Fig. 56.1B)
- Lift clear.

### Removing Michel clips

- Hold the clip remover as if a pair of scissors
- Insert the narrow blade under the clip
- Squeeze the handles together; the clip will be lifted from the skin as it concertinas (Fig. 56.1C).

### Removing Kifa clips

- Place the forceps over the wings of the clip
- Squeeze the wings together
- The clip will be lifted from the skin as it concertinas (Fig. 56.1D).

**Figure 56.1** (A) Removing sutures; (B) removing staples; (C) removing Michel clips; (D) removing Kifa clips (Fig. 56.1A and D adapted with kind permission from Jamieson et al 1997; Fig. 56.1B adapted with kind permission from Lammon et al 1995; Fig 56.1 C adapted with kind permission from Jamieson et al 2002)

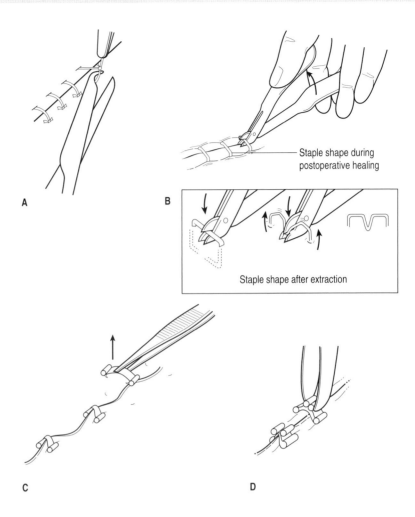

A

B

Staple shape during postoperative healing

Staple shape after extraction

C

D

---

PROCEDURE    removing sutures, clips and staples

- Gain informed consent and gather equipment:
    — sterile gloves and plastic apron
    — suture removal pack/dressing pack with scissors, stitch cutter, staple or clip remover (includes receiver to place clips or staples in)
    — disposable bag
- Position the woman to expose the wound, maintaining privacy and dignity
- Apply apron and wash hands
- Open the pack and cutter/remover
- Apply gloves
- Assess the wound; if healing is evident remove the suture(s), clips or staples as described above, placing sutures into the refuse bag, clips or staples into receiver. If in doubt as to wound healing,

consider removing every other. Refer early in the procedure if it is clear that healing is not complete
- Assist the woman to be comfortable
- Dispose of equipment correctly
- Wash hands
- Document findings and act accordingly.

## Care of wound drains

A wound drain reduces the dead space and decreases the likelihood of haematoma formation, but can increase the risk of wound infection by supplying a route for microorganisms to track deeply into the tissue (Briggs 1997). A wound may be drained by using either an open or a closed drainage system; a closed system is usually vacuumed (which 'pulls' the exudate from the tissues) whereas an open drain drains with gravity. The nature of the surgery determines whether a drain is inserted, and if so, which type.

Postoperatively, wound drains are observed for their drainage and must be kept positioned so that they are able to drain correctly and do not pull or fall to the floor. Any drainage from the wound drain should be recorded on the fluid balance chart. Briggs (1997) suggests that the optimal time for removal is after 24 hours.

### Emptying a wound drain

Care should be taken to maintain the integrity of the closed drainage system to reduce infection risks; however, the drain should be emptied if the vacuum is reduced or lost, or if the drain is to be retained for longer than 24 hours.

Drains vary; the midwife will need to be familiar with individual types. Most drains have the vacuum mechanism integral to them, by compressing the drain or an attachment. Occasionally external suction may be required. The principles of emptying a wound drain are:

- It is an aseptic procedure in which the midwife wears sterile gloves, cleanses the emptying port with an alcohol-impregnated wipe before and after emptying the drain, and empties it into a sterile receiver
- Once the drain is emptied the vacuum is achieved and the drain sealed
- There is minimal disruption for the woman.

### Dressing a wound drain

If required for longer than 24 hours, the drain may require re-dressing. Asepsis is required; the area may be cleansed with 0.9% sodium chloride and a hole is cut into the non-adherent dressing so that it sits snugly around the drain (Fig. 56.2) and is secured with tape.

**Figure 56.2** Dressing a wound drain (Adapted with kind permission from Jamieson et al 1997)

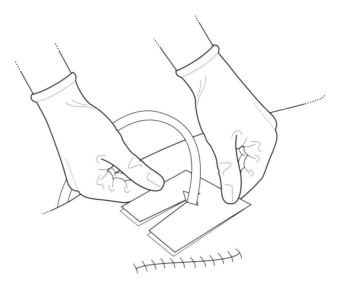

### Removal of a wound drain

Asepsis is indicated as there will be a small open wound when the drain has been removed. The drain should have its vacuum released before it is removed, and the woman should be aware that removal is an uncomfortable procedure. After removing the stitch, one hand supports the skin gently, while the other removes the drain. The area is cleansed and an appropriate dressing is applied. The amount that has drained is recorded on the fluid balance chart and the drain is disposed of in the clinical waste. The tip of the drain may be sent for laboratory investigation if required. The woman may need analgesia before or after the procedure. The site will need assessing the following day.

---

**Role and responsibilities of the midwife**

These can be summarised as:

- evidence-based practice to minimise the risks of wound infection, including education of the woman
- use of correct equipment and techniques to undertake procedures safely
- correct documentation.

---

## Summary

- Promoting healing and preventing infection includes care during the pre-, intra- and postoperative periods
- For clean sutured wounds, daily assessment is necessary, but cleansing and redressing will do more damage than good if not needed

- Many aspects can be carried out as clean techniques; asepsis is reserved for wound infections. Nevertheless, hand hygiene remains essential
- A wound that needs cleaning aseptically may be irrigated or cleaned with foam using warmed saline or tap water, and an appropriate dressing applied
- There are aspects of wound management that are still unanswered.

| Self-assessment exercises | The answers to the following questions may be found in the text: |
|---|---|

1. Discuss the factors that reduce wound infection.
2. Describe the management of the wound following caesarean section.
3. List the equipment required for redressing a surgical wound.
4. Describe how to remove sutures correctly. Compare and contrast the removal of clips and staples with sutures.
5. Describe how to empty, dress and remove a wound drain.

## REFERENCES

Briggs M 1997 Principles of closed surgical wound care. Journal of Wound Care 6(6):288–292

Briggs M, Wilson S, Fuller A 1996 The principles of aseptic technique in wound care. Professional Nurse 11(12):805–810

Bucknall T 1981 Abdominal wound closure: choice of suture. Journal of the Royal Society of Medicine 74:580–585

Byrne D, Phillips G, Napier A et al 1991 The effect of whole body disinfection on intraoperative wound contamination. Journal of Hospital Infection 18:145–148

Cruse P, Foord R 1980 The epidemiology of wound infection. Surgical Clinics of North America 6(1):27–40

Cunliffe P, Fawcett T 2002 Wound cleansing: the evidence for the techniques and solutions used. Professional Nurse 18(2):95–99

Dale J 1997 Wound dressings. Professional Nurse Study Supplement 12(12):S12–S14

Dealey C 1999 The care of wounds: a guide for nurses. Blackwell Science, Oxford

Dougherty L, Lister S 2004 The Royal Marsden Hospital manual of clinical nursing procedures, 6th edn. Blackwell Publishing, Oxford

Enkin M, Keirse M J N C, Neilson J et al 2000 A guide to effective care in pregnancy and childbirth, 3rd edn. Oxford University Press, Oxford

Flanagan M 1997 Wound management. Churchill Livingstone, Edinburgh

Fletcher J 1997 Wound cleansing. Professional Nurse 12(11):793–796

Jamieson E M, McCall J M, Blythe R et al 1997 Clinical nursing practices, 3rd edn. Churchill Livingstone, Edinburgh

Jamieson E M, Mc Call J M, Whyte A W 2002 Clinical Nursing Practice, 4th edn. Churchill Livingstone, Edinburgh

Krasner D 1992 12 commandments of wound care. Nursing 92(22):12, 34–41

Lammon C B, Foote A W, Leli P G et al 1995 Clinical nursing skills. W B Saunders, Philadelphia

Meers P, Jacobsen W, McPherson M 1992 Hospital infection control for nurses. Chapman and Hall, London

Morison M 1992 A colour guide to the nursing management of wounds. Wolfe Publishing, London

NICE (National Institute for Clinical Excellence) 2004 Caesarean section: Clinical Guideline 13. NICE, London

Nicol M, Bavin C, Bedford-Turner S et al 2000 Essential nursing skills, 2nd edn. Mosby, Edinburgh

Noe J, Keller M 1988 Can stitches get wet? Plastic and Reconstructive Surgery 82:205

Simmons M 1998 Preoperative skin preparation. Professional Nurse 13(7):446–447

# Chapter 57

# Principles of restricted mobility management — pressure area care

This chapter focuses on the principles of pressure area care, an important aspect of care for a woman with restricted mobility. Women may have restricted mobility for many reasons – bed rest due to antepartum haemorrhage, pre-eclampsia, during and following epidural anaesthesia, general anaesthetic, following a postpartum haemorrhage or post-operatively, etc. – making them vulnerable to or at an accelerated risk of pressure ulcer formation. Babies who are unwell, particularly the very preterm babies, are also vulnerable to or have an elevated risk of developing pressure ulcers. Damage to skin and underlying fatty tissues from pressure ulcers causes pain. If the ulcer becomes infected, septicaemia and/or bone infection can ensue. Muscle or bone may be destroyed in severe cases (NICE 2001). These complications of restricted mobility, although they are not commonly seen within the midwifery setting, increase morbidity and mortality but are often avoidable; it is important that the midwife develops the knowledge and skills to reduce their incidence. NICE (2003) recommends that all health care professionals undergo relevant training and education in both pressure ulcer assessment and prevention.

| **Learning outcomes** | Having read this chapter the reader should be able to: |

- discuss why pressure ulcers occur
- identify factors that increase the risk of pressure ulcer formation
- describe the four stages of pressure ulcer formation
- undertake assessment of the skin, recognising normal and abnormal changes resulting from pressure
- discuss the principles of pressure area care.

# Pressure area care

Pressure area care attempts to reduce the incidence of pressure ulcer formation. A pressure ulcer is a skin ulceration that forms due to localised tissue necrosis, commonly found on the parts of the body that have received unrelieved pressure or friction, or both. It may have been referred to as a decubitus ulcer, pressure sore or (less commonly) a bedsore. A variety of risk assessment tools are available for use in the clinical setting (e.g. the remodified Norton Scale, Braden Scale, RAPS scale). NICE (2003) recommend these should not replace clinical judgement, but should be used only as an aide-mémoire.

## Aetiology of pressure ulcers

Pressure ulcers develop as a result of two processes, occurring either separately or together:

1. unrelieved pressure
2. shearing and friction.

### Unrelieved pressure

Pressure within the capillaries varies from 30 mmHg (arterial) to 10 mmHg (venous). External pressures can increase this to above 32 mmHg (Ayello 1999), resulting in occlusion of the capillaries. If the pressure is prolonged, even with low-intensity pressure, the resulting anoxia causes tissue ischaemia and necrosis. Necrosis may begin in the muscle that lies over the bone. The length of time the pressure needs to be applied for damage to occur will vary from person to person, but there is a critical period of 1–2 hours before pathological changes occur (Dougherty & Lister 2004).

Healthy lightly pigmented skin with a good circulation blanches when blood flow is restricted (e.g. fingertip pressure). The skin whitens, replacing the usual red/darker skin tones. The effects of pressure can be seen when the pressure is removed and a sudden, large increase in blood flow occurs, up to 30 times the normal resting value. This results in a normal 'reactive hyperaemia', when blanching is replaced by a bright red flush, lasting usually less than 1 hour. Providing the lymphatic vessels are not damaged and excess interstitial fluid is removed, there is no permanent damage. However, if there is lymphatic vessel damage, tissue changes occur and large amounts of interstitial fluid are squeezed out. The cells rub together and the cell membranes rupture, releasing toxic intracellular material and normal skin colour is not restored. A deep pressure ulcer can arise when the lymphatic vessels and muscle fibres tear.

With excessive pressure, abnormal reactive hyperaemia and induration can occur, causing the affected area to appear darker than surrounding skin. Absence of blanching with a fingertip may also be seen.

These effects can last for more than 1 hour after the pressure has been removed, possibly up to 2 weeks (Ayello 1999).

Darkly pigmented skin does not blanch or change colour when pressure is applied, making it more difficult to recognise impending tissue damage.

### Shearing and friction

A shearing force is the pressure exerted against the skin in a direction parallel to the body's surface, occurring when the body moves up or down the bed while in an upright position. As the layers of muscle and bone slide in the direction of the body movement, the skin and subcutaneous layers stick to the bed surface, causing the bone to slide down into the skin, with a force exerted onto the skin. A shearing force results at the junction of the deep and superficial tissues. The microcirculation is compressed and damaged, causing microscopic haemorrhage and necrosis deep within the tissues. This is compounded by the decreased capillary blood flow resulting from the external pressure pressing against the skin. Eventually, a channel opens through the skin and the necrotic area drains through this. The areas commonly affected by shearing forces are the sacrum and coccygeus. Shearing forces can be reduced if the head is kept below 30° (Ayello 1999), i.e. place the chin on the chest when moving.

Friction is the mechanical force that is exerted when the skin is dragged across a coarse surface (e.g. bedding). The epidermis is rubbed away, giving the appearance of a shallow abrasion injury, often on the elbows and heels.

Pressure ulcers can form on any part of the body, the commoner sites being the heels, toes, knees, buttocks (sacral and coccygeal area, ischial tuberosities and greater trochanters), shoulders, elbows and ears (Fig. 57.1). Preterm babies can develop friction injuries when their delicate, immature skin rubs against bedding. The elbows and knees are primary sites for this to occur. Pressure may also occur from drainage tubes, indwelling catheters (against labia), nasogastric tubes (nasal passages), nasal oxygen cannulae and antiembolic stockings.

# Stages of pressure ulcer formation

There are four recognised stages of pressure ulcer formation related to the depth of tissue damage and recognisable by changes seen to the skin and underlying tissues.

Stage I: Intact skin showing non-blanchable erythema – the early sign of potential ulcer formation

Stage II: Partial thickness skin loss of epidermis and/or dermis – a superficial ulcer that presents as an abrasion, blister or shallow crater

**Figure 57.1**   Pressure area sites

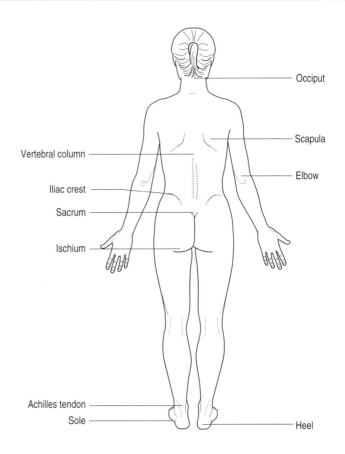

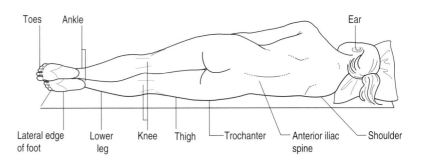

Stage III: Full thickness skin loss and damage/necrosis of subcutaneous tissue which does not extend through the underlying fascia – presents as a deep crater that can also undermine adjacent tissue

Stage IV: Full thickness skin loss with damage/necrosis to underlying muscle, bone or supporting structures, e.g. tendon.

## Factors influencing development

- Impaired sensory input – an altered sensory perception resulting in decreased or no experience of pressure and pain, with no awareness of the need to move, e.g. epidural
- Impaired motor function produces an inability to move despite the presence of pain or pressure, e.g. epidural
- Immobility, e.g. bed rest/reduced mobility
- Decreased circulation
- Altering levels of consciousness
- Severe/chronic illness
- Previous history of pressure damage
- Oedema – reduces blood circulation in affected tissues and impairs clearage of waste products
- Anaemia
- Infection
- Obesity may accelerate the development; adipose tissue may have an inadequate blood supply and be more susceptible to ischaemia
- Inadequate dietary intake of protein, carbohydrate, fat, vitamins and trace elements, all of which are necessary for collagen synthesis and maturation, promoting healthy skin and wound healing. May also influence amount of subcutaneous fat which acts as padding between bone and skin
- Excessive moisture on the skin – e.g. urine, sweat, liquor, wound exudate, faeces – decreases skin's resistance to physical factors such as shearing forces and pressure
- Temperature changes
- Immunosuppression
- Increasing age resulting in loss of subcutaneous fat and skin elasticity and generalised skin atrophy.

## Assessment of skin integrity

The midwife, using good (preferably natural) lighting, should inspect the skin and potential pressure ulcer sites. The frequency is determined by individual needs and influenced by the presence of risk factors. For those women who are willing and able, the midwife can show them how to inspect their own skin and that of their baby (NICE 2003).

The presence of hyperaemia should be noted when it first appears and steps taken to minimise pressure on the affected area. The area should be rechecked after 1 hour to determine if hyperaemia is still present. The midwife should look for persistent erythema and the absence of blanching on fingertip pressure in lightly pigmented skin by depressing the skin firmly but gently with a clean fingertip. When the pressure is removed the colour of the skin is noted. In darkly pigmented skin the colour should be observed; purplish/bluish discolouration that is darker than the surrounding skin is abnormal. The location, size and colour of the affected area should be recorded; Ayello (1999) recommends using a marker pen to outline the area to make reassessment easier and more accurate.

The skin is also assessed for other signs of potential damage:

- localised heat over the affected area; with further tissue damage this heat is replaced by coolness, a sign of tissue devitalisation
- localised oedema – the area will feel spongy and the skin may appear shiny and taut
- localised induration
- break in the skin integrity, e.g. blister, pimple.

## Principles of pressure area care

The aim is to prevent the development of pressure ulcers by:

- identifying those who are either vulnerable to or at an elevated risk of pressure ulcer development and undertake a risk assessment within 6 hours (NICE 2003)
- regular assessment of the skin, noting the colour, integrity, presence of blanching or oedema, heat
- relieving pressure by assisting the woman or baby to change position on a regular basis (depending on the condition of the individual and the duration of hypoxia; with lightly pigmented skin the duration of redness is approximately half that of the duration of hypoxia). A turning chart may be used to record the time of turning and the positions used
- use of high specification foam mattresses with pressure-relieving properties for women and babies at elevated risk (NICE 2003)
- raising the bedclothes from the body, e.g. bedding should be loosened at the end of the bed or left untucked, or using a bed cradle
- placing a pillow between the knees of the woman when lying laterally to reduce the pressure from the top leg
- removing all creases, crumbs, etc. from the bedding as these can exert unnecessary pressure
- increasing circulation by passive or active exercises (Ch. 58)
- ensuring the woman or baby is adequately hydrated; a fluid balance chart may be required
- ensuring the diet is well balanced, referring to the dietician if there are any difficulties
- ensuring the woman has her head below 30° if she is moving up or down the bed to reduce the shearing forces
- use of appropriate equipment for manual handling to prevent friction
- good hygiene, especially if incontinent or sweating profusely, but avoiding soap as it is usually alkaline and can dry the skin; after washing, the skin should be dried with gentle patting motions

- use of moisturisers for dry skin areas
- use of soft cotton bedding in preference to synthetic fibres.

## Role and responsibilities of the midwife

These can be summarised as:

- identifying women and babies who are vulnerable to and at elevated risk of developing pressure ulcers
- assisting the woman and baby with measures to reduce pressure ulcer formation
- referral as appropriate
- correct documentation.

## Summary

- Pressure ulcers develop as a result of unrelieved pressure, and shearing and friction
- They are avoidable; the midwife needs to be aware of who is vulnerable or at elevated risk and to assess the skin condition regularly
- There are a number of measures that can be taken to reduce the likelihood of pressure ulcer formation; the midwife should be familiar with these.

## Self-assessment exercises

The answers to the following questions may be found in the text:

1. How do pressure ulcers arise?
2. What factors predispose to pressure ulcer formation?
3. Describe the different stages of pressure ulcer formation and how these are recognised.
4. What is the midwife looking for when an assessment of the skin is undertaken?
5. How can the midwife provide pressure area care to reduce the risks of pressure ulcers forming?

## REFERENCES

Ayello E A 1999 Skin integrity and wound care. In: Potter P A, Perry A G (eds) Basic nursing: a critical thinking approach, 4th edn. Mosby, St Louis, ch 38

Dougherty L, Lister S E 2004 The Royal Marsden Hospital manual of clinical nursing procedures, 6th edn. Blackwell Publishing, Oxford

NICE (National Institute of Clinical Excellence) 2001 Pressure ulcer risk assessment and prevention. NICE, London

NICE (National Institute of Clinical Excellence) 2003 Pressure ulcer prevention, including the use of pressure-relieving devices (beds, mattresses and overlays) for the prevention of pressure ulcers in primary and secondary care. NICE, London

Chapter **58**

# Principles of restricted mobility management — prevention of thromboembolism

This chapter focuses on the principles of preventing the formation of thromboembolism, specifically on two areas – exercises and graduated compression stockings. Women with restricted mobility are at risk of thromboembolism formation and, less commonly, joint and muscle contracture, increasing morbidity and mortality.

**Learning outcomes**

Having read this chapter the reader should be able to:

- describe the exercises that can be undertaken following an operative delivery
- discuss the role and responsibility of the midwife in relation to the use of graduated compression stockings.

## Exercises

Passive and active exercises are movements of the muscles and joints through their normal range, undertaken with the aim of promoting circulation, maintaining and improving muscle tone and preventing the development of joint contracture. Passive exercises imply the woman is assisted to undertake the exercises until such time as she is able to undertake active exercises herself. The midwife is rarely required to undertake passive exercises. If there is an occasion where the woman is immobile for a prolonged period of time, the midwife should refer to the obstetric physiotherapist. The midwife can encourage women with restricted mobility to undertake a limited number of exercises that will promote circulation, with the aim of reducing the formation of thromboembolism. Following a general anaesthetic, breathing exercises should also be undertaken to promote full ventilation of the lungs, assist with the removal of anaesthetic gases and promote venous return. Exercises should be undertaken with caution in the woman with pre-eclampsia, in consultation with the obstetric team.

## Exercises to promote circulation

These exercises are easy to undertake, aim to promote circulation, decrease the risk of thrombus formation and reduce oedema of the feet and ankles.

- Foot exercises – the woman should sit or lie with her knees straight, then flex and extend her ankles by moving her feet towards and away from her body at least 10 times (Fig. 58.1). She should then circle her ankles by moving her feet in a clockwise direction at least 10 times, then in an anticlockwise direction, keeping her hips and knees still (Fig. 58.2). These exercises are particularly important for the postoperative woman (Brayshaw & Wright 1994)
- Leg tightening – the woman should sit or lie on the bed with her legs straight. As she pulls her toes towards her legs, the back of her knees should press down towards the bed and the position held for 4 seconds, then relaxed. This exercise should be repeated five times (Brayshaw & Wright 1994).

## Deep breathing exercises

These are undertaken to promote circulation and assist with ventilating the lungs:

- The woman should preferably be sitting and take two to three deep breaths to improve ventilation and repeat frequently. The woman should also be encouraged to follow the deep breathing with short forced expirations, referred to as 'huffing', to loosen secretions. This reduces the risk of a chest infection developing.

**Figure 58.1** Foot exercises – flexing the feet

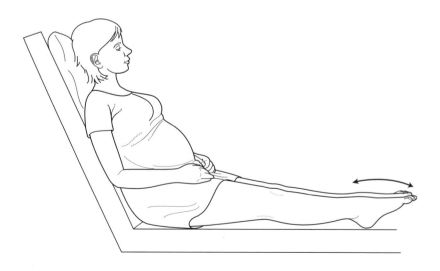

**Figure 58.2**   Circling the ankles

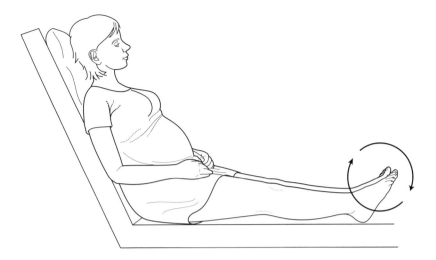

Women with restricted mobility should be actively discouraged from crossing their legs, as this can impede circulation. Oedematous legs can be raised slightly, provided they are well supported.

### Thrombus formation

Deaths from pulmonary embolism remain one of the major causes of maternal mortality. During the 3-year period 1997–1999 there were 31 deaths in the United Kingdom from pulmonary embolism, secondary to deep vein thrombosis. This rate of 1.45 deaths per 100 000 maternities has decreased 50% from the previous 3-year period, when the rate was 2.1 per 100 000 maternities (CEMD 2001). Pregnant and postnatal women are at risk of thrombus formation, particularly the latter, due to impaired circulation, hypercoagulability and potential tissue and blood vessel damage resulting from birth. The DoH (1998) identified particular risk factors:

- increasing age, over 35 years
- obesity, above 80 kg
- para 4 or higher
- gross varicosities
- current infection
- pre-eclampsia
- major current illness
- emergency caesarean section in labour
- immobility prior to surgery of more than 4 days.

The presence of one of these risk factors indicates the woman is at moderate risk of thrombus formation, whereas high risk is indicated if:

- three or more factors are present
- major abdominal or pelvic surgery occurs

- there is a personal or family history of thromboembolism or thrombophilia
- the woman has paralysis of the lower limbs
- the woman has antiphospholipid antibody, e.g. lupus anticoagulant.

The Royal College of Obstetricians and Gynaecologists also add further risk factors (RCOG 2002):

- surgical procedure during pregnancy or the postnatal period
- excessive blood loss
- sickle cell disease
- dehydration.

Women at risk of thrombus formation may be given heparin (an anticoagulant) and advised to wear graduated compression (e.g. TED) stockings. If a thrombus is suspected or confirmed, both of these treatments are required. The RCOG (2002) recommend that graduated compression stockings be worn on the affected leg for 2 years following a thrombus formation to reduce the risk of post-thrombotic syndrome.

## Graduated compression stockings

External compression applies controlled pressure to the skin, which helps to reduce oedema and promote venous return (Armstrong 1998); graduated compression stockings can apply this compression. Graduated compression stockings are often made of nylon with elastane or lycra (other mixes are available), in two main lengths – full length and below knee. They are classified according to the degree of compression they apply, from light support (14–17 mmHg at the ankle, suitable for mild varicosities and venous hypertension in pregnancy), to medium support (18–24 mmHg, suitable for mild oedema and moderate to severe varicosities) to strong support (25–35 mmHg, for use with severe varicosities).

Graduated compression stockings should fit the leg that is wearing them, which means the midwife is required to measure the woman's legs. This is undertaken in the morning ideally, before the effects of oedema are evident. The woman should stand with her feet flat on the floor; both legs should be measured as size differences between the legs can occur. The leg measurements should be reviewed on a regular basis as changes may occur (e.g. occurrence of or disappearance of oedema).

If below knee stockings are used, three measurements are required (Fig. 58.3):

1. the narrowest point around the ankle, above the ankle bone
2. from the base of the heel to just below the knee
3. the widest part of the calf.

**Figure 58.3**   Below knee
stockings measurements

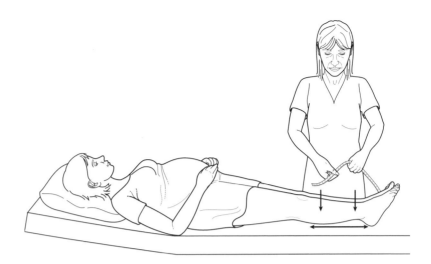

If full length stockings are used, two further measurements are necessary (Fig. 58.4):

4. the widest part of the thigh
5. from the base of the heel to the gluteal fold.

If the legs are not measured, the graduated compression stockings are
unlikely to be a good fit. If too loose, compression will not be applied
and they are likely to roll down. If too tight, they can be uncomfortable
and cause trauma, possibly increasing the risk of thrombus formation.

It is important that the stockings are applied correctly, ensuring
there are no wrinkles and that the bands over the feet and at the top are
not so tight as to apply excessive pressure. They should be put on first
thing in the morning before getting out of bed to dry legs and feet. To
apply the stockings:

**Figure 58.4**   Full length
stockings measurements

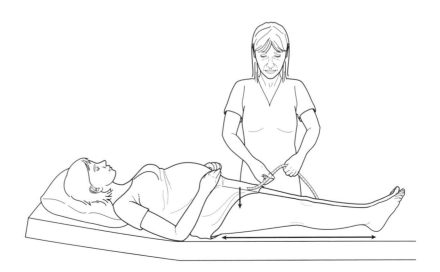

- A hand is inserted into the stocking up to the seamed heel
- The heel is held between the forefinger and thumb and the stocking turned inside out, until the heel pocket is seen
- The stocking is placed over the foot, with the heel pocket positioned over the heel
- The stocking is pulled over the foot and up the leg.

If the stockings are difficult to apply, moisturising the legs before putting the stockings on may help. Wearing rubber gloves may make it easier to grip the stocking. As pregnancy progresses, the woman may find it increasingly difficult to apply the stockings herself and may require assistance with this. Graduated compression stockings should be washed according to the manufacturer's recommendations.

### Role and responsibilities of the midwife

These can be summarised as:

- assisting the woman to undertake exercises to promote circulation and ventilation
- identifying women for whom graduated compression stockings are appropriate
- measuring the leg accurately to ensure the graduated compression stockings are a good fit
- advising the woman on how to apply graduated compression stockings
- referral as appropriate
- correct documentation.

## Summary

- Exercises are passive (whereby the woman is assisted to undertake the exercises) or active (the woman undertakes them herself)
- Gentle foot and leg exercises, combined with deep breathing, can reduce the likelihood of thrombus formation
- Thromboembolism is a major cause of maternal mortality; the use of graduated compression stockings can reduce the incidence of thrombus formation
- Graduated compression stockings must be fitted correctly to be effective.

### Self-assessment exercises

The answers to the following questions may be found in the text:

1. What exercises should women be encouraged to do to promote venous circulation?
2. How would the midwife ensure that a below knee compression stocking is the right size?

3. How are compression stockings applied?
4. What are the role and responsibilities of the midwife in relation to the prevention of thromboembolism in a woman with restricted mobility?

## REFERENCES

Armstrong S 1998 Compression hosiery. Professional Nurse 14(1):49–56

Brayshaw E, Wright P 1994 Teaching physical skills for the childbearing year. Books for Midwives, Hale

CEMD 2001 Why mothers die. The Confidential Enquiries into Maternal Deaths in the United Kingdom 1997–1999. RCOG Press, London

DoH (Department of Health) 1998 Why mothers die. Report on Confidential Enquiries into Maternal Deaths in the United Kingdom 1994–1996. The Stationery Office, London

RCOG (Royal College of Obstetricians and Gynaecologists) 2002 Thromboembolic disease in pregnancy and the puerperium: Acute Management Clinical Green Top Guidelines. www.rcog.org.uk 14 March 2002

Chapter **59**

# Principles of cardiopulmonary resuscitation — maternal resuscitation

This chapter considers effective cardiopulmonary resuscitation for a childbearing woman. The reader is encouraged to read this chapter in conjunction with Chapter 60 (neonatal resuscitation) to compare and contrast the resuscitation skills.

**Learning outcomes**

Having read this chapter the reader should be able to:

- discuss in detail the role and responsibilities of the midwife when resuscitating a pregnant woman
- describe the equipment and how it is used
- demonstrate/simulate a maternal resuscitation technique.

Resuscitation is the means by which life is supported in the event of sudden apnoea or cardiac arrest. In a maternity setting where women are healthy and undergoing a physiological process, collapse is both rare and unexpected. The potential for complications does exist, some of which can be life threatening or fatal (CEMD 2004). There are two implications for the midwife:

- the skills of managing maternal cardiopulmonary resuscitation are rarely used
- the need to maintain these skills for use at a moment's notice remains a priority, wherever the arrest may occur (Morris & Willis 1999, Nolan 1998).

## Considerations for childbearing

In its simplest form resuscitation follows the ABC format – A for airway, B for breathing and C for circulation. Resuscitation techniques are modified for the childbearing woman to accommodate the physiological body changes (Table 59.1); the principles are the same as for any

Table 59.1 Pregnancy physiological differences and adaptation for resuscitation

| Physiological difference | Resuscitation modification |
| --- | --- |
| Gravid uterus: potential for massive internal concealed haemorrhage | Observations to detect haemorrhage. Prompt infusion using at least two wide bore cannulae, rapid request for cross-matched blood, stat. infusion I.V. fluid up to 2 L, but with careful fluid balance. Use of CVP monitoring |
| Additional circulation (fetal) | Caesarean section within 5 minutes if resuscitation not successful |
| Aortocaval occlusion when supine | Wedge firmly to the left or manual displacement of the uterus |
| Splinting of diaphragm | May be harder to ventilate the lungs, requiring higher ventilatory pressures |
| Relaxation of cardiac sphincter of the stomach, silent regurgitation and aspiration of stomach contents a possibility | Application of cricoid pressure, use cuffed ET tube when intubated |
| Oedema of glottis, neck obesity, larger breasts | More difficult to intubate, call a skilled anaesthetist who is likely to be successful on the first attempt |
| Increased oxygen requirements | Begin resuscitation quickly using 100% oxygen |

other resuscitation. The essential difference is that the fetus is also compromised, but the presence of the fetus with its additional circulation may further compromise the mother and make resuscitation more difficult. Successful resuscitation of the mother becomes the priority, such that an emergency caesarean section may be carried out swiftly in order to improve the success of the resuscitation, whatever the gestation of the fetus (Mitchell 1995).

A lesser number of modifications will be required for a newly delivered woman, but some of the physiological changes will remain. Silent regurgitation of the stomach contents is still a possibility until progesterone levels have returned to their pre-pregnant state. Cricoid pressure (gentle pressure on the cricoid cartilage to occlude the oesophagus) is a valuable means of preventing regurgitation of the stomach contents and should be considered for a childbearing woman from the moment of collapse (Fig. 59.1). CEMD (2001) indicates that postpartum fatality occurs from many of the same complications as in pregnancy (e.g. pulmonary embolism, haemorrhage and eclampsia).

Senior skilled staff should attend the woman quickly, working together as a team. This will include obstetricians, physicians, midwives, anaesthetists and haematologists. The midwife should always be familiar with the quickest way to summon help: in the hospital setting this is likely to be one particular emergency number; in the community it may be to telephone 999 and request paramedic assistance.

**Figure 59.1** Application of cricoid pressure (Adapted from Fraser & Cooper 2003)

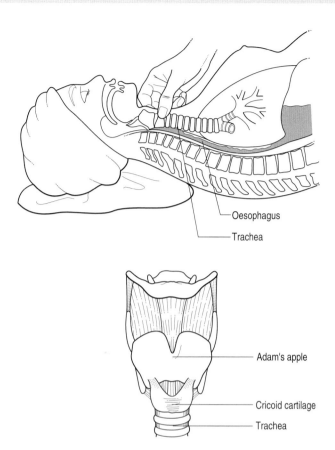

Oesophagus

Trachea

Adam's apple

Cricoid cartilage

Trachea

Resuscitation is tiring for one resuscitator working alone; two or more people are helpful, and additional people can be usefully deployed. Intensive care facilities should be available and used, and quick access to blood for transfusion must be available if required (CEMD 2001).

## Anticipation and recognition of collapse

The midwife should be aware of the potential situations when apnoea and/or cardiac arrest may occur. These include:

- pulmonary embolism
- amniotic fluid embolism
- massive ante- or postpartum haemorrhage
- eclampsia
- existing medical disorder, e.g. cardiac disorder, epilepsy
- trauma, e.g. road traffic accident
- drug toxicity, e.g. drug abuse, use of epidural or spinal analgesics, use of magnesium sulphate, general anaesthesia.

This is not an exhaustive list. Arrest can sometimes be averted by administering 100% oxygen, repositioning into a left lateral position, giving a bolus of intravenous (I.V.) fluid and then calling medical assistance.

In the event of collapse, the midwife will make an assessment initially based on colour, movement, breathing and heart rate. There may be some variations according to the cause of the arrest, but generally the following features will be noted:

- colour: pale, cyanosed (heavily so if amniotic fluid embolism), clammy
- movement: no response to stimulation; midwife may have observed seizure or twitching immediately prior to arrest; woman will be slumped as if fainted
- breathing: absent, no rise and fall of the chest, no breath sounds heard or felt
- heart rate: absent (use major pulse, e.g. carotid).

An emergency call is sent instantly upon recognising that cardiac or respiratory arrest has occurred. This should indicate where the arrest has occurred, including the name of the ward and specific location (e.g. first side room) or, if at home, the room the woman is in.

## Equipment

While some basic equipment is desirable, it is possible to complete a successful resuscitation without any equipment; however, the midwife usually has access to some equipment. Wherever the setting, protection from contact with body fluids is indicated by using facemasks rather than undertaking mouth-to-mouth resuscitation. Equipment should be checked regularly to ensure that it is present and working effectively. Cleaning and maintaining equipment is indicated according to manufacturer's instructions. A wedge is required for the pregnant woman; this should be firm enough to permit effective chest compression. Adaptations may be made in the home using books, files or other appropriate items.

Standard equipment includes:

- oxygen
- suction apparatus
- bag and facemask for ventilation (with oxygen reservoir) or pocket mask
- wedge
- Guedel airways, sizes 2 and 3
- resuscitation drugs
- stethoscope
- laryngoscope
- cuffed endotracheal (ET) tubes size 7–9 mm and 10 mL syringe
- introducer

- connectors and bag for ventilator
- CVP line
- cannulae, I.V. lines and blood bottles
- defibrillator and cardiac monitor.

In hospital the equipment is usually stored on a trolley in an accessible place. The defibrillator is usually plugged in, and has to be unplugged before the trolley can be moved! Defibrillation is only required to correct certain cardiac arrhythmias. In the event of it being used all personnel must stand away from the woman in order that they also do not receive an electric shock. Care must be taken if the defibrillator is used in a wet environment (e.g. a bathroom).

## Initial assessment

On finding a collapsed woman, the midwife should quickly assess the area to ensure there are no dangers to the midwife or to the woman. The midwife should approach the woman from the side and establish whether she is conscious by asking the woman a question and firmly touching the shoulders. This should evoke a response; if none is forthcoming help should be sought immediately and resuscitative measures commenced. The woman should be turned onto her back, pillows removed (if present) and a wedge positioned under the right side. Resuscitation then follows the ABC format.

### Airway

Opening the airway may be sufficient for the woman to re-establish respiration and prevent further compromise. Tilting the head backwards by applying pressure on the forehead with one hand and supporting the chin in position will facilitate this by positioning the head into a neutral position. Any obvious obstructions seen within the mouth should be removed but the midwife should not perform a finger sweep of the mouth. If there is concern about regurgitation of stomach contents in the pregnant unconscious woman, cricoid pressure should be applied when she is supine and maintained throughout the procedure or until intubation has occurred. There are three options:

**Chin support** The midwife should place two/three fingers over the bony part of the tip of the chin, avoiding pressure on the soft tissues and hold the chin in position, or;

**Jaw thrust** Using both hands, the midwife should place two/three fingers either side of the bony part of the lower jaw to lift the lower jaw forwards. Avoid pressure on the soft tissues as this can occlude the airway, or;

**Use of oropharyngeal (Guedel) airway** If there is difficulty maintaining the chin support/jaw thrust while undertaking other resuscitation manoeuvres an appropriately sized airway (usually 2 or 3) inserted into the oropharynx will maintain the patency of the airway by pushing the tongue forwards, negating further manual assistance.

Airway size is assessed by holding the flange of the airway against the mid-point of the woman's lips, with the airway held horizontally so that the curved part of the airway curves around the woman's jaw; it should end at the angle of the jaw.

Prior to inserting the airway, it may be necessary to use a wide bore suction catheter to remove secretions/debris from the woman's mouth.

To insert the airway, the head should be tilted backwards and the airway held in the inverted position, i.e. the opposite way up to its final position within the oropharynx, to allow the curved part of the airway to depress the tongue, preventing it from being pushed backwards. The airway is inserted following the curve of the woman's airway. As it reaches the junction of the hard and soft palate, the airway should be rotated 180° to turn it to the correct position while continuing to move it further into the mouth. When the airway is lying in the oropharynx the flange should sit between the woman's teeth. The tilted, neutral head position should be maintained and chin support given as required. The position of the airway should be assessed intermittently to ensure it has not been dislodged. If the woman begins to breathe, oxygen should be administered.

### Breathing

When the airway is clear, breathing may follow spontaneously. To assess whether the woman is breathing, the midwife's head should be positioned close to the woman's head. This will ensure the midwife's eyeline is in line with the woman's chest so that chest movement can be looked and felt for. The midwife may also feel the woman's breath on her face when this close to the woman's nose and mouth.

If no effective breathing is seen, it is important to fill the lungs with air or oxygen as quickly as possible, usually via a facemask. Two effective rescue breaths are needed.

The facemask should have a deformable rim that will fit snugly around the woman's mouth and nose when even pressure is applied to form an airtight seal. The correct size should be used so that it does not extend over the end of the chin or into the eye sockets. Fingertips are used to support the jaw and seal off the mask (grasping under the chin will also occlude the airway). An airtight seal is essential to ensure adequate ventilation, and the head should be maintained in the neutral position.

The facemask can be attached to a self inflating bag–valve–mask (BVM) system. If using a BVM, the blow-off valve should be tested before use by occluding the outlet and squeezing the bag. As the pressure rises, the blow-off valve makes a noise that confirms it is working and is safe for use. A good seal is needed from the mask; the bag is squeezed slowly for 2–3 seconds (the valve will begin to blow when the correct pressure is reached) and the chest should rise as air enters the lungs. The bag is then released to refill and the process repeated until two rescue breaths have been given.

This technique can be difficult for one person to manage as keeping the head and mask in position while squeezing the bag can be complex and requires practice. Ideally one person will hold the mask and head while another squeezes the bag (Fig. 59.2). The person supporting the airway should ensure that the chest rises with each inflation.

A pocket mask can also be used and should be placed over the nose and mouth with the head in the neutral position and the jaw pulled upwards and forwards. The midwife blows through the opening on the pocket mask to inflate the lungs (a normal expiratory breath of approximately 400–600 mL) (Fig. 59.3).

Alternatively, mouth-to-mouth resuscitation can be undertaken if no other equipment is available; however, this increases the risk of coming into contact with bodily fluids. The nose should be pinched with the thumb and forefinger to prevent air escaping through the nasal passages. The midwife should then place her mouth over the woman's mouth with a good seal and blow into her lungs as for the pocket mask.

If no chest movement is seen, the head and mask position should be checked and corrected, obvious obstructions removed and the two rescue breaths reattempted. There should be no more than five attempts to achieve the two effective rescue breaths.

**Figure 59.2** Bag–valve–mask ventilation using two resuscitators (Adapted with kind permission from Morris & Willis 1999)

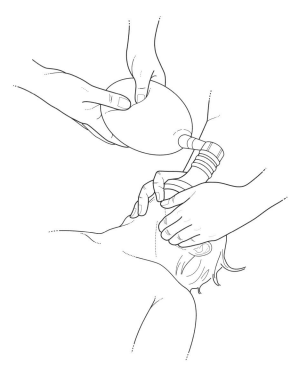

**Figure 59.3** Using a Laerdal pocket mask (Adapted with kind permission from Morris & Willis 1999)

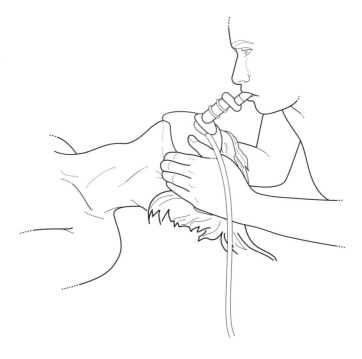

## Circulation

After two rescue breaths (or five failed attempts) the carotid pulse should be felt to assess the heart rate. This should take no longer than 10 seconds. If a pulse is present, with no respiratory effort, rescue breaths should be continued and the carotid pulse rechecked every minute (after every 10 breaths). Rescue breaths should continue until the woman shows signs of spontaneous respiration.

If no carotid pulse is found, the midwife will need to commence chest compression which should be undertaken in conjunction with further rescue breaths.

**Chest compression** The xiphisternum should be located and the heel of one hand positioned two fingers' width above it (Fig. 59.4A). The other hand is placed over the first hand and the fingers interlocked. With both arms straight, the midwife should lean over the woman, depress the sternum 4–5 cm and then release the pressure (maintaining the hand position over the sternum) (Fig. 59.4B). This is repeated until 15 chest compressions are completed and is followed by two rescue breaths. The compression and release of the chest should take the same length of time and the midwife should aim to achieve 100 compressions per minute. Chest compression and ventilation are continued at a rate of 15:2.

Resuscitation can be tiring on the individual and where there are several people involved in the resuscitation, it can be helpful to take turns with the different manoeuvres.

**Figure 59.4** (A) Positioning the hands for cardiac compression; (B) cardiac compression (Adapted with kind permission from Peattie & Walker 1995)

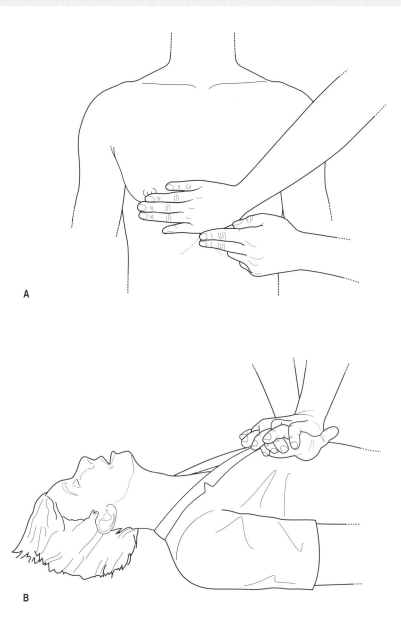

A

B

As further personnel and equipment arrive to assist with the resuscitation, ECG leads may be applied to the chest to obtain an indication of cardiac rhythm. Once chest compression has been commenced, the pulse is not reassessed as it is assumed that the heart will not restart spontaneously unless this is seen on the ECG or the woman shows signs of movement or breathing.

A senior member of the emergency team will take overall control of the resuscitation and will make the decisions. Drugs will be administered as requested; adrenaline (epinephrine) is often the drug of choice, but sodium bicarbonate and atropine may also be used. Such drugs are usually issued in a 'ready to administer' form. The midwife must be familiar with these and their dosages, mode of action and side effects.

Other personnel can be usefully deployed to insert I.V. lines, request blood, care for the woman's family, prepare for theatre, and keep a records of events and times, drugs, etc. The midwife may be required to assist with but should not undertake defibrillation unless competent to do so.

If the woman is pregnant an emergency caesarean section may be required in an attempt to save the woman's life and resuscitation should continue while surgery is happening.

If successful it is likely that the woman will be cared for in an intensive care unit until such time as she is able to be transferred back to maternity care. If unsuccessful, the most senior member of the medical staff will decide at which point the resuscitation is abandoned. This is often in consultation with other members of the team.

## PROCEDURE    maternal resuscitation

- Recognise the arrest and assess the situation for any potential dangers
- Assess the level of responsiveness
- If unresponsive, call for emergency assistance
- Turn the woman on her back with a wedge under her right side and tilt her head back to the neutral position
- Ensure the airway is open, using chin support, jaw thrust and/or an oropharyngeal airway as necessary, and remove obvious obstructions
- Apply cricoid pressure until intubation has occurred (see Fig. 59.1) if required
- Assess breathing; if no spontaneous respiration give two effective rescue breaths using a bag facemask system, pocket mask or mouth-to-mouth resuscitation
- If the chest wall does not rise, reassess the head and equipment position and adjust accordingly
- Undertake two effective rescue breaths (up to five can be attempted)
- Assess the carotid pulse; if present, continue with rescue breaths, reassessing carotid pulse each minute until spontaneous respirations occur
- If no pulse present, commence chest compression at a rate of 100 beats per minute (bpm) (Nolan 1998)
- Synchronise the compressions and ventilations at a rate of 15 chest compressions to 2 ventilations (15:2)
- Continue with resuscitation until spontaneous respiration or movement seen, or until told to stop by the senior person present (or if

too exhausted to continue and there is no one to take over from you)

- If after 5 minutes there is minimal success, preparation should begin for caesarean section (if pregnant)

## Role and responsibilities of the midwife

These can be summarised as:

- responses to avert the collapse if possible
- swift recognition and response in the event of arrest
- familiarisation with resuscitation techniques, including adaptations for the pregnant woman
- familiarisation with equipment, its use and maintenance
- awareness of other aspects of care, e.g. care of the family
- appropriate team work
- consultation with others, e.g. risk manager, supervisor of midwives, especially if resuscitation is unsuccessful
- detailed contemporaneous records.

## Summary

- The skills of maternal resuscitation are not often needed, but are skills that should be practised and adapted according to venue and available equipment.
- The standard format of ABC is indicated, with some adaptations for the physiological changes of pregnancy: a wedge or manual displacement of the uterus, cricoid pressure and preparation for caesarean section within 5 minutes.

## Self-assessment exercises

The answers to the following questions may be found in the text:

1. State a rationale for each of the necessary adaptations when resuscitating a pregnant woman.
2. List the essential equipment required and indicate how and when each piece would be used.
3. Describe, in order, the actions taken when finding a woman in a state of collapse.
4. Discuss how effective lung ventilation may be achieved.
5. Draw a diagram to indicate the correct positioning of the hands for chest compression.
6. Summarise the role and responsibilities of the midwife when resuscitating a pregnant woman.

## REFERENCES

CEMD 2004 Why mothers die. The Confidential Enquiries into Maternal Deaths in the United Kingdom 2000–2004. RCOG Press, London

Fraser D M, Cooper M A (eds) 2003 Myles textbook for midwives, 14th edn. Churchill Livingstone, Edinburgh

Mitchell L 1995 Cardiac arrest during pregnancy: maternal–fetal physiology and advanced cardiac life support for the obstetric patient. Critical Care Nurse 15(1):56–60

Morris S, Willis B A 1999 Resuscitation in pregnancy. In: Colquhoun M, Handley A, Evans T (eds) ABC of resuscitation, 4th edn. BMJ Publishing Group, London, ch 7

Nolan J 1998 The 1998 European Resuscitation Council guidelines for adult single rescuer basic life support. British Medical Journal 319(7148):1870–1876

Peattie P I, Walker S 1995 Understanding nursing care, 4th edn. Churchill Livingstone, Edinburgh

Chapter **60**

# Principles of cardiopulmonary resuscitation — neonatal resuscitation

Resuscitating the baby incorporates some of the fundamental principles used when resuscitating an adult but requires a different approach. However, the predisposing factors may be very different, often because the baby has not yet established respiration in the extrauterine environment. The aim of neonatal resuscitation is to initiate or sustain extrauterine life, limiting any cerebral damage.

This chapter focuses upon recognition and action, suggested equipment and the midwife's role and responsibilities. The reader is encouraged to compare and contrast the care given when resuscitating an adult (Ch. 59).

**Learning outcomes**

Having read this chapter the reader should be able to:

- discuss in detail the role and responsibilities of the midwife prior to, during and following a neonatal resuscitation
- describe the signs that indicate that resuscitation is required
- describe the equipment and how it is used
- demonstrate/simulate a neonatal resuscitation technique, discussing how effective resuscitation is achieved.

## Anticipation

The midwife may recognise the potential for neonatal compromise according to the known maternal or fetal risk factors. Such examples include:

- prematurity
- known malpresentation, e.g. breech
- maternal disease, e.g. hypertension, diabetes mellitus
- previous poor obstetric or neonatal history
- abnormalities of the fetal heartbeat indicative of fetal compromise

- instrumental or operative delivery, especially under general anaesthetic
- obstetric emergency, e.g. prolapsed cord, antepartum haemorrhage, shoulder dystocia, eclampsia
- precipitate delivery
- heavy maternal sedation, e.g. drug overdose
- fresh meconium within the amniotic fluid.

However, the need for neonatal resuscitation can occur without any warning, predisposing factors or obvious cause. The presence of two midwives at delivery (wherever the venue) is a safeguard that allows one to care for the woman, and the other to begin resuscitation of the baby. However, the first element of resuscitation must be to call for appropriate assistance. The midwife must know how to do this, whether in hospital or in the community. In hospital it may be one emergency number to ring; in the community the paramedic service may be called using 999 and the midwife must be familiar with their local arrangements.

A baby may require resuscitating at other times in the postnatal period; the fundamental principles of resuscitation apply in the same way. Examples include:

- occlusion of the airway, e.g. choking, feeding problems or mucus
- undetected congenital abnormality
- retained effects of respiratory depression after the effect of naloxone has subsided
- infection.

### Pathophysiology of asphyxia

Asphyxia occurs when there is insufficient oxygen and excessive carbon dioxide and lactic acid in the blood. The consequence of this is a failure to breathe, which ultimately causes the baby's metabolism to shift from aerobic to anaerobic respiration. A metabolic acidosis is created. An anoxic baby may be in any one of four phases depending upon the level of intrauterine hypoxia:

1. hyperventilation
2. primary apnoea
3. gasping
4. terminal apnoea

but it is rarely possible to assess at birth which of these phases the baby is in. It is necessary to respond and then to assess the measures of progress.

## Equipment

Resuscitation can be successfully completed with a minimal amount of equipment, in any environment, whether home or hospital. In the hospital environment it is likely that a standard resuscitaire with additional equipment will be available. At home a chest of drawers or table may be utilised, but care should be taken to avoid draughts.

Ideal requirements include:

- a flat surface
- towels and gloves (somewhere to wash hands if time permits)
- a radiant heater
- a clock, with a second hand
- stethoscope
- oxygen/air source with flow regulation, reservoir and adjustable pressure relief valve (these should be checked prior to the delivery to ensure they are working correctly)
- T-tube or self-inflating resuscitation bag with valve and assorted size face masks 00, 01
- Guedel airways sizes 0, 00, 000
- laryngoscopes (with spare bulbs and batteries)
- tracheal tubes, introducers and connectors
- suction apparatus with tubing and catheters
- drugs
- needles, syringes, scissors, tape, other extras, e.g. umbilical catheterisation pack.

Adaptation for the home includes a basic portable kit that can be utilised effectively. Maddy (1998) provides such an example, where suction, ventilation and oxygen apparatus for both the woman and baby are contained within one bag.

If resuscitation is anticipated the equipment should be prepared in advance of the delivery so that the baby can be delivered onto warmed towels, taken to a resuscitation area with a good heat and light source and where equipment is readily to hand. If resuscitation is unexpected this preparation occurs concurrently with the resuscitative measures used.

# Principles of resuscitation

The principles are summed up as ABCD: airway, breathing, circulation, drugs. However, for the newly delivered wet, hypoxic baby, the principles begin with the need to dry thoroughly, remove the wet towel and cover the baby while assessing the colour, tone, breathing and heart rate of the baby, calling for appropriate help and noting the time (if a stopwatch is available, this should be started at the time of birth or at the beginning of the resuscitation period).

Drying the baby provides tactile stimulation and reduces further heat loss and hypoxia. It is important to discard the wet towel and wrap the baby in a warm dry towel. This measure should be undertaken immediately and as the baby is being transferred to the resuscitation area.

As this is being undertaken the midwife should assess the baby, taking into account the colour of the trunk, lips and tongue, muscle tone, respiratory pattern and heart rate. Blue hands and feet should never be mistaken for cyanosis in the newborn; assessment of cyanosis should be made by observing the baby centrally, even when the baby has pigmented skin. The mucous membranes (inside of the lips), tongue and trunk are alternative sites to assess. Mildly hypoxic babies usually respond well to drying; if the colour and tone are good, the baby is breathing regularly with a fast heart rate, no further measures are required and the baby can be returned to his mother. However, if this is not the case, further resuscitation and assistance are required.

## Airway

The airway must be open to facilitate air entry into the lungs. Loss of pharyngeal tone can occur in the floppy baby, causing the tongue to fall back and occlude the airway. To prevent this, the baby's head is placed in a neutral position, causing it to neither flex nor extend. The prominent occiput can cause the neck to flex; to minimise this a folded towel approximately 2 cm in depth should be placed under the shoulders of the baby to bring the head and neck in alignment to keep the trachea straight (Fig. 60.1). Further support may be required in the floppy baby with the use of chin support or jaw thrust to maintain the upward and outward position of the chin. After each manoeuvre, the midwife should reassess the baby (colour, tone, breathing, heart rate) as the baby may begin to breathe spontaneously when the airway is open.

### Chin support

The midwife should place a finger over the bony part of the tip of the chin, avoiding pressure on the soft tissues and hold the chin in position.

Figure 60.1 Neutral position

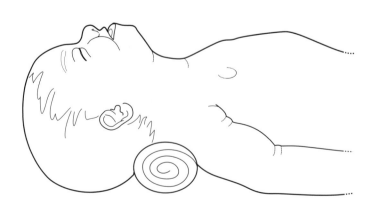

### Jaw thrust

Where there is little or no tone, the midwife may need to place one or two fingers on either side of the lower jaw (at the angle of the jaw and avoiding soft tissues) to push the jaw outwards and forwards.

### Tracheal suction

If the midwife is concerned that the airway is blocked, a direct visual assessment can be undertaken using a laryngoscope. A suction catheter should not be used unless the area is seen first and a blockage visualised, as inadvertent stimulation of the posterior pharynx and larynx with the suction catheter can result in severe vagal bradycardia, quickly exacerbating the situation. Although meconium can cause tracheal obstruction, routine suctioning is not recommended for babies born through meconium-stained liquor. Only someone experienced with intubation should undertake tracheal suction.

### Use of oropharyngeal (Guedel) airway

This may be required when the baby has an abnormality of the face or mouth (e.g. cleft palate, micrognathia) or when there is difficulty maintaining the chin support/jaw thrust while undertaking other resuscitation manoeuvres. An appropriately sized airway (0, 00 or 000) inserted into the oropharynx will maintain the patency of the airway by pushing the tongue forwards, negating further manual assistance.

Airway size is assessed by holding the flange of the airway against the mid-point of the baby's lips, with the airway held horizontally so that the curved part of the airway curves around the baby's jaw; it should end at the angle of the jaw.

To insert the airway, hold the airway in the position it will sit within the oropharynx. Open the baby's mouth by depressing the chin and slide the airway over the baby's tongue, avoiding pushing the tongue backwards. The airway should slide easily into position. A laryngoscope can also be used to depress the tongue during airway insertion.

## Breathing

When the airway is clear, breathing may follow spontaneously. If no effective breathing is seen, it is important to fill the lungs with air or oxygen as quickly as possible, usually via a facemask. Prior to the first breath, the baby's lungs are filled with fluid; physiologically the pressure required to inflate the lungs for the first time is higher than with subsequent breaths. Once the alveoli have been inflated, the presence of surfactant maintains the inflation. Inflation breaths are used to assist with removing the lung fluid; these are followed by ventilation breaths.

Practically this means that if mechanically ventilating the lungs the initial pressures should be 30 cm $H_2O$ lasting 2–3 seconds for the first five inflation breaths. This is as effective as using a higher pressure for a shorter period and easier to achieve. The chest may not rise effectively until much of the fluid has been expelled from the lungs, usually within the fourth to fifth inflation breath.

If no chest movement is seen, the midwife should ensure that both the neutral position and the airway are correct, using methods described above, then repeat the five inflation breaths.

### Facemask

The ideal facemask is circular with a deformable rim that will fit snugly around the baby's mouth and nose when even pressure is applied to form an airtight seal. The correct size should be used (00 or 01) and should not extend over the end of the chin or into the eye sockets (Fig. 60.2). Fingertips are used to support the jaw and seal off the mask (grasping under the chin will also occlude the airway). An airtight seal is essential to ensure adequate ventilation, and the head should be maintained in the neutral position.

The facemask can be attached to a T-piece connected to a supply of oxygen or air (with a pressure dial and pressure release valve to ensure correct pressures used) (Fig. 60.3) or attached to a self-inflating bag–valve–mask (BVM) system.

**Figure 60.2** Correct positioning of the facemask (Adapted with kind permission from RCPCH, RCOG 1997)

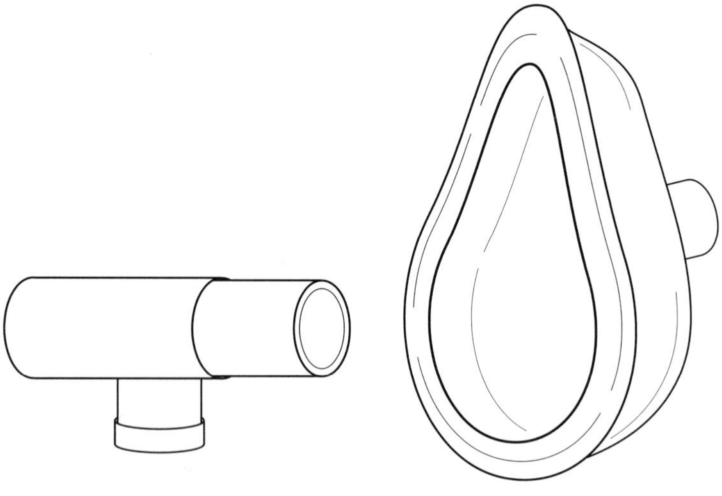

Correct          Incorrect          Incorrect          Incorrect

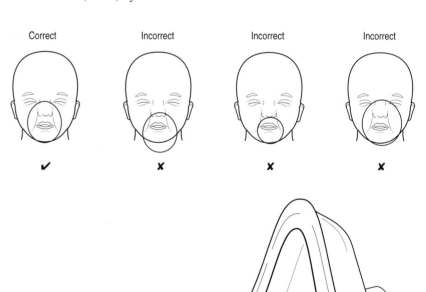

**Figure 60.3** T-piece and mask

When using a T-piece to inflate the lungs, the open end is occluded by the resuscitator's thumb (the fingers are usually keeping the face-mask in position) for 2–3 seconds then removed for the five inflation breaths and occluded and removed at a rate of 30 breaths for the ventilation breaths.

If using a BVM, the blow-off valve should be tested before use by occluding the outlet and squeezing the bag. As the pressure rises, the blow-off valve makes a noise that confirms it is working and is safe for use. The principles of using BVM are similar to the T-piece in that a good seal is needed from the mask; the bag is squeezed slowly to produce a pressure of 30 cm $H_2O$ for 2–3 seconds (the valve will begin to blow when the correct pressure is reached). The bag is then released to refill and repeated until five inflation breaths have been given.

If the midwife has no equipment available, she can use mouth-to-mouth breathing. The baby's head should be in the neutral position and the airway patent. The baby's mouth and nose are sealed with the midwife's mouth and air from the midwife's cheeks is gently breathed into the lungs to provide inflation then ventilation breaths.

With effective ventilation the chest can be seen to rise. If this does not occur, the airway should be reassessed to ensure it is patent, and the position of the facemask/mouth should be reassessed to ensure there is an airtight seal, and the five inflation breaths repeated.

Following the five inflation breaths the colour, tone, respiratory effort and heart rate should be reassessed. With effective ventilation the heart rate usually increases within 20–30 seconds as the baby responds to the resuscitation. If the heart rate increases and chest movement is achieved with the inflation breaths, the midwife should continue to provide ventilatory support via ventilation breaths at around 30 breaths per minute until the baby is able to breathe unaided. If spontaneous respiration does not occur, the presence of other complications should be considered and treated (e.g. effect of maternal opioid/drugs, neurological compromise) by the paediatrician. Assessment of the colour, tone, respiratory effort and heart rate should be undertaken following every 30 ventilation breaths. In practice the colour, tone and respiratory effort are usually assessed continually during the procedure and the manoeuvres adjusted according to the response shown by the baby to the resuscitation measures used.

If, during ventilatory support, chest movement reduces or the heart rate decreases, the midwife should reassess the airway to ensure it is still patent and the seal on the mask is still airtight. The eyeline of the midwife should be level with the baby's chest to visualise the chest movements more easily. The midwife's position should be adjusted to facilitate this.

If the heart rate has not increased quickly despite effective inflation and ventilation breaths, cardiac compression is necessary.

## Circulation

Prior to commencing chest compression, the midwife should ensure that:

- the baby's head and jaw are in the correct position
- the mask is the correct size, with a good seal against the face
- the air/oxygen supply is working
- the inflation breaths have been given correctly.

It is easier to undertake chest compressions with two people, but if help is not immediately available, the midwife should continue on her own.

The most effective method of compressing the chest is to hold the baby's chest with both hands, placing the fingers over the spine and the thumbs together on the sternum just below an imaginary line between the nipples (Fig. 60.4). It is important to avoid pressing on soft tissue or the ribs as this will result in ineffective chest compression and damage, which may exacerbate the situation.

A less effective method of chest compression is to use the index and middle fingers positioned centrally on the sternum immediately beneath the imaginary line (Fig. 60.5). The other hand should be used to support the baby's back.

The chest is compressed quickly and firmly to a depth of one-third of the anteroposterior diameter of the chest (1–2 cm). Time must be allowed for the chest to re-expand after each compression to enable the heart to refill.

It is important that *effective* ventilation of the lungs continues and that the cardiac compression is synchronised with it. The synchronised rate is three compressions to one ventilation (3:1). In a 6-second

**Figure 60.4**   Two-handed chest compression

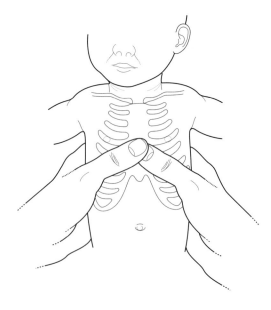

**Figure 60.5** One-handed chest compression

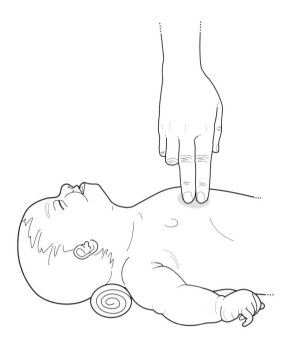

period three cycles should be completed (a heart rate of approximately 90 beats per minute – bpm) but this may be difficult to sustain. Where two people work together, one of them should count aloud, to maintain concentration.

The heart rate usually responds rapidly to effective ventilation and chest compressions. The midwife should recheck the heart rate every 30 seconds to determine if there is a response. Chest compressions should be stopped when the heart rate is responding.

Should the heart rate not respond, despite correct ventilation and compressions, drug therapy and transfer to a high dependency unit may be required.

## Drug therapy

Prescription and administration of drugs in this setting is the responsibility of the paediatrician who may administer them via an umbilical catheter. The midwife may assist in the checking and drawing up of such drugs, although many are pre-prepared. Drugs commonly required are sodium bicarbonate 4.2% (1–2 mmol/kg), adrenaline (epinephrine) 1:10 000 (10 mcg/kg) (this can be administered via the tracheal tube) and dextrose 10% (250 mg/kg). If a volume expander is needed, a bolus dose of 10 mL/kg 0.9% saline may be given.

## After the resuscitation

A successful resuscitation may mean that the baby will either remain with his parents or, if unwell, be transferred to neonatal intensive care. Body temperature should be maintained and feeding is essential due to the use of glucose during anaerobic respiration. The parents will need support and information to understand what has occurred and to appreciate whether any further dangers exist. The midwife will document all of the resuscitation details including the time the emergency call was made and when staff arrived, time of onset of respiration, nature of resuscitation, drugs administered and personnel present.

If the resuscitation is unsuccessful the paediatrician will make the decision to halt the resuscitation. Local protocols will vary, but it is often abandoned after 20 minutes without a heart rate but with full resuscitation support during that time (RCPCH, RCOG 1997). Considerable care of the parents will be required. The staff involved are also encouraged to gain support for themselves; the risk manager or supervisor of midwives may be instrumental in this.

## PROCEDURE    neonatal resuscitation

1. Move the baby to the resuscitation area. At the same time:
   — assess the colour, tone, respiratory effort and heart rate
   — send out an emergency call for appropriate personnel (if an anticipated problem the paediatrician should already be present)
   — set the clock and note the time
   — switch on the heater and light if not undertaken prior to delivery
2. Dry the baby thoroughly and remove the damp towel; wrap in a clean warm towel, with the chest exposed
3. Position the baby's head in the neutral position (see Fig. 60.1)
4. Assess the colour, tone, respiration rate and heart rate (these are reassessed every 30 seconds):
   4.1 If pink, with a heart rate above 100 bpm and breathing spontaneously, keep the baby warm and return him to his parents
   4.2 If breathing irregularly (shallow or slow), but a heart rate above 100 bpm, provide tactile stimulation, keep the baby warm and the head in the neutral position. It can take some healthy babies up to 3 minutes to establish respiration (Resuscitation Council (UK) 2001). Continue to assess the colour, tone, respiratory effort and heart rate, returning the baby to his parents when breathing spontaneously, with good colour, tone and heart rate
   4.3 If no response from the actions described in 4.2 or if there is no respiratory effort:
       a. Ensure a neutral position and an open airway, using chin support, jaw thrust or an oropharyngeal airway as necessary
       b. Inflate the lungs using a facemask and T-piece or BVM system, providing five effective inflation breaths and looking

for chest movement. If no chest movement is seen, check head position and repeat inflation breaths

c. After effective inflation breaths assess the heart rate by feeling it over the apex (the base of the umbilical cord can be palpated but this may be difficult on some babies and, if slow, the apex beat should always be counted). Count for 6 seconds then multiply by 10 to calculate the beats per minute (if the rate is low a stethoscope should be used to listen for the heart beat). Where more than one person is involved in the resuscitation, the heart rate should be tapped out so that everyone is aware of the rate

d. Continue ventilation breaths until spontaneous respiration occurs if the heart rate is more than 100 bpm. Reassess the colour, tone, respiratory effort and heart rate following every 30 ventilation breaths (continue the ventilation while counting the heart rate)

5. If the heart rate is decreasing or is below 60 bpm commence chest compression with ventilation at a rate of 3:1

6. Reassess the heart rate every 30 seconds (while continuing ventilatory support) and stop chest compressions when the heart rate is above 60 bpm and increasing. Colour, tone and respiratory effort are assessed throughout the resuscitation. Ventilatory support is stopped when the baby is breathing adequately without assistance.

Resuscitation is summarised in Figure 60.6.

## Role and responsibilities of the midwife

These can be summarised as:

- anticipation of potential problems and preparation of the environment and equipment
- recognition of the need to resuscitate
- competent resuscitation skills, including correct use of equipment and maintenance of the skill (regular updates and practice)
- recognition of the need to call for appropriate medical/newborn life support (NLS) trained assistance
- ability to support and assist the person called
- accurate contemporaneous record keeping
- information for, and support of, the parents during and following the event
- appropriate transfer of the care of the woman and baby
- familiarity with local resuscitation protocols.

**Figure 60.6** Summary of neonatal resuscitation

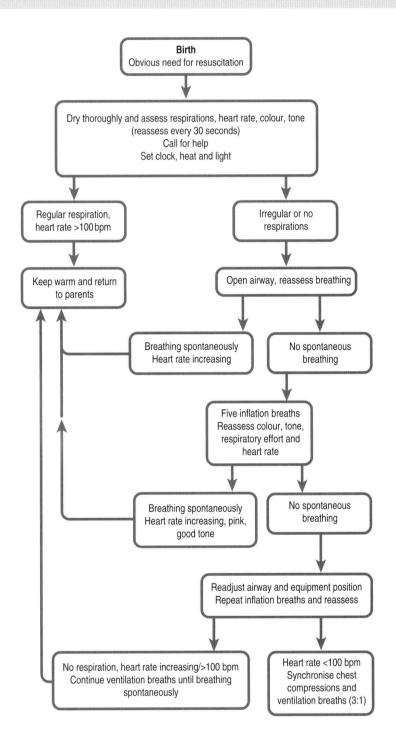

**Summary**

- The midwife has a responsible role in the recognition and management of neonatal resuscitation. Equipment should be accessible and the midwife should be familiar with its use
- Appropriate help should be sought quickly. Management includes drying the baby and assessing colour, tone, respiratory effort and heart rate. Manoeuvres to open the airway, ventilate the lungs and chest compression should be undertaken efficiently when required. Drug therapy may be required when the response is poor.

**Self-assessment exercises**

The answers to the following questions may be found in the text:

1. How is the need to resuscitate a baby recognised?
2. Which predisposing conditions may alert the midwife to the need to prepare for resuscitation?
3. List the equipment required for neonatal resuscitation, indicating how each piece is used.
4. What measures can the midwife take to ensure the airway is open?
5. If a baby has a heart rate of 60 bpm, is pale and is gasping, what action should be taken?
6. List the responsibilities of the midwife:
   a. when anticipating the need to resuscitate
   b. during a neonatal resuscitation situation
   c. following a successful resuscitation
   d. following an unsuccessful resuscitation.
7. Demonstrate/simulate a neonatal resuscitation, giving verbal explanations for the actions taken.

## REFERENCES

Maddy B 1998 The vital components of a resuscitation kit. British Journal of Midwifery 6(4):256–258

RCPCH, RCOG (Royal College of Paediatrics and Child Health, Royal College of Obstetricians and Gynaecologists) 1997 Resuscitation of babies at birth. BMJ Publishing Group, London

Resuscitation Council (UK) 2001 Resuscitation at birth: newborn life support manual. Resuscitation Council (UK), London

# Glossary

**Abduction** – movement away from the midline of the body

**Adduction** – movement towards the midline of the body

**Agglutination** – clumping together

**Aortocaval occlusion** – occlusion of the inferior vena cava and aorta by the pregnant uterus. Tends to occur if a heavily pregnant woman is asked to lie flat. Avoided by adopting a lateral position or using a wedge under the right hip. Also known as supine hypotension

**Apical** – the apex of the heart

**Apnoea** – absence of respiration for >20 seconds

**Bacteriuria** – the presence of bacteria in the urine

**Bilirubinuria** – the presence of bilirubin in the urine

**Biparietal diameter** – the distance between the parietal eminences, usually 9.5 cm in the term baby. This is the widest transverse diameter of the fetal skull to pass through the pelvic brim (during engagement) and to distend the perineum (during crowning)

**Bishop's Score** – a scoring assessment used to assess the favourability (or ripeness) of the cervix prior to induction of labour. Considers the position, consistency, length and dilatation of the cervix and station of the presenting part within the pelvis. Each factor is awarded a score accordingly; the dose of Prostin may be adjusted according to the total score. A Bishop's Score of 6 or more considers the cervix to be favourable

**Blanching** – colour changes in the skin with fingertip pressure, turning the skin white. The colour should quickly return to normal as capillary refill occurs

**Bradycardia** – a slow heart rate, <60 bpm for an adult, <80 bpm for a baby

**Constipation** – infrequent or difficult defaecation, caused by decreased motility of the intestines in which faeces remain in the colon for prolonged periods. Greater quantities of water are absorbed making the faeces hard and dry. It may be caused by improper bowel habits, spasms of colon, insufficient bulk in diet, lack of exercise and emotions

**Cyanosis** – bluish appearance of skin and mucous membranes caused by reduced oxygenation

**Cystocele** – bulging of the bladder into the upper part of the anterior vaginal wall

**Denominator** – the leading part of the fetus, likely to meet the pelvic floor first. For a flexed vertex presentation it is the occiput, for the buttocks it is the sacrum

**Diarrhoea** – frequent defaecation of liquid faeces caused by increased motility of the intestines. There is not enough time for absorption and it can lead to dehydration and electrolyte imbalance. Diarrhoea has several causes, e.g. infection, stress. Diarrhoea overflow may also occur in the presence of constipation

**Diuresis** – increased formation and excretion of urine

**Dysuria** – difficult or painful micturition

**Erythema** – redness

**Erythema toxicum** – a blotchy red rash, sometimes with yellowish pinhead papules, which occurs usually between days 2 and 8. Cause unknown, no treatment required

**Extravasation** – escape of fluid from the vessels into the surrounding tissues

**Extubation** – removal of the tube inserted during intubation

**Fetal lie** – relation of the long axis of the fetus to the long axis of the uterus. Where the two are parallel it is a longitudinal lie. Variations include transverse or oblique

**Fetal pole** – an extremity or end, e.g. skull or buttocks (when in flexed position)

**Fetal position** – the relation of the denominator on the fetus to a landmark on the fetal pelvis, e.g. occiput facing the left iliopectineal eminence equates to left occipitoanterior (LOA)

**Fever** – a cause of hyperthermia, produced in response to the presence of pyrogens in the blood

**Fistula** – an abnormal connection between two hollow organs or between a hollow organ and the body surface

**Haematuria** – the presence of blood in the urine

**Haemorrhoids** – varicosities of the rectal vein. Can occur as a result of chronic repetitive straining to defaecate, resulting in enlargement of the venous plexuses

**Hydronephrosis** – a collection of urine in the pelvis of the kidney

**Hyperthermia** – an increase in the core body temperature to above 37.5°C. Also referred to as pyrexia – low grade pyrexia is classified as a temperature up to 38°C, a moderate to high pyrexia is 38–40°C and hyperpyrexia is an excessively high temperature above 40°C

**Hyperventilation** – increased rate and depth of respiration that results in excess carbon dioxide retention

**Hypoglycaemia** – a lowered level of glucose in the blood

**Hypothermia** – a decrease in the core body temperature to 35°C or below

**Hypovolaemia** – a reduction in the circulating blood volume

**Induration** – an area of localised oedema under the skin, often occurring with abnormal reactive hyperaemia

**Intrathecal** – within the meninges of the spinal cord

**Intubation** – the introduction of a tube into part of the body, e.g. for anaesthesia – introduction of an endotracheal tube into the trachea

**Laxative** – a medicine that helps loosen the contents of the bowel and encourages evacuation. Those with a mild action are referred to as aperients; those with a stronger action are called purgatives

**Micrognathia** – a receding jaw

**Milia** – blocked sebaceous glands that appear as small white spots over the nose and cheeks

**Nocturia** – excessive urination at night

**Occiput** – the back of the head

**Oliguria** – diminished capacity to form urine. In the baby, this is a urine output of less than 0.5 mL/kg/hour after 48 hours

**Oxytocin** – a hormone released by the posterior lobe of the pituitary gland, responsible for contraction of the myometrium and epithelial cells within the breast

**Parenterally** – administered by any route other than through the mouth

**Paronychia** – a staphylococcal infection of the nailbed, often associated with hangnails

**Pharmacokinetics** – the way the body affects the drug, e.g. absorption, distribution, metabolism and excretion

**Phimosis** – a condition where the foreskin is retracted back from the glans penis and becomes obstructed, causing swelling and pain

**Phlebitis** – inflammation of a vein

**Polydactyly** – extra fingers or toes

**Polyuria** – voiding large amounts of urine

**Postural hypotension** – lowering of blood pressure occurring during a change of position from sitting to standing, or lying to upright. Frequently accompanied by dizziness and light-headedness, and sometimes syncope

**Proteinuria** – the presence of protein in the urine

**Pruritus** – itching caused by localised irritation of the skin, nervous disorders, infection, e.g. fungal infection of the vulva, haemorrhoids, intestinal worms and some forms of jaundice

**Rectocele** – a prolapse of the lower posterior vaginal wall

**Rigors** – uncontrollable, involuntary episodes of intense shivering during which the temperature rises rapidly, and then decreases after a short period of time. Often associated with the presence of bacteria or toxins within the blood, it may occur with severe cases of pyelonephritis in pregnancy

**Shoulder dystocia** – occurs when the normal mechanism of labour stops as the shoulders attempt to enter the pelvic brim but are unable to do so. Occurs with pelvic abnormalities reducing the pelvic diameters or increased bisacromial diameter (distance between the shoulders). This may be due to one (unilateral dystocia) or both (bilateral dystocia) shoulders becoming impacted at the brim or, with a large baby, delay occurs because of the tight fit

**Sternal recession** – occurs when the alveoli fail to remain inflated and the compliant chest wall begins to collapse around the stiff lungs. The sternum is seen to recess in, rather than expand out, with breathing movements

**Stress incontinence** – as a result of reduced control of the internal and external sphincter, involuntary voiding of small amounts of urine occurs when the intra-abdominal pressure increases, e.g. during bouts of coughing, laughing or sneezing

**Subinvolution** – the uterus is involuting at a slower rate than expected or remains at the same size for several days. This may be due to the presence of retained products of conception, blood clots within the uterus, uterine fibroids or infection. It predisposes to postpartum haemorrhage and is considered a deviation from the normal

**Surfactant** – a phospholipid present in the lungs of the mature newborn that reduces surface tension in the alveoli permitting the lungs to expand and the alveoli to remain inflated

**Syndactyly** – webbing between the fingers or toes

**Tachycardia** – a fast heart rate, >100 bpm for an adult, >160 bpm for a baby

**Tachypnoea** – abnormally rapid rate of breathing, >20 per minute

**Terminal digit preference** – occurs when a person recording blood pressure rounds the measurement to a digit of their preference, most commonly zero

**Threshold avoidance** – occurs when the blood pressure is recorded as being lower than the threshold for implementing treatment, when the actual measurement is at or above that level

**Thrombophlebitis** – inflammation of a vein with clot formation

**Trisomy 21** – a condition where there is an extra chromosome 21 present, resulting in three chromosome 21s in each cell. Also referred to as Down's syndrome

**Urgency** – the need to micturate immediately

**Urinary frequency** – increased need to micturate, often voiding small amount of urine

**Urinary retention** – the inability of the bladder to empty resulting in an accumulation of urine in the bladder

**Urticaria** – a skin rash characterised by the recurrent appearance of an eruption of wheals (raised stripes of skin, similar to whiplash marks) which results in severe skin irritation

# Index

Page numbers in *italics* refer to figures or tables.